PROSTATE
CANCER

Understand, Prevent and Overcome

Professor Jane A. Plant

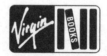

First published in Great Britain in 2004 by
Virgin Publishing Ltd
Thames Wharf Studios
Rainville Road
London
W6 9HA

A catalogue record for this book is available from the
British Library.

ISBN 1 85227 188 4

Typeset by TW Typesetting, Plymouth, Devon
Printed and bound in Great Britain by
Creative Print & Design Wales, Ebbw Vale

Contents

Author's Note

The diagnosis and treatment of medical conditions is a responsibility shared between you and your medical advisors. All diets should begin with a medical check-up to make certain that no special health problems exist and to confirm that there are no medical reasons why you should not undertake a change of diet.

Acknowledgements

I would like to thank my husband Peter Simpson for his support and practical help with the book and the Director of the British Geological Survey Dr David Falvey and Gill Tidey for their encouragement. I should also like to thank Professor Jonathan Waxman from Imperial College for his help, especially with Chapter 1. I am most grateful to Henry Haslam for his assistance with the book.

Also by Professor Jane Plant

YOUR LIFE IN YOUR HANDS: UNDERSTANDING, PREVENTING AND OVERCOMING BREAST CANCER

With Gill Tidey

THE PLANT PROGRAMME

UNDERSTANDING, PREVENTING AND OVERCOMING OSTEOPOROSIS

Welcome

It is now more than ten years since my breast-cancer secondaries disappeared following a fundamental change in my diet and lifestyle. In spite of a radical mastectomy, three further operations, 35 radiotherapy treatments, irradiation of my ovaries to induce the menopause and several chemotherapy treatments my cancer had spread to the lymph nodes in my neck. Despite all this treatment, my doctors had given me only three months to live. I then recalled that people in rural China, where I had worked, had a very low incidence of breast (and prostate) cancer. At that point I changed my diet and lifestyle and, to everyone's amazement, including I have to admit my own, the large cancerous lump in my neck disappeared within five weeks.

Since that time I have not even had a scare, and my annual check-ups at Charing Cross Hospital have tended to focus more on my diet and lifestyle than on my cancer.

I have talked to senior doctors who have said that they personally have not met anyone who has survived such serious illness and had been very sceptical about my book until they had talked to me.

My experience, and that of many other women who had followed my diet and lifestyle, led me to write *Your Life in Your Hands*,[1] which was published in 2000. In this book I used the term 'the Plant Programme' for the diet and lifestyle that I recommended, and this became the title of my next book: *The Plant Programme*,[2] written with Gill Tidey and published in 2001, is a cookbook to help you follow the dietary advice in *Your Life in Your Hands* and this book about prostate cancer.

In the first edition of *Your Life in Your Hands* I gave some information about prostate cancer because whenever and wherever I looked for information on breast cancer the same factors kept emerging as factors for prostate cancer too. I therefore included the data and information about prostate cancer in the book – and I included more in the second edition, published in September 2003.

I know, from the many communications I have had with men and women who have complemented their conventional medical treatment with the dietary and lifestyle factors that I recommend that I am now far from unique. Many people contact me, telling me they are now healthy and cancer free. Indeed, when I attend functions these days I am always surprised by the number of men who come bounding up to me and the first thing they want to tell me is how good their test results are now!

Since the first edition of *Your Life in Your Hands* was published, more than three years ago, more and more scientific evidence has appeared to support its recommendations. It is perhaps worth noting that, despite the press seizing on one or two of the most easily grasped recommendations of the book – eliminating dairy produce and reducing exposure to hormone-disrupting and hormone-mimicking chemicals – there were seven food factors and five lifestyle factors to be addressed. There are now eight and eight, respectively, for prostate cancer.

Examples of new supporting evidence include the results of studies conducted by eminent epidemiologists showing the link between prostate cancer and dairy and calcium intake. There is also more and more evidence that the disease is associated with high circulating levels of a chemical messenger in the body called IGF-I and new evidence that this is linked to food factors identified in *Your Life in Your Hands*, especially high dietary intakes of dairy produce, as well as trans-fatty acids and refined carbohydrate and low dietary intakes of vegetables and fruit.

Also, there is further evidence of the importance of the correct balance of oils in the diet, as well as increasing evidence against consuming man-made vitamins and supplements, including megadoses of vitamin C.

The reason all the recently published science has confirmed the recommendations in my books and shown them to be soundly based is not because I am clairvoyant or indeed particularly clever. It is simply because both books were based on research into the peer-reviewed scientific literature. Because of my scientific training, I was able to read information in publications written in the sort of scientific shorthand that all scientists tend to use to communicate with other specialists in their field, and translate it into simple straightforward English to make it accessible to a wider readership. This is something that I have found some people have apparently misunderstood. In reply to those who have made such arm-waving statements as 'There is no scientific basis' or 'Give me the evidence', I say that most of the science in my books is from the mainstream scientific literature – presented in the context of the story of my personal battle with cancer so as to make it more readable. I have been shocked to discover that some of the senior cancer specialists invited to debate my views on TV or radio do not know enough chemistry to explain, for example, what a free radical is, or had not heard that 100 per cent of the male fish in some British rivers are feminised because of our emissions of endocrine-disrupting chemicals which alter the way hormone systems work. I have also come to realise that the gulf between scientific researchers and many medical clinicians is far greater than I had imagined. The extent to which medical practice is influenced by vested-interest groups is something that many others, including the *British Medical Journal (BMJ)*, now take very seriously indeed. The *BMJ* now requires that authors of any paper published by them should declare the funding sources of their study or other potential conflicts of interest. For this reason, many of the references in this book are from the *BMJ*. I am not alone in being concerned about such issues, particularly in relation to our food. In *Save Yourself From Breast Cancer*[3] by Robert D Kradjian, head of the breast-surgery division at the Seton Medical Centre, Daly City, California, the problem is clearly stated:

> The issue is clear. Much of our highly varied, desired, and profitable food supply has been found to be dangerous. The people who furnish this food and who are enriched by its sale do not want you to know this. They have generously contributed to scientists who have supported, and are willing to continue to support, their products. If those scientists suddenly have a change of heart, and seriously challenge the safety of that food, you may be certain that the bulk of the food-industry financial support will promptly disappear.
>
> Whom are you going to believe? Those with no financial gain from the sale of food and with the backing of the world's scientific literature? Or are you going to follow those who have at times devised flawed studies and reaped millions of dollars in support of the industries that they fail to seriously criticize? You must decide, and your health will be substantially determined by your decision.

Happily, many medical professionals and scientists have been supportive of my work. I am aware that many are now recommending my books to their prostate-cancer and breast-cancer patients. Increasingly, I am invited to address medical societies and cancer support groups, with very positive feedback.

Perhaps it's worth mentioning that the diet will NOT cause osteoporosis. Quite the reverse. The new book *Understanding, Preventing and Overcoming Osteoporosis*,[4] which I have written with Gill Tidey, provides the scientific evidence that this disease, like breast cancer and prostate cancer, is strongly linked to the Western diet. The book also contains many delicious, healthy recipes, which complement those in *The Plant Programme*.

Prostate cancer is an important illness: it is currently the second most common cause of male cancer deaths in the West, and death rates from it have trebled over the last thirty years. For a long time, the disease was surrounded by silence, but recently it has moved more into the public domain.[5] The fact that it is now talked about more openly has been helped by high-profile men such as former Mayor Giuliani of New York and the former Archbishop of Cape Town, Desmond Tutu, being prepared to admit publicly to having prostate cancer.

This new book aims to bring you the most up-to-date scientific information on the disease. I look first at new developments in the conventional medical diagnosis and treatment of prostate cancer – though even screening and diagnosis are controversial, and this is one of the reasons the disease is such a problem. Many men have non-malignant but enlarged prostates, others have very slow-growing cancer which could continue for ten or fifteen years before any treatment is really needed, while others may have more aggressive disease. There is a serious need for better funding for prostate cancer studies, to identify and optimise the best methods of diagnosis and treatment. Some aspects and types of diagnosis and treatment of prostate cancer can be unpleasant and have damaging short-term and long-term side effects. No man would want to go through all this unless it is essential.[6] This is definitely a case of prevention being better than cure, and the main message of this book is ... prevention ... prevention ... prevention.

I go on to describe some of the latest research findings into growth factors and endocrine-disrupting chemicals in our food, drink and environment. I take forward the debate on chemopreventive substances in our diet and I provide simple, practical advice on how to reduce your risk of suffering from prostate cancer – advice that will also help to treat the disease in those already affected. I look again at the politics of the problem, such as links between the pharmaceutical industry and medical clinicians.

Finally, I should like to reassure readers that I wrote this book in my own time, with no funding or influence from any vested-interest group, and have done my best to ensure that the science on which it is based is, to the best of my knowledge, objective, authoritative and as free as possible from commercial, political or other such influences.

I hope very much that you can put the information in this new book on prostate cancer to the best possible use in your life.

Professor Jane A Plant CBE, FRSE, FRSA, BSc (Geochemistry: Class 1), PhD, D Univ (Hon), DSc (Hon), DSc (Hon), FIMMM, CEng, FGS, CGeol, Freeman of the City of London

(I am not normally someone who uses titles. Everyone I know quickly calls me just 'Jane' and that is how I like to be addressed. However, I am a scientist and this book is based on what I believe to be sound science, so I include here my academic and professional qualifications and honours in order to reassure you, the reader, of my scientific credentials.)

1 Problems with the Prostate?

In this chapter, I explain why, as a natural scientist, my approach to the problem of prostate cancer is different from that of many orthodox medical researchers. I then go on to examine the orthodox approach to prostate cancer. I review the conventional risk factors for the disease, the value and reliability of different diagnostic tests, the advantages and disadvantages of the various treatment options that are now available . . . and much, much more. I include three brief case histories, examples of the many men who have been in touch with me about their disease after reading my first book, Your Life in Your Hands.[1] *By observing what has happened to all of them, I am convinced that the best outcome is achieved if the conventional medical treatments described in this chapter are combined with the dietary and lifestyle advice given later in the book.*

It was my hope that my first book, *Your Life in Your Hands*, would serve two purposes. First, I wanted it to be directly useful to other people. I wanted to make the information I had access to as a scientist available to them as simple, straightforward advice, told in the context of my own story – a detective story centred on my own breast cancer, the findings of which, I believe, saved my life. In this book I hope to do the same for men affected by prostate cancer, using my experience of helping many to overcome their disease since *Your Life in Your Hands* was first published.

The straightforward advice and simple lifestyle suggestions described here will, I hope, be of practical benefit to men in significantly reducing their risk of developing prostate cancer. If you happen to be that one man in about twelve in the UK who has been diagnosed with prostate cancer, then you will also find much information here which will give you a better chance of survival and help you to cope with the rigorous treatment methods.

Secondly, it is vitally important that this book takes forward the debate within the scientific and medical communities – a debate that was ignited by *Your Life in Your Hands*. Science is, at heart, an adversarial process. This new book on prostate cancer backs up the evidence and hypotheses on the cause of the disease with the mounting evidence from the scientific literature on factors that promote it, especially the most dangerous form of the disease – metastatic prostate cancer. The inescapable conclusion is that relatively small augmentations to the orthodox medical therapies currently being used in clinics and hospitals would result in major improvements in patient survival. Providing prostate-cancer patients with sound dietary advice (common in cases of heart disease and diabetes) could greatly increase survival rates. Prostate cancer appears to be a particularly cruel disease, and I believe that so much suffering could be prevented, and so many lives could be saved, if the new evidence I have compiled in this book is acted on.

HOW ON EARTH CAN A NATURAL SCIENTIST CONTRIBUTE TO PREVENTING AND TREATING PROSTATE CANCER?

I am trained in a subject called geochemistry – a combination of geology and chemistry aimed at understanding the chemistry of the Earth. My speciality is in understanding the chemistry of the surface of the Earth, especially concentrations of chemicals where these occur either as natural concentrations in ore deposits or as a result of man's activity, for example, where there are landfill sites or contaminated land. When I studied this subject at university I had no idea how useful it would be in helping to deal with problems of human health (especially in developing countries), agricultural animals and the environment generally.

I have frequently worked with biochemists, veterinarians, epidemiologists and medical geographers looking at the impact of chemicals in the environment on the health of humans, animals and crops. Early in my career, between 1975 and 1977, I served on a Royal Society committee concerned with geochemistry and health.[2] Since that time, I and my team of scientists at the British Geological Survey (BGS), often working in collaboration with Imperial College, London, where I am now a professor, have been concerned with a wide range of human health problems related to the environment. Some of the methods we have developed allow us to make high-resolution maps showing the distribution of chemicals over the Earth's surface. We are able to look on our computer screens at the distribution of, say, cadmium or lead (as potentially toxic chemical elements) or copper or cobalt (elements essential to animal and human health in trace amounts) in the same way people can look at the Earth's physiography – using remotely sensed photographs from space.[3]

Almost from the beginning and initially to our great surprise, these images, although intended for geologists, created a lot of interest from veterinarians, who found them helpful in diagnosing environmental and nutritional animal diseases. For example, the veterinarians had an experimental farm to identify the levels of copper needed as a supplement in the diets of sheep and cattle in the north of Scotland. They could not understand why, when they gave the copper supplements developed on this farm to animals elsewhere, the animals quickly showed symptoms of copper poisoning. When they saw the maps we had produced, all became clear: their experimental farm contained soils with very high concentrations of another trace element, molybdenum, which blocks the uptake of copper, so the copper supplements they had developed contained far too much copper for general use. Seeing the natural variation in these two elements helped them to work out more appropriate doses of copper and other trace elements in relation to the natural variability of the soil. It was by working with veterinarians that I first began to learn of some of the amazing connections between geochemistry and biochemistry. I also learned, when I was ill, that veterinary rather than medical literature frequently provided the most fundamental answers. Eventually, I established a team that is regarded as one of the best in the world in tackling health problems related to the levels of trace elements in the environment: some, such as arsenic and fluoride, can occur at levels so high that they cause diseases like cancer or severe bone deformity, while others, such as selenium, iodine, zinc and cobalt, can occur at such low levels that they cause ill health in both man and animals. This is a particular problem in many developing countries.

Very recent work by the BGS team has included studies of iodine deficiency and fluoride toxicity. The latter can lead to severe bone deformity and may be caused by the burning of poor-quality coals (in parts of China, for example) or by the presence of naturally high levels of fluoride in drinking water.[4]

What I had learned as a result of this type of environmental detective work, time and time again, was that until you had identified the fundamental cause of such problems there was little or nothing that could be done to help the affected individuals. And until you've found the cause (whether it's of prostate cancer or any other disease) and effectively neutralised it, then you can never, ever claim to have 'cured' the problem.

HOW SCIENCE SERVES US – AND
WHY SOMETIMES IT DOESN'T

A good scientist will see things a little bit differently. I'd like to tell you something about the way that science works, which will help you to make sense of the differing approaches that scientists from different disciplines adopt when trying to treat diseases such as cancer. Also why any good scientist will want to probe and know *why* something such as a disease has occurred.

I also want to look at why, despite vast expenditure, we have made so little progress against cancers such as those of the prostate.

Not seeing the wood for the trees

There is a word to explain this situation, which also sums up what has happened to many branches of science in recent decades. This word, which is increasingly used pejoratively, is reductionism, which I would define as a rush to premature specialisation.

Let me quote from David Horrobin's article 'Not in the Genes', published in the *Guardian* on 12 February 2003, shortly before his death. Dr Horrobin was a prestigious medical researcher, and author of more than 800 papers. In the *Guardian* article he states:

> Starting in the 1960s, molecular biologists and genome specialists took over biomedical science. Journals and grant-giving bodies came to be dominated by reductionists, who were scathing about the complexity of the whole organ, whole animal and especially whole human studies which were seen as too full of uncontrolled variability to be interpretable. Now we have an almost wholly reductionist biomedical community which repeatedly makes exaggerated claims about how it is going to revolutionise medical treatment, and which repeatedly fails to achieve anything.

For some time this reductionist approach dominated my own subject of earth sciences in the UK and it is difficult to think of any memorable scientific breakthrough from that period. We have now returned to a systems-based approach, whereby all the Earth's complex interactions and feedbacks are taken into account to understand likely outcomes, as demonstrated in a recent lecture by Professor John Lawton, Head of the UK Natural Environment Research Council. In the case of global climate change, he showed how models are being developed at a global scale that take account of earth movements – for example the continuous rise of the Tibetan plateau and its influence in drawing the monsoons over India while keeping the Mediterranean supplied with warm air. He also discussed the interaction of greenhouse gases (released from natural sources and pollution) and the organisms at the Earth's surface and in the oceans that help to lock them away, and much, much more. We now grandly refer to our new approach as Earth Systems Science. In fact this is not new. In his 1991 book *Gaia: The Practical Science of Planetary Medicine*, the great natural scientist James Lovelock explains 'To understand the physiology of the Earth as a whole system we need science, but it must grow from the top down as well as from the bottom up!'

Of course reductionist science is vital. It provides the pieces of the jigsaw, but too great a reliance on reductionism can lead to so many pieces of the puzzle that it serves only to confuse.

Reductionist science produces masses and masses of data, but there are too few people to read and digest it. What happens to all the data that is generated by this work? Well, it gets published in learned journals, helping to create scientists' reputations and win more funding for yet more research. But how much of this work is directly beneficial to cancer patients? Disappointingly little, I suspect.

A better balance is needed, with the sort of science that involves analysing, synthesising or reviewing the work of others – putting the pieces of the jigsaw together. This is now highly unfashionable. It is thought not to be creative and not to provide the original cutting-edge ideas that 'bottom-up' science produces. Hence there are few prizes or distinctions for scientists carrying out such tasks and it is difficult for them to find sources of funding. Also, review papers are generally not welcomed by the prestigious research journals and they count for little on the curriculum vitae of an individual scientist.

The implied aim of reductionist science, in the case of cancer, is to find the single 'magic bullet'. Hence modern medical research in general, and especially in cancer research, is aimed at trying to find a pure form of a chemical compound which has a clearly defined (stoichiometric) chemical formula which can be administered in quantitative doses and shown in statistically designed clinical studies to have a significant and reproducible effect on the outcome of the disease. This approach falls under the worthy-sounding title of 'evidence-based medicine'.

But what if such a magic bullet doesn't exist? In that case, no amount of scientific research and no amount of expenditure will ever find it. We will have wasted many fortunes, many decades and many lives for little or nothing.

In the meantime, we are left with surgery, radiotherapy and chemotherapy – albeit improved and refined – as the main front-line treatments against prostate cancer, as they have been since the 1950s, together with hormone-based methods. True, there have been small improvements in survival, but the reported incidence of prostate cancer continues to rise (*see* Chapter 3, p. 95). If I am feeling at my most cynical, I cannot help thinking how this must be the best of all possible worlds for those involved in 'the cancer industry'.

Too great an emphasis on a reductionist approach towards cancer research also, sooner or later, runs into the law of diminishing returns, whereby we have to spend more and more to achieve less and less. That's why all the cancer charities you know seem to have an inexhaustible appetite for money and why many of them are the best-funded charities in existence. In *Your Life in Your Hands*, I complained that the only message we all seem to receive loud and clear is: 'Give us another billion or so, and give us another decade . . . and then we may finally have a cure that works.' Only the other night, when I was listening to the BBC, I heard the Head of the Medical Research Council in the UK ask for a substantial increase in government funding to take forward [reductionist] medicine. In this way, he said, many chronic illnesses would be treatable in *twenty years time*!

But, even if a cure were identified, would we be able to afford to prescribe it to cancer sufferers? The National Health Service in the UK is already in difficulty because of the cost of prescribing expensive new drugs which cost a lot of money to develop.

The high-technology approach to developing drugs for cancer is leading to many new drugs that are extremely expensive – which are then strongly marketed, often directly to patients via the Internet – although they may prolong life for only a few weeks or months. Hence there are increasingly highly charged emotional debates between individual patients and their families, who, understandably, wish to have the latest treatment, and health authorities and organisations that find it difficult to justify the large aggregated bills for groups of patients for marginal benefit. Is this approach really helpful except in the very short term?

The modern era in cancer research really began in America more than thirty years ago when President Richard Nixon proclaimed 'war' on cancer in his State of the Union address in

1971. And right from the beginning, it was dominated by reductionist scientific thinking, with its requirement for large-scale funding, extracted with the beguiling promise of a cure 'just round the corner'. 'Many people anticipated swift victory' recounts the news magazine *US News & World Report*, 'with the taming of the dread disease likened to a moon landing. Even as recently as 1984, the National Cancer Institute's director predicted that cancer deaths could be halved by the year 2000 in America.'

Such optimism was, of course, unjustified. Despite massive expenditure, the cancer death rate has continued to rise inexorably, and is now predicted by the World Health Organization (WHO) to double worldwide by 2020.[5]

Certainly, there have been some success stories: for example, childhood cancers, particularly some leukaemias, can now be treated and cured effectively. But such bright spots are too few and far between.

So what, you may be wondering, is the alternative to relying so heavily on reductionist science? And is it any more effective in delivering tangible benefits to ordinary people?

The benefits of a more holistic approach

Let me give you a couple of examples to explain how really significant medical breakthroughs have been made in the past with minimal resources but with great intellect and flair and a large measure of common sense. Most doctors would agree that the greatest contribution to all mankind in overcoming infectious diseases came not from the use of antibiotics but from improvements to public health: a clean water supply, improved sanitation, better nutrition and proper housing. These improvements came about as we gradually increased our understanding of why and how infectious diseases were transmitted. An early example of this type of work was carried out by Dr John Snow, who showed the value of studying the pattern of occurrence of disease. He made the famous dot map that showed the location of deaths from the epidemic of cholera which occurred in central London in September 1854. Deaths were marked by dots and, in addition, the area's eleven water pumps were located by crosses. Examining the scatter over the surface of the map, Snow observed that cholera occurred almost entirely among those who lived near (and drank from) the Broad Street water pump. He had the handle of the contaminated pump removed, ending the neighbourhood epidemic which had taken more than 500 lives.

This 'scientific detective work' is called epidemiology – literally the study of epidemics – and it has been used successfully many times to identify the cause of disease and, through public health medicine, to correct the things society was doing wrong.

In the case of cancer, Professor Sir Richard Doll's epidemiological study of lung cancer in the 1950s was one of the most significant advances in understanding cancer this century. He demonstrated beyond any shadow of a doubt the relationship between lung cancer and smoking tobacco, something human beings were doing to themselves. For the first time we had a modern rationale and scientific understanding of the cause of a common type of cancer. Following Doll's work, we can now choose whether to smoke or not in the knowledge that by doing so we shall significantly increase our risk of getting lung cancer. Moreover, identifying the cause of lung cancer has led to people quitting the habit, approximately halving the death rate from the disease.[6] Since that time, rational explanations have been found for many other types of cancers. For example, mesothelioma – a type of chest-wall cancer – is now known to be caused by exposure to asbestos dust, skin cancer to be caused by exposure to ultraviolet light or arsenic poisoning, and cervical cancer is known to be caused by infection by the sexually transmitted human papilloma (wart) virus, to give but a few examples.

Many doctors tend to see non-communicable diseases like prostate cancer as simply an inevitable result of ageing. For example, a 1999 article in the *British Medical Journal* (*BMJ*) spoke of '. . . the growing burden of non-communicable disease – in both developed and developing countries – as a consequence of population ageing. Cardiovascular disease, cancer, neuro-psychiatric conditions, and injury are fast becoming the leading causes of disability and premature death in most regions.'[7] There is no mention in the article of the influence of 'Western diet and lifestyle' or other possible underlying causes of non-communicable diseases. According to this line of reasoning, age is a primary cause of cancer. I, for one, think this is far too simplistic.

Before we proceed, let me tell you a little more about the scientific method and the way I was trained to approach problems.

This involves five stages:

1. **Gather existing information.** Previous facts and theories are reviewed as objectively and impartially, but as critically, as possible.

2. **Produce new information.** This is collected by experiment or observations, without emotional involvement. In some cases new ideas are produced by analysis and synthesis of information produced by other scientists. To be a good scientist you must be prepared to admit you are wrong: arriving at the truth is what is important, not personal prestige. If you raise a question, even if you arrive at the wrong answer, you will be respected if you work with honesty and openness. At the beginning of my science career, I learned a saying that has always stayed with me and guided my work: 'the person who asks the questions solves the problem'.

3. **Evaluate.** The new results are evaluated in relation to existing theories, and new insights or ideas are identified.

4. **A new hypothesis is proposed.** Speculation must be identified as such and clearly separated from facts.

5. **Test the hypothesis.** If the hypothesis works, submit it for further testing and validation until you have a new theory. If it doesn't work, begin again.

The characteristic values to which scientists have traditionally aspired are:[8]

- Honest experimentation.
- Meticulous respect for evidence.
- Candid admission of mistakes or error.
- Pursuit of truth.
- Moral and intellectual independence of all political authority and economic power.
- Openness to the public scrutiny of research by one's peers. (You will see that throughout the book I use the term 'peer reviewed' to indicate science published after it has been critically reviewed by other scientists. This type of information is distinguished from newspaper reports and other sources of information.)

This logical and ethical framework has been successfully used by scientists (whether they realised it or not) for centuries. It is how I and my team have successfully solved many human-health problems related to environmental factors, and it is precisely how I approached the challenge of my own breast cancer and also now prostate cancer.

There is a wealth of research – some of which goes back many decades – on the factors involved in prostate cancer. As you read the chapters that follow, I am sure you will be just as astonished as I was to learn how much has been discovered already but has not reached the public. While it is true that some of the risk factors for prostate cancer – such as increasing age or a family history of prostate cancer – are completely outside our control, there are many other risk factors that we can control – easily. These 'controllable' risk factors readily translate into simple changes that all men can make in their day-to-day lives to help prevent or treat the disease.

My message is: even advanced cancer can be overcome.

I know, because I've done it – and I have helped many, many prostate-cancer (and breast-cancer) sufferers to do the same.

RISK FACTORS

A risk factor is something that increases your chance of getting cancer. Different cancers have different risk factors. For example, smoking is a risk factor for cancers of the lung, mouth, larynx, bladder, kidney and some other organs.

But having a risk factor, or even several, does not mean that you will automatically develop cancer. Some men who have one or more prostate-cancer risk factors never develop the disease, while many men with prostate cancer have no known risk factors.

According to the University of Michigan website,[9] the following are the key known risk factors for prostate cancer in the USA:

- **Age.** Prostate cancer is found mainly in men over age 55. The average age of patients at the time of diagnosis is 70. (In the UK, the average age at diagnosis of prostate cancer is 72.[10])
- **Family history of prostate cancer.** A man's risk of developing prostate cancer is higher if his father or brother has had the disease.
- **Race.** This disease is much more common in African-American men than in white men. It is less common in Asian and native American men.

Scientists have studied whether benign prostatic hyperplasia (BPH), obesity, lack of exercise, smoking,[11] radiation exposure or a sexually transmitted virus might increase the risk for prostate cancer. At this time, there is little hard, validated evidence that these factors contribute to an increased risk.

In the UK, the following risk factors for prostate cancers have been suggested:

Factor	Variable
Demographic	Increasing age
	Place of residence
Genetic	Family history of prostate cancer
	Family history of breast cancer
	Race – black
Dietary	High fat consumption
	Low green-vegetable consumption
Occupational	Cadmium exposure
	Radiation exposure
	Farming

Source: Factsheet 20.3 1994 (Cancer of the Prostate) of the Cancer Research Campaign, adapted from Dearnaley, DP, 1994. Cancer of the prostate. *BMJ*, 308, 780–784.

One authority, Professor Jonathan Waxman of Imperial College, London, a distinguished oncologist specialising in prostate treatment,[12] points out that the Chinese diet, rich in soya, has been shown to be protective.

I am impressed that at least some dietary and lifestyle factors are mentioned in the factsheet above and by Professor Waxman; I have yet to see such factors included in most discussions of breast cancer.

In the section that follows I shall explain the reasoning and rationale for current cancer therapy.

One of the first questions that I think everyone asks when they are diagnosed with cancer is 'Why me? Why has this awful thing happened to me?' Eventually, I believe I found the answer to this question for breast-cancer and prostate-cancer sufferers, and it is very disquieting, because it brings home the high risk that people living a Western lifestyle are taking – a risk that increases more and more each year, despite the fact that, like me, most of the sufferers I know thought they were living a healthy lifestyle.

Throughout the West, prostate cancer is one of the most commonly occurring cancers affecting men. In the UK, for example, it is the commonest cancer in men, with a lifetime risk of being diagnosed of 1 in 14; it is rare under the age of 50.[13] In the US it is now the most commonly diagnosed cancer among men, with a lifetime risk of 1 in 6; one man there loses his life to the disease every 20 minutes.[14]

No man living a Western lifestyle should be surprised, therefore, to be one of those affected. The odds are high. However, what struck me very forcibly when I first became aware of these figures was the contrast between the comparatively high risk Western men and women run of contracting prostate or breast cancer, compared with the much lower risk of people living in the East (*see* Chapter 3). This was the first suspicion that there might be a cause for such cancers, just as there is a specific cause for the high risk of lung cancer that smokers run. In the following chapters I will tell you what I think that is, but first let us look at how to equip yourself to fight against the disease.

HOLDING YOUR GROUND

The typical route through cancer treatment is surgery, radiotherapy and chemotherapy. Many people use the analogy of cancer treatment as a battle between the disease and the treatments – with the patient as the battlefield. Although this analogy is unpopular with cancer charities or doctors, one of the things you must realise from the outset is the heavy toll that surgery, anaesthesia, radiotherapy and chemotherapy will take on your body. Many people have to take breaks or give up treatments, especially chemotherapy courses, because they become too ill – for example, if their blood-cell counts fall to too low a level. To cope with treatment you need to ensure you are equipped physically, emotionally and practically. Dietary and other methods to keep my body as well nourished as possible helped me cope physically (*see* Chapter 5 and *The Plant Programme*[15]). Using my scientific knowledge I developed other coping strategies to ensure that radioactive substances (used for diagnosis) or chemotherapeutic substances (used for treatment) were removed from my body as soon as possible after they had done their job. I outline these coping strategies in a tips section at the end of the chapter. I have found that other cancer sufferers find such tips very helpful. One of the first and most crucial things you have to do is to understand how to work with your doctor.

A GOOD DOCTOR-PATIENT RELATIONSHIP

Cancer patients often feel as if the disease is their 'fault' – either a genetic defect, something to do with 'blocked emotions' (research shows that there's no such thing as a 'cancer personality' – *see* Chapter 6) or the result of some other personal failing. This isn't true. Additionally, conventional cancer therapy can 'process' patients to the extent that they no longer understand what is really being done to them. A cancer patient is a vulnerable person and the relentless procedures may induce a feeling of loss of control. But it is vitally important to retain control and develop a constructive working partnership with all your medical team. Let me show you, particularly, how to work with your doctors and set out to recover your health.

In the case of cancer it is important to understand the different roles of research scientists and clinical doctors. Scientists are generally trying to answer the question 'why?' Doctors are professional human biologists who have taken an oath – the Hippocratic oath – which requires that they follow a strict code of ethical and professional behaviour. They tend to use only orthodox procedures established by clinical trials usually based on pure chemical substances or standardised technical pro-cedures validated by controlled, statistically based experiments using cell cultures or laboratory animals and, finally, patients. The growing threat of litigation against medical practitioners is making it more and more difficult for them to depart from orthodox medicine – though some alternative medicine is gaining acceptance by a profession that is necessarily conservative. Our GP recently treated my daughter Emma's repetitive strain injury with acupuncture rather than pills, for example. Emma said she felt a bit achy the following evening but was fine the next morning and has had no recurrences after more than two years.

Like most groups of professionals, doctors range in their ability from excellent to poor. My experience with medical doctors encompasses both and is probably typical. I was fortunate, in some ways, because right from the beginning, I was not in awe of them as many patients are. Even before I embarked on a career in science, I had developed something of a questioning approach towards medical custom and convention.

Your relationship with your doctor, be it your GP or cancer specialist is crucial to how well you manage the disease. Although it is only natural to be anxious and afraid (and, believe me, I was terrified), try to show your doctors that you will work with them to recover your health and that you wish to be fully involved in decisions.

How can you quickly tell whether your doctor is going to be a good bet? Here's a quick-and-easy ready reckoner I use: it makes no claim to be scientific, but it will help you focus your mind on the most important issues.

A CHECK-UP FOR YOUR DOCTOR	
Possesses lots of common sense and explains things clearly and effectively	Treats you arrogantly or impatiently and falls back on confusing jargon if questioned
Follows his or her chosen vocation because s/he obviously cares about people	Authoritarian – gets a kick out of telling you what to do, gets angry when you ask questions or suggest what is wrong with you
Demonstrates s/he is up to date in their knowledge	Indicates s/he is ignorant of subjects that they should understand. Dismisses information, even from the peer-reviewed scientific literature
Technically skilful, e.g. knows how to carry out a thorough physical examination	Fails to give a thorough examination or to come up with a meaningful diagnosis
Prepared to discuss your health with you on a partnership basis and to recommend dietary, lifestyle or other factors you can change yourself	Uninterested in underlying cause and displays a clear preference for empirical (suck it and see) methods to suppress symptoms; reaches for the prescription pad or computer keyboard almost before you have started your second sentence

Interestingly, a systematic review of the literature on patients' priorities for general-practice care, conducted as part of a project by a European task force,[16] raises similar points. The most highly rated aspect of care was 'humaneness', followed by competence and accuracy. Provision of information and opportunities for participation also featured highly in most studies of patient satisfaction. It was noted that patients increasingly expect to participate in decisions about their care, but these aspirations are rarely met. Most patients want to be able to trust the health professionals they consult, but this did not mean they wanted to be deceived about the nature of their illness or the risks and potential harms of medical treatment. The authors suggest that in order to avoid putting greater burdens on doctors' time, they should provide information and educational packs and help patients to think through their preferences with training to manage their condition by nurses, counsellors, information officers or fellow patients.[17] The success of the approach centres on having access to and understanding information.

In an article in the *BMJ*, the Chief Medical Officer of the Department of Health, Dr Liam Donaldson, wrote 'The patient as expert and partner in care is an idea whose time has come and has the potential to create a new generation of patients who are empowered to take action to improve their health in an unprecedented way.'[18]

Of course, this is the whole principle behind this book and my previous books, *Your Life in Your Hands*, *The Plant Programme* and *Understanding, Preventing and Overcoming Osteoporosis*,[19] and I am aware that these books, or references to them, are included in patient packs provided by good GPs and hospitals.

Another factor of particular relevance in prostate cancer, with a possible bearing on the relationship between patient and health professional, is gender. Initial statistics suggest that men are significantly less likely to visit their GP than women and anecdotal evidence suggests that they are more likely to present with their disease at a more advanced stage. The reasons for this are not known. According to some doctors, many men are reluctant to accept personal vulnerability and this may affect their judgment. It may also mean that they prefer not to see their own GP, or even attend their own practice, about 'embarrassing problems'.[20] On the other hand, many patients would prefer to see the same doctor all the time. While some general practices regard this as the preferred procedure, this is by no means always the case. If you have cancer and insist that you need this kind of support and your practice refuses, you might wish to consider changing your practice. Discussing a diagnosis of prostate cancer with elderly men (aged 65 or more) may require considerable care, since it has been reported that serious physical illness, including cancer, is associated with increased risk of suicide, especially in men.[21] Patients in emotional distress who find it difficult to talk to friends and family may find it helpful to talk to the Samaritans, a charity devoted to providing a free 24-hour telephone counselling service.

According to the Director of the Patients Association,[22] there are some key things that patients want from their doctor.

- **Eye contact.** Apparently some doctors continue to look at their computer screen while greeting their patients.
- **Partnership.** Patients want to be people who doctors do things with, not people that doctors do things to. They want to be consulted about their condition and treatment [including more information about the possible side effects of any drug they are prescribed[23]].
- **Communication**. Communication from doctor to patient and vice versa is the key to a successful consultation. In many cases patients are scared and don't understand (or can't take in) what the doctor is saying. With the shock that follows a diagnosis of cancer, the doctor's description of the illness may have been inaccurately heard or misrepresented. It may even be remembered variably, with the patient repeating their description of events in different ways, depending on who they are talking to. For these reasons it is important that patients who may receive a diagnosis of cancer are accompanied by a friend or companion who can sit in and, if possible, make written notes of the conversation.[24]
- **Time.** Patients want to spend more time with their doctor.
- **Appointments.** Patients want to see their doctor within a reasonable time.

It is also considered important, in the case of prostate cancer, to understand fully the patient's main goal, which may be survival, postponing or relieving symptoms, or minimising the side effects of treatment such as incontinence or impotence.[25]

Medical professionals are now being advised to:[26]

- Build the doctor-patient relationship.
- Develop a shared understanding of the situation.
- Agree a way forward.

On the other hand patients should realise that many doctors will find it difficult to tell them of a diagnosis of prostate cancer and to discuss aspects of the disease that are important but uncomfortable to discuss, such as incontinence and other possible side effects. People who have had such cancer describe how sexual difficulties were ducked and how they struggled to maintain their previous persona.[27]

A frequent problem that patients encounter is the use by the medical profession of language that seems calculated to be obscure. Before medical students can become doctors, they must be initiated into a language which, it has been estimated, contains 10,000 new words – words that, to most of us, seem just as dead as the Greek or Latin from which they originated.[28] Why, for example, should itching be called 'pruritis' or a runny nose 'rhinorrhea'? Although it is easy to see why the term 'idiopathic hypercalcuria' (too much calcium in the urine, of unknown origin) is used to describe this condition! These are extreme examples, it is true, but they make a useful point.

With the increasing bureaucratisation of the NHS, even English is being turned into gobbledegook. Describing the aims of the new Commission for Patient and Public Involvement in Health, the chief executive is quoted as saying 'We would want to have highly effective knowledge databases that people could draw on so that they could have constructive, meaningful debate that moves the agenda forward in a constructive way. What we're talking about are intelligent, informed, democratised challenges that provide better outcomes for everyone'. The new body's aims are therefore described in anything but lucid terms.[29]

Always insist on fully understanding what your doctor or other health professional is saying to you, and if they start to use new and alarming-sounding words, ask them to explain precisely what they are trying to tell you in simpler language. Clarify any details by asking them to draw you a diagram, for instance. Then you will be in a much stronger position to evaluate, influence and, if necessary, query your diagnosis and treatment. Once my doctors realised I was a scientist, they tolerated my questions and tried hard to answer and reassure me. But even then I felt I didn't know enough. It wasn't that they were holding anything back: it's just that their approach seemed so different from mine.

THE PROVINCE OF THE PROSTATE
As there was in the case of breast cancer,[30] there remains great controversy among health professionals about the value of screening and early detection.

The common-sense thing to do is to learn about your own body. It always amazes me how little men know or understand about the prostate gland until it causes trouble. A survey in *The*

1 8   P R O S T A T E   C A N C E R

Times, for example, found that 89 per cent of men did not know where their prostate is located (www.healthandnutrition.co.uk/articles/prostate/htm). We should all learn the basics of our anatomy and how our body feels normally and examine ourselves regularly to find out when things are wrong – especially when they are seriously wrong. Although self-examination is out of the question in the case of prostate cancer, there are several symptoms to be aware of, as discussed below. Let us first learn a little more about the prostate gland.

Looking at the simplified drawing of male reproductive organs and urinary tract (Figure 1.1 overleaf), you will see that the prostate gland is situated between the pubic bone and the rectum, and surrounds the urethra, the tube through which urine passes from the bladder to the penis. The tubes of the reproductive system through which the sperm pass meet the urethra in the prostate. The prostate gland provides the fluid in which sperm are carried and it contracts at orgasm to propel the sperm out of the penis. Hence its function is connected with the whole urinary and male reproductive system.[31]

In a young boy, the gland is the size of a pea, growing at puberty to the shape and size of a walnut. At the same time growth within the prostate leads to the development of microscopic glands that produce the prostatic secretion called prostate-specific antigen (PSA). This fluid, which is rich in sugar and enzymes, is important in sexual activity. The PSA, which drains through tiny prostatic ducts, provides the fluid in which sperm are carried. The sperm is nourished by the sugar-rich fluid. PSA also clears residual matter left in the prostatic ducts after orgasm.[32] The level of PSA normally present in the bloodstream reflects the activity and health of the prostate gland. This can be measured in a PSA test (*see* pp. 24–29).

The development and growth of the prostate at puberty are influenced by the pituitary gland, the master gland of the body, which sits in the centre of the brain and produces growth hormone and another important hormone called prolactin and orchestrates thyroid hormone production, all of which are important in the development and growth of the prostate gland.[33]

Certainly in the West, however, the prostate seems to grow again in men in their late forties, and herein lies the problem.[34] Prostate growth increases with age, and enlargement of the gland in older men can cause significant difficulties with urination, including as a result of obstruction of the neck of the bladder by an enlarged prostate.[35]

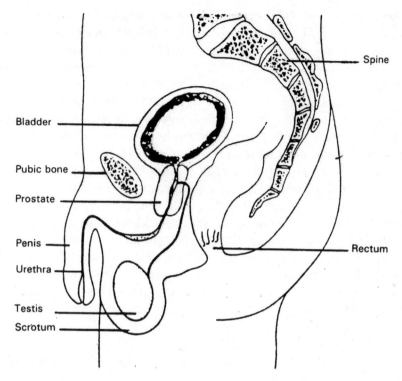

Bladder

Pubic bone

Prostate

Penis

Urethra

Testis

Scrotum

Spine

Rectum

Figure 1.1: Male urino-genital tract, showing position of the prostate gland.

PROSTATE CONDITIONS[36]

Let us now look at diseases of the prostate generally.

Benign prostatic hyperplasia (BPH)

Benign enlargement of the prostate, otherwise known as benign prostatic hyperplasia (BPH; sometimes also known as benign prostatic hypertrophy) is the most common cause of prostate problems and is considered a condition of ageing. Treatments to limit the size of the prostate include surgery such as transurethral prostatectomy (TURP) in which a tube is inserted through the penis along the urethra to remove physical obstruction. Alternatively, drug treatments can be used to reduce the size of the prostate. Because prostate enlargement can be a slow process, taking many years, medical treatment is generally less effective than surgery and often takes a considerable time to improve symptoms; it is usually reserved for patients who are unfit for surgery. A TURP will lead to an improvement in nearly all patients. Drug treatments are hormonal and include the LHRH agonists (*see* p. 51). Herbal medicines can also help (*see* p. 59).

More than half of the men in the United States between the ages of 60 and 70 and as many as 90 per cent between the ages of 70 and 90 have symptoms of BPH. For some men, the symptoms may be severe enough to require treatment.[37] The symptoms of BPH and cancer are very much the same and are principally the symptoms of enlargement of the gland.[38]

According to Wilt, treatment options for BPH depend on how men, in discussion with their doctor, balance the bother of lower urinary tract symptoms with the relative effectiveness and likely adverse effects of various types of treatments.[39] For men with mild to moderate urinary symptoms, management by GPs is appropriate. Alpha-blocking drugs are the preferred pharmacological treatment for improving symptoms and urine flow, regardless of the extent of prostate enlargement, although they are associated with side effects such as dizziness and headaches. Combining these drugs with another drug, finasteride (which inhibits the activity of an enzyme that converts the androgen testosterone into its active form dihydrotestosterone (DHT) (see p. 52), provides no greater improvement in symptoms than alpha-blockers alone. Alpha-blockers have not been clearly shown to prevent complications from BPH or the need for surgery in the long term.

A study to compare two drugs doxazosin and finasteride, alone and in combination, for the treatment of symptoms of BPH showed results for finasteride that were not significantly different from the placebo. Doxazosin was effective in improving urinary symptoms and urinary flow rate, and was more effective than finasteride alone or a placebo. The addition of finasteride did not provide further benefit to that achieved with doxazosin alone.[40]

Another study showed that a drug called tamsulosin was more effective than finasteride for short-term treatment of BPH, with a better safety profile.[41]

Men with severe symptoms (see below) should be referred to a urologist. If the conditions are due to BPH, surgery is thought to result in a lower incidence of complications, including the need for blood transfusions and hospital stays. Another systematic review compared surgery with laser treatment for BPH and showed that the former led to greater improvement in urinary symptoms than either contact or non-contact laser therapies. However, men treated with lasers had fewer complications (although many trials did not report adverse events). There were no differences between the groups in the incidence of sexual problems or incontinence.[42]

In another study, comparing TURP, non-contact laser therapy and watchful waiting, Brookes and colleagues[43] found that older men needing treatment for urinary symptoms but wanting to retain sexual function should consider standard surgery rather than non-contact laser therapy.

Prostatitis

Prostatitis is an inflammation of the prostate gland and can be caused by infection or, sometimes, sexual activity. Symptoms include significant pain, usually with a temperature and frequency of urination. Treatment with antibiotics, in some cases intravenously, may be required. Prostatitis can be a recurring problem for some men, requiring repeated courses of antibiotics.

Prostate cancer

Prostate cancer can vary from a relatively harmless condition to a serious illness, and its frequency increases with age. A small amount of prostate cancer is commonly found in older men who have died from other causes, with up to 80 per cent in 80 year olds. According to Waxman, little spots of cancer occur in 70 per cent of 70 year olds, 60 per cent of 60 year olds and 50 per cent of 50 year olds, but their relationship with the development of aggressive cancer is unknown.

A non-aggressive type of prostate cancer is known as prostatic intra-epithelial neoplasia, or PIN. Some doctors regard PIN as being a precursor of cancer, likely to lead to the development of an invasive tumour, although most remain unconvinced that PIN is related to overt prostate cancer. If you are diagnosed with PIN, you should be reassured that it is unlikely to progress to invasive cancer, but you will be advised to have an annual check-up including PSA testing (see p. 24).

Difficulties with urination caused by prostate cancer can be due to the physical enlargement of the gland or to the invasion of the prostatic urethral valves by cancer so that they are unable to open and shut normally. In serious cases, it becomes impossible to pass urine; this causes considerable pain, because of the pressure on the bladder, and requires catheterisation to remove the obstruction.

SYMPTOMS OF PROSTATE CANCER

Remember that, although any of the symptoms listed below can indicate cancer, they are more likely to be caused by a non-cancerous disease. In any case, if you find any of the symptoms described, see your doctor as soon as possible. Even if you are reassured that nothing is wrong, monitor changes and return to the doctor and press for a referral if you think there is a problem, certainly if any of your symptoms become worse. Such symptoms include:[44]

- difficulty or pain when passing urine
- the need to pass urine more often
- broken sleep due to the need to pass urine
- waiting for long periods before urine flows
- dribbling during urination
- incomplete emptying of the bladder, which may lead to urinary infection accompanied by pain in the penis and a high temperature

These symptoms are the same as those for BPH. Prostate cancer may additionally cause:

- blood in the urine and/or semen

This and associated symptoms can be caused by other factors such as bacterial infection.[45]

Other symptoms of advanced prostate cancer can include:

- swollen lymph nodes in the groin area
- impotence (difficulty having an erection)
- pain in the pelvis, spine, hips, or ribs

These symptoms, too, may be due to other diseases (for example, pain in the spine, pelvis or hips frequently reflects arthritis, especially in older men) and do not necessarily mean that a man has prostate cancer.[46]

A TESTING TIME

The time taken to diagnose prostate cancer in the UK is longer than for any other tumour type, for a range of reasons, one of the most significant being the non-specific nature of the symptoms of the disease.[47] Urinary frequency, for example, the commonest symptom of prostate cancer, can also reflect BPH, and hence affects almost all older men. Typically, the symptoms will have developed gradually over many years and may be ignored until the problem becomes critical. For the same reasons, GP referrals of their patients to hospitals may fail to indicate any need for urgency.

Another problem is that even if the tumour is cancerous, to date there is no way of telling how aggressive the growth will be. The problem is that some men with small yet rapidly growing cancers have not been spotted in time. Others with enlarged and malignant prostates may have had slow growth for ten years or more, with no spread to other tissues.[48]

In America, the American Cancer Society (ACS) recommends that a PSA test and a digital rectal examination (DRE) should be offered annually beginning at age fifty to men who have a life expectancy of at least ten years. Men at high risk (see p. 10) should be tested beginning at age 45. Some men, apparently, ask their doctor to make the testing decision on their behalf, and they should be tested.[49] A clinical policy of not offering testing, or discouraging testing in men who request early prostate cancer detection tests, is considered inappropriate in the US. It is recommended, however, that if healthcare professionals offer men the option of PSA and/or DRE tests they should, prior to testing, discuss the potential benefits, side effects, and uncertainties regarding early detection and treatment to help them make an informed decision.[50] In the UK, advice is more equivocal but if you are concerned you should go to see your GP.

On visiting your GP to discuss symptoms, give the fullest, clearest information possible. They should listen to an account of your symptoms, assess your general physical condition, check for bladder enlargement, perform a DRE and blood tests for blood count, kidney function and PSA levels (see below). During the DRE, you will be asked to lie on your side and adopt a foetal position, drawing your legs up to your stomach. The doctor will insert a gloved finger coated with lubricating jelly into the rectum to determine the size and shape of the prostate, which is likely to be much bigger with BPH and become knobbly if cancer is present.[51] Be reassured that even abnormal findings on DRE, such as nodularity or induration of the prostate, lead to a diagnosis of prostate cancer as a result of biopsy in only 15 to 25 per cent of cases. This compares with prostate cancer prevalence of less than 5 per cent among men of similar age without abnormal DRE. Although neither accurate nor sensitive for prostate cancer detection, abnormal DRE is associated with a five-fold increased risk of cancer present at time of screening.[52]

PSA TEST

As discussed earlier, PSA is produced by the normal prostate and secreted in the seminal fluid in large quantities. Prostate cancer changes the cellular barriers that normally keep PSA within the ductal system of the prostate and causes it to be released into the bloodstream. The PSA test measures the level of PSA in the blood. The result is reported in ng/ml (nanograms per millilitre – very tiny amounts).

Doctors have had a hard time establishing an absolute cut-off level at which more testing is needed. Most (but not all) doctors agree that PSA levels below 4 are normal and levels over 10 indicate that a prostate biopsy (in which tissue is removed and examined under a microscope) is needed. But a grey zone exists for levels between 4 and 10. About one in four men whose PSA is in this range have prostate cancer and in such cases some doctors recommend that a biopsy should be performed immediately. But the biopsy can be uncomfortable and carries a risk of infection and bleeding, so other doctors suggest repeating the PSA test at a later date or using other tests.[53]

In the US,[54] many doctors now recommend a biopsy when PSA levels are higher than 4. But there is controversy about the exact cut-off point that separates 'normal' from 'abnormal' PSA levels, and some doctors use 3.0 or 2.5 as the upper limits of normal.

PSA levels can be used together with clinical examination results and the tumour's Gleason score from biopsy samples (*see* p. 32) to decide which additional tests are needed. The PSA test is also used to monitor the effectiveness of treatments and indicate evidence of recurrence.[55]

Since the first use of the PSA blood test in the 1980s, doctors have been able to detect many more cases of prostate cancer at an earlier stage and, unlike mammography for breast cancer detection, which involves irradiation, the PSA test has no effect on the body. But the test is not perfect, and several important questions have yet to be answered. For example, it is not yet known if screening with the PSA test will save lives or prolong patients' survival. Prostate cancer is thought to be more curable if detected at an early stage. But some doctors argue that the test may be detecting some cancers that would never cause symptoms in a normal lifetime because they are so slow growing.[56] This is important because some treatment for prostate cancer can have lasting adverse side effects, and patients with abnormal PSA, particularly those who have no other symptoms, should weigh their options carefully before proceeding with radical forms of treatment. Certainly, a biopsy must be performed before proceeding with treatment, but even this carries a risk of infection since it is generally carried out through the rectum, which is full of bacteria.

Let us look further at some of the pros and cons of the PSA test to help you and your doctor decide what is best for you.

The pros of the PSA test

According to a recent article in *The Times* by Dr Thomas Stuttaford,[57] evidence in the US and in most of the developed world, where most doctors recommend regular testing with the PSA blood test, strongly suggests that this policy is paying off. The PSA reading for those with a prostate gland-confined cancer is vital. The chances of long-term survival fall dramatically if the PSA is over 10 (not my experience of communicating with prostate-cancer sufferers who follow my diet and regime). It is therefore important to have regular testing so that any cancer can be detected while the PSA is still low. In the US, doctors consider the PSA to be fundamental. In the UK, research has shown that if the PSA is over 10 only 34 per cent of the patients treated do not have evidence of a spreading tumour after 5 years.

A qualitative study by Chapple and colleagues[58] shows that the reasons why men with prostate cancer advocate screening include beliefs about the benefit of early diagnosis and the need to have responsibility. Policy makers, politicians, and doctors, the authors say, need to understand why people want wider access to PSA testing.

Herxheimer and Ziebland also found that men with prostate cancer felt strongly that healthy men should be offered PSA testing, despite the false positives (high PSA results for patients who turn out not to have prostate cancer) and the fact that earlier diagnosis has not been shown to lead to more effective treatment. They believed that early diagnosis would reduce mortality, improve quality of life and save the NHS money. They argued that testing should be available because 1) symptoms can be ambiguous, 2) screening is seen as responsible health behaviour and would encourage men to look after their health, and 3) there is equivalent screening for women's cancers.[59] A related finding was that many men for whom 'watchful waiting' (*see* p. 41) would have been an appropriate option would not contemplate it, and indeed few of those who might have chosen it remembered any mention of it in discussion with their doctor.[60]

In Europe, unlike the USA, a system of screening men for prostate cancer once in every four years is considered sufficiently effective in catching nearly all tumours in time. Researchers on the ongoing European Randomised Study of Screening for Prostate Cancer studied more than 17,000 men and reported that 'very few, if any, aggressive prostate cancers escape the screening'.[61]

It has also been pointed out by one patient that had he not had a PSA test his prognosis might have been worse than others who presented with bone metastases and high PSA values. He points out that during his decision-making process he came across a paper on dilemmas in treating early prostate cancer.[62] It was easy, he said, to work out that there just aren't enough experienced urologists (able to carry out this tricky operation successfully) to carry out the number of radical prostatectomies that early detection by PSA screening would require. A sample of 244 urologists had a mean of 14.1 years experience, and 130 of them managed 100 patients or more with prostate cancer. Expertise in performing radical prostatectomy was restricted to comparatively few – 98 reported having ever performed the procedure and only 12 (14 per cent) that they performed 20 or more operations yearly. He also suspects that the UK is far short of the number of three-dimensional conformal radiotherapy machines (*see* p. 45) needed to offer that treatment option.[63]

The cons of the PSA test

Opponents of PSA testing claim that the use of this test is responsible for the observed increase in incidence of the disease. It is also claimed that PSA screening causes over-diagnosis in about 29 per cent of white men and 44 per cent of black men in the USA who would otherwise have died of another cause, without their prostate cancer being detected in their lifetime.[64] One recent study compared data on prostate-cancer mortality in the Seattle–Puget Sound area of the USA, where screening and aggressive treatment were adopted early, with Connecticut, where adoption of these procedures was slower. In 1987–1990, men aged 65 to 79 in Seattle were 5 times as likely to undergo PSA testing and twice as likely to undergo biopsy, and rates of radical prostatectomy and radiotherapy were also substantially higher. Nevertheless, through eleven years of follow-up, prostate-cancer mortality was similar in the two areas.[65]

A high PSA test result suggests that cancer may be present, but similar results can also be caused by inflammation of the prostate, urinary retention, prostatic infection, BPH, and prostatic manipulation. According to some authors, neither the DRE nor the PSA test is accurate, nor are they adequately sensitive for prostate-cancer screening.[66]

Factors found in the blood from high dairy consumption and some medications increased PSA levels, as well as vigorous exercise (though bike riding has been suggested not to influence PSA levels[67]). Moreover, it has been stated that the test does not seem able to distinguish between malignant and non-malignant prostate tumours, and one USA report concluded that as many as two thirds of those testing positive probably do not have cancer.[68]

Physicians have speculated that PSA screening may be responsible for the reduction in prostate-cancer deaths observed in the late 1990s, but the results of a recent survey suggest that, for the study population, PSA screening cannot explain the decline in prostate-cancer mortality.[69]

Another study reported that only 15 to 25 per cent of cases with PSA greater than 4.0 were found to have prostate cancer on biopsy.[70]

An editorial in the *Journal of the National Cancer Institute* commented on the PSA controversy under the title, 'The More We Know, the Less We Understand'. 'Only one man in four with a PSA level greater than 4.0 is found to have prostate cancer on biopsy,' it noted, 'and about one-third of prostate cancers are detected in men with a normal PSA level'[71] (the problem of false positives and false negatives respectively).

In a review article in the *BMJ* entitled 'The PSA Storm', Yamey and Wilkes describe how questioning cancer screening can be a risky business in America.[72] They conclude that they angered a group of urologists who are protagonists of the PSA test by challenging its 'wishful thinking'. They also suggest that they 'stepped on the toes of a very wealthy and powerful pro-screening lobby that stands to make money from encouraging men to get tested. Even some of the patient-support groups in this lobby have a conflict of interest, since they rely on pharmaceutical company support. With the widespread belief in America that every man should know his PSA, a belief driven by politics and not evidence,' Yamey and Wilkes fear that 'sceptical voices like theirs will always be drowned out.'

Improved methods of testing
Efforts are underway to improve the reliability of the PSA test. Scientists have discovered variations in a gene that controls levels

of PSA in men – a finding that could make PSA screenings for prostate cancer more accurate.[73]

One new study shows that genetic variations can directly influence levels of PSA that can be detected in a man's bloodstream. It is estimated that 29 million men may have the genes that produce levels of PSA about 30 per cent higher than average. PSA levels are generally higher in African-American men.[74] It is too early to know whether men with higher levels are at higher risk for cancer. It is also too soon to know whether men with lower-than-normal PSA levels are at risk of having their cancer remain undiagnosed.

If the results of the study are confirmed it is suggested that $12 billion a year could be saved in unnecessary biopsies. Testing for the newly discovered gene variants is quick and inexpensive and could become a part of the PSA screening regimen.[75]

In another study, scientists have reported that measuring a precursor form of PSA called proPSA improves the accuracy of testing. By measuring the proportion of proPSA relative to PSA they were able to identify the men with aggressive cancer earlier and they believe this method could also reduce the number of unnecessary biopsies.[76]

Some PSA circulates unbound to other substances in the blood and is called the per cent free PSA. PSA results between 4 and 10 combined with a low per cent free PSA means that a prostate cancer is more likely to be present. The laboratory doing the testing will provide this information to your doctor. Another refinement uses the PSA velocity (the increase in PSA level over time), which is calculated from the results obtained from three specimens over at least an eighteen-month period. A PSA velocity over 0.75 per year is considered high and suggests the need for a biopsy.

Other, less common, methods of using PSA results include PSA density, to adjust for men who have large prostate glands, and age-specific PSA levels. Doctors are looking at whether the latter may be a more accurate indicator of the presence of cancer, because levels increase naturally with age. Neither of these methods has yet been validated.[77]

The PSA test – some suggestions

In summary, according to the ACS,[78] there are many uncertainties regarding the early detection and treatment of prostate cancer. Cancers found by PSA testing and/or DRE are, on average, smaller and have spread less than cancers discovered because of the symptoms they cause. But prostate cancer is unlike many other cancers in that it often grows very slowly.

For men with cancer that has not spread beyond the prostate, the five-year relative survival rate is almost 100 per cent, whether or not they are treated. On the other hand, before early detection tests were widely used, most men with prostate cancer were diagnosed with advanced disease and most died within a few years of the diagnosis.

Although early diagnosis and treatment of prostate cancer can help some men to live longer, it may not affect the life span of other men. For a man who has poor health or other serious medical illnesses and is not likely to live more than ten years, there may be no benefit in an early diagnosis of prostate cancer, and it may do more harm than good, by affecting his quality of life.

Certainly I think the suggestion that a high PSA test result should be repeated at least once before an invasive biopsy is performed[79] is sound advice. The lead author of the study is quoted as saying, 'Even if the repeat test shows an elevated level, prostate cancer will only be discovered in about one quarter of men who undergo biopsy . . . A single elevated PSA level does not automatically warrant a prostate biopsy'. Yet another study found that the PSA results may fluctuate from year to year. In some cases, levels that were abnormally high returned to normal on their own, avoiding the need for immediate biopsy.[80]

There are certain measures you can take to make your PSA test as accurate as possible. Because ejaculation can cause a temporary increase in blood PSA levels, abstinence from sexual activity is recommended for two days before the test is performed. Also, urinary tract infections, BPH and inflammation of the prostate can all elevate PSA levels. On the other hand, several medicines (including finasteride and some anti-androgens) and herbal preparations (such as PC-SPES, a herbal mixture that contains Saw Palmetto, see p. 61) can lower PSA levels **so that early prostate cancer is undetected**.[81] Ask your doctor for advice on the length of time you should stay off such drugs and preparations before having your PSA test.

REFERRAL

If your GP finds significant evidence of prostate disease, after due consideration of your symptoms and test and examination results, you will be referred to a consultant urologist, or to an oncologist if a diagnosis of cancer is suspected. Most patients will be found to have BPH and their care will remain with the urologist.[82] Those with suspected cancer will generally be referred to an oncologist specialising in prostate cancer, and usually the same examination, tests and case histories that their GPs carried out will be repeated at the hospital.

If you are referred to a hospital consultant, my general advice to all UK patients is to obtain treatment for serious illnesses such as cancer at NHS centres of excellence. I am aware of several people whose cancer remained undiagnosed by their private hospitals or physicians and by the time they attended NHS clinics their cancer was very far advanced. A recent study has shown that patients in for-profit hospitals in the USA are more likely to die than those in non-profit hospitals (approximately 2200 extra deaths a year – about the same number as die from suicide, colon cancer or traffic accidents in Canada each year).[83]

Most good hospitals treating prostate cancer now have a specialist unit with a team that includes oncologists, radiotherapists and chemotherapists. I still hear from men who have been treated, some of them privately and expensively, by general surgeons using an approach which can only be described as in the best tradition of 'muddling through', with no attempt to assess the nature and scale of the problem at the outset. Being treated by a specialist team is essential. Ensure your GP knows your views and refuse to be fobbed off with anything less than treatment at a specialist centre of excellence. Your life, quite literally, may depend on it. In the case of surgery, for example, ensure you are treated by a surgeon who carries out at least thirty such operations a year, and ask about his or her success rates compared to the national average. Also ask about survival rates generally at the centre at which you are being treated. (Asking for such information is particularly important for men having prostate operations, because this operation is quite complicated.) Such statistics need to be treated with caution, however, because some doctors will treat patients whom others regard as incurable. I remember asking senior doctors at Charing Cross at what point did they give up – was it when patients had less than a 50:50 chance of survival? I found their reply very moving. They said that, providing the patient wanted to survive, they would never give up.

BIOPSY

A *core-needle biopsy* is the main method used to diagnose prostate cancer accurately. The doctor will commonly use TRUS (*see* p.

34) for guidance.[84] Biopsies are performed using fine, spring-loaded needles inserted into the prostate through the wall of the rectum. Six to ten core biopsies may be taken, from different places in the prostate. A local anaesthetic is normally used. Some patients find the procedure painless, others report some discomfort, while some experience severe pain. The biopsy procedure can leave some patients in pain for quite a time. It results in infection (since the needle passes through the rectum) in 1 to 2 per cent of patients in the UK, and it may even lead to incontinence and impotence for a time. The specimens taken should be examined by a pathologist experienced in staging and grading prostate cancer (*see* below).[85] Some blood in the urine or in bowel movements is common for two to three days following the biopsy. Blood may occur in the semen for up to two to three weeks.[86]

Lymph-node biopsy may also be performed to find out if cancer has spread from the prostate to nearby lymph nodes. This is done in, for example, men with a high Gleason score (*see* below) or young men with a high PSA level. A specially trained radiologist may take a small sample of cells from lymph nodes using a technique called *fine-needle aspiration*, using a computed tomography (CT) scan image to guide insertion of the long, thin needle.[87] If cancer cells are found in the lymph-node biopsy specimens, treatment options other than surgery are likely to be used.

STAGING AND GRADING

The **stage** of a prostate cancer indicates how far it has spread within the gland, neighbouring tissues and other organs. It is an important factor in selecting treatment options and considered to be highly significant in predicting outcome. The TNM System of the American Joint Committee on Cancer (AJCC) is the most commonly used system in the US and is the basis for the WHO system. It describes the extent of primary tumour (T), the presence or absence of spread to nearby lymph nodes (N), and the presence or absence of spread (metastasis) to distant organs (M). The stages described here are generalised from the 1992 version of the AJCC staging manual. Ensure that your doctor is using the 1992 version before trying to apply it to the guidelines below – but note that it predates the widespread use of the PSA test.[88]

T stages   There are two types of T classifications for prostate cancer: the *clinical* stage, based on DRE, needle biopsy and TRUS findings (*see* p. 34), which is used in making treatment decisions; and the *pathological* stage, following surgery, which is based on full investigation of the entire prostate, the seminal vesicles (two small sacs next to the prostate that store semen) and, in some cases, nearby lymph nodes, and is therefore more accurate in prognosis. There are four T stages. T1 refers to a cancer that is not felt during a DRE, although cancer cells are found in a prostate biopsy or prostatectomy specimen. T2 means that the doctor can feel the prostate cancer by DRE and that the cancer is thought to be confined to the prostate gland. T3 cancers have spread beyond the outer rim of the gland and have reached the surrounding tissue and/or the seminal vesicles, but do not involve any other organs. T4 cancers have spread to tissues next to the prostate.

N stages   N0 means that the cancer has not spread to any lymph nodes. N1 indicates spread to one lymph node in the pelvis, but its size is less than 2 cm in diameter. N2 means that the cancer has spread to one lymph node, and is between 2 and 5 cm in diameter; or that it is in more than one node, but none is larger than 2 cm. N3 means that there is at least one lymph node larger than 5 cm. Nx means that tests to detect lymph node spread have not been done.

M stages   M0 means that the cancer has not metastasised beyond the regional nodes. M1 means that metastases are present in distant (outside the pelvis) lymph nodes, in bones, or in other distant organs such as liver, lungs or brain. Mx means that tests to find distant spread have not been done.

GLEASON RATING[89]

One system used to assess the severity of prostate tumours, known as the Gleason rating system, can be used by doctors when discussing treatment options with their patients.

Gleason scores are determined by examining prostate biopsy samples, or by examining the entire prostate after surgical removal. Since biopsy samples represent only a small portion of the entire prostate, they may not be representative of the gland as a whole. The Gleason score as determined from the biopsy specimen, however, has been shown to be one of the best methods of predicting how prostate cancer will progress. An accurate Gleason score can help decide on the best treatment options.[90]

The Gleason score indicates the aggressiveness of the tumour, according to how well it is differentiated (cells that are completely differentiated are good, healthy cells). Gleason Patterns 1 and 2 are well differentiated; Pattern 3 is moderately differentiated; and Patterns 4 and 5 are poorly differentiated. Perfectly differentiated prostate cells are happy to go about their business in the prostate making PSA and ejaculatory fluid. They look and act like the mature prostate cells they are. They interact with other perfectly differentiated prostate cells to create the tiny tubular structures that the prostate requires to deliver its product to the urethra. Once they become malignant, however, they become less differentiated and start behaving badly. The tubules they make with other malignant cells are distorted and arranged haphazardly, and they may eventually form solid clumps and even go off on their own to make new colonies elsewhere in the body. See further in Chapter 2.

The Gleason score, which should always be calculated by a pathologist with considerable experience in examining samples of prostate tissue, is written as the sum of the two most prominent Gleason patterns. So a Gleason score of $2+3=5$ has a dominant well-differentiated pattern (i.e. pattern 2) and a less dominant moderately differentiated pattern (pattern 3). A score of $4+3=7$ means that a poorly differentiated component (pattern 4) is dominant. If 95 per cent or more of the tumour is composed of one pattern, the corresponding number is counted twice; thus, a wholly moderately differentiated tumour would be scored $3+3=6$. Ask to see your score, and check that it adds up: e.g. $2+3=5$, not some other number. Mistakes can happen!

Ensure that you thoroughly understand the difference between the Gleason pattern and the Gleason score, before discussing such information with your doctor, and remember that other terms such as 'Gleason grade' or 'Gleason degree' are meaningless.

Among untreated patients with clinically localised prostate cancer, those with a low Gleason score (5 or less) have a very small risk (4 to 7 per cent) of dying of their cancer within 15 years, even if their cancer is never treated. Men with cancers with a Gleason score 6 have a 15 to 30 per cent risk of cancer death if untreated for 15 years. Those with cancers with a Gleason score 7 have a 50 per cent risk of cancer death if untreated for 15 years. Those with poorly differentiated tumours (Gleason scores 8 to 10) have an 87 per cent risk of dying from the disease within 15 years if untreated.[91] (Remember that these are just statistical risks, and all my experience of communicating with prostate-cancer sufferers indicates that you can greatly improve your odds by following the Plant Programme diet and lifestyle factors.)

OTHER SCREENING TECHNIQUES, INCLUDING SCANNING

Blood tests

A **full blood count** (FBC) determines whether the patient's blood has the correct number of various types of blood cells. Abnormal test results may suggest spread of cancer to the bone marrow, where blood cells form, but doctors repeat this test regularly in patients being treated with chemotherapy because the drugs used affect the bone marrow temporarily. Spread of prostate cancer to the bones or liver can be detected by other blood tests. Some of the drugs used in hormone therapy can interfere with liver function and are also identified by blood tests.[92]

Recently, researchers in the United States have developed a simple blood test that can be used to identify which patients with prostate cancer need the most aggressive treatment, even among those whose tumours seem to be at the same stage of development. The research is published in the journal *Cancer*,[93] and the authors include Donald Gleason, who developed the Gleason system. The new test involves measuring the level of an enzyme (cathepsin beta) involved in the progression of cancer cells and the level of natural inhibitors of the enzyme (called stefins). The researchers found that more aggressive types of prostate cancers showed a higher ratio of the cathepsin beta to stefin A than less aggressive types.[94]

Scanning

Several types of imaging tests may be used to look for cancer that has spread beyond the prostate gland, but all have imperfections:[95]

Transrectal ultrasound (TRUS)   This uses sound waves to create a computer image of the prostate on a video screen. In addition to providing information about the configuration of the prostate, the ultrasound probe gives an idea of the shape of the structures around the gland. It can also establish if there are changes in the capsule of the prostate suggesting that it may have been breached.[96] Note, however, that a biopsy is the only way that prostate cancer can be diagnosed definitively.[97]

If the specialists feel that the cancer may have spread, they may also suggest a CT scan, an MRI scan or a bone scan, which provide additional information of the extent of the cancer. Remember, though, that a CT scan and a bone scan use ionising radiation (*see* pp. 44–5).[98] The choice between MRI and CT scans depends on the physician's preference and the availability of scanners.

Radionuclide bone scan   The bone scan involves injection with a radioactive substance called technetium in a phosphate compound designed to 'stick' to the bones. The radioactivity of the technetium decays quickly and the total amount of radioactivity is low compared with the much higher doses used in radiation therapy, so the scan generally does not cause side effects. The radioactive substance is attracted to diseased bone cells throughout the skeleton and can therefore be seen on the bone-scan image. These areas may suggest that metastatic cancer is present, but arthritis, bruises or other bone diseases can give the same pattern.[99,100] If required to have such a scan, do follow the instructions carefully so that the procedure does not have to be repeated and you minimise your exposure to any unnecessary ionising radiation. After the test, drink several glasses of a well-known cola which contains phosphoric acid to try to encourage your body to exchange the radioactive phosphates for the non-radioactive phosphate compounds in the cola as soon as possible. (Otherwise I never drink such products.)

Computed tomography (CT)   Commonly referred to as a CT or CAT scan, this test uses a rotating X-ray beam to create a series of pictures of the body from many angles. A computer combines the information from these pictures, producing a detailed cross-sectional image. The CT scan may reveal abnormally enlarged pelvic lymph nodes, which could be a sign of a spreading cancer (or a sign that the immune system is fighting an infection). The CT scan can also detect cancer that has spread to other internal organs, such as the liver, and is frequently performed prior to treatment, especially if there is evidence of lymph-node involvement.[101]

Magnetic resonance imaging (MRI)   MRI is like a CT scan except that magnetic fields are used instead of X-rays to create detailed cross-sectional pictures of selected areas of your body. These pictures can identify cancer that has spread from the prostate, and, as with the CT scan, may be performed if there is evidence of lymph-node involvement.[102]

Some new techniques
A new advanced technique of high-resolution magnetic resonance computerised imaging that uses magnetic nanoparticles that

seek out lymph nodes is being developed.[103] This method should help doctors to distinguish more accurately between normal nodes and those affected by cancer. The studies reported found detectable metastases, confirmed by pathological examination, and also showed that some lymph nodes, which might otherwise have been removed, contained no cancer. Forty-five of the 63 malignant nodes were so small they would not have been identified as malignant by conventional imaging techniques.[104]

ProstaScint scan   This is still a relatively new type of test, which, like the bone scan, uses low-level radioactive material to find cancer that has spread. In this test, the radioactive material is attached to a type of antibody engineered in the laboratory to recognise and stick to a particular marker on cancer cells. The disadvantage of this method is that it often suggests spread when there is none.[105]

Sentinel lymphadenectomy   This is a new method of identifying the spread of cancer into the lymph nodes. The sentinel node is defined as the first node to receive drainage from a tumour and is identified by injecting a special substance around the primary tumour and noting its spread via lymphatic channels. This method has been reported to have a 95 per cent success rate in identifying cancer spread to lymph nodes.[106] It is replacing removal and pathological examination of lymph nodes and is suitable for many, but not all, patients. This method may reduce the incidence of lymphoedema (build-up of fluid due to disruption of normal lymph drainage following surgical removal of the lymph node).

Positron emission tomography   This is a relatively new method of detecting cancer spread, based on radioactive labelling of glucose which is taken up more readily by cancer cells than normal cells. Again, it depends upon computer images of radioactive emissions from high-energy short-lived radioactive isotopes such as fluorine-18. Presently it is used only for the early detection of lung and brain cancer.

DIAGNOSIS AND PROGNOSIS IN LOCALISED PROSTATE CANCER

According to Dr Stuttaford, research has now shown convincingly that in the great majority of cases there are four factors that are fundamental in assessing risk in those patients in whom the tumour hasn't already spread beyond the prostate gland (which form a different group):[107]

1. The PSA reading.
2. The Gleason score.
3. The age of the patient.
4. The extent of tumour spread within the prostate.

There are now tables taking these factors into account, which estimate the average survival time. Medicine isn't an exact science. Some patients do better than the average, others worse.[108]

I think Dr Stuttaford should add a fifth point: the extent to which men are keeping closely to my diet and lifestyle recommendations. These are the men bounding up to me or emailing me to tell me how low their PSA test results are – in some cases having fallen from above 100 to below 1.

WHAT NEXT?

In the UK, it is common for all tests and scans to have been carried out before treatment options are considered, although this may not always be the case. I think that it is essential that you have the fullest possible information before making any decisions about your treatment options with your doctors.

Generally, you will be seen by a consultant oncologist or urologist to be given your diagnosis and the results of all the tests and scans.

In cases of cancer I think it important that doctors are compassionate but honest and that this is preferable to giving false reassurances.

The mainstays of prostate-cancer treatment continue to be surgery; radiotherapy (the use of radioactive rays – usually high-energy X-rays – to destroy cancer cells); chemotherapy (the use of chemicals to disrupt the physiology and biochemistry of the cancer cells); or hormone treatment to prevent the androgen hormones, especially testosterone, from reaching the receptor cells in the cancer or prostate-tissue cells generally. The problem with some of these treatments (mainly radiotherapy and chemotherapy) is that they can give rise to side effects so harmful that they compromise the benefits of the treatment (in some extreme cases causing other different types of cancer such as leukaemia to arise). Also, they can, for reasons which are not understood, fail in a significant proportion of cases. Hence doctors can only quote survival statistics to their patients. They cannot offer any assurance of a cure to an individual. Remember that your body is as unique as your personality and your fingerprints. Although understanding your cancer's stage and learning about your treatment options can help predict what health problems you may face, no one can say precisely how you will respond to cancer or its treatment.[109]

It is important for patients to understand that medical procedures can often be the subject of far more controversy within the medical profession than the public usually realises. Different specialists may have very different views about the best treatment options.

Professor Waxman points out that the efficacy of a particular course of treatment is arrived at from an analysis of the results of different clinical trials. In the case of prostate-cancer treatment, however, the relative advantages of different types of treatment have often not been clinically proven. In other words, there is, as yet, no proof that there is one certain and 'correct' way to manage the disease. As a result, opinions sometimes differ as to which might be the best course of treatment for the individual patient.[110]

Moreover, it has been argued that any figures comparing different outcomes and side effects are of questionable validity because there is a significant bias in the selection of patients for trials. All of this uncertainty can cause understandable anxiety in some patients.[111]

Before agreeing to any invasive procedure, it would be wise to ask these questions (some of which are taken from a prostate-cancer website[112]):

- Is my cancer only in the prostate or has it spread?
- Will I need additional tests? What are the purposes of the tests?
- What are my treatment options? How long does treatment last?
- What is the overall success rate for the procedure? (and how is 'success' defined?)
- What other therapies are available, and how do they compare?
- What is the likely outcome in my own situation?
- What is the individual success rate of the specialist/surgeon involved?
- How does this compare with other specialists in the same field?
- What are the side effects (both common and rare) and their chance of occurring?

- Will the treatment cause serious bone thinning and hence osteoporosis?
- What are the chances that I will have problems in urinating?
- What are the chances of my becoming sexually impotent following treatment?
- What are the chances of chronic colitis and diarrhoea?
- What is the quality of my life going to be after the procedure?
- What are the chances of my cancer coming back?
- What are the new and promising drugs and treatment for prostate cancer management?
- Is there anything else I should know?

A good doctor will take the time to answer these questions for you.

One issue you should also discuss with your doctors before undertaking any treatment is methods to prevent blood clots developing. Many oncologists underestimate the risk of these blood clots, despite the vulnerability to the condition of many patients with cancer. Most oncologists included in a recent survey reported not using preventive methods routinely in chemotherapy, hormone therapy, or radiotherapy.[113] The authors of the report say that national guidelines are needed for this.

While I think it wise that you should tell your oncologist and other health professionals if you are following the dietary and lifestyle factors I recommend, if you wish to do so, do not be put off if they are not convinced. Try to persuade them to read the book and show them the lists of references from the peer-reviewed science it is based on. Many doctors have been persuaded of the value of my approach by their patients, some of whom are doctors or other health professionals themselves, thereby helping other sufferers. If you cannot persuade them, then do not worry. Make your own decision, bearing in mind that all my recommendations are based on sound science and dietary principles based on thousands of years' experience (see p. 140).

THE HALF-TIME SCORE

Some questions to ask yourself at this stage. Have you:

- Found the strength to admit to yourself that you have a prostate problem?
- Sought medical advice as soon as possible and obtained information to calm your fears and reassure yourself as much as possible?

- Ensured that your GP has sent you to a specialist hospital, not to a general surgeon, and that you have confidence in the team who will be treating you?
- Involved your friends and family who are prepared to help (*see* further in Chapter 6)?
- Attended for all the tests and followed instructions closely?
- Listened to people with a positive supportive approach?
- Tried to remove old wives' tales and irrational fears from your mind and developed a more rational, less frightening concept of prostate cancer based on scientific understanding (*see* Chapter 2)?

Or have you:

- Panicked and scared yourself by thinking of all the awful things that could happen?
- Listened to people with scary stories?
- Gone alone to be given the diagnosis or the results of tests and become confused and frightened?
- Been influenced by too many different doctors? Take the advice of the consultant in charge of your case. They will have treated the most cases and will have the greatest real experience rather than simply theoretical knowledge of prostate cancer.

TREATMENT OPTIONS

If you are diagnosed with prostate cancer and have had all of the tests, the next step is to decide with your oncologist which is the most appropriate course of treatment for you. Modern doctors will try to involve you in such discussions. It does not mean they do not know their facts and have their own views. It simply means they wish you to engage with them and work together to decide on treatment options to defeat your prostate cancer.[114]

The result of early screening, particularly in Europe and the USA, means that more and more men are receiving early diagnosis of prostate cancer, and more and more patients are therefore faced with the dilemma of deciding on treatment options.[115]

Also do try to bear in mind that today a diagnosis of cancer no longer equates to a death sentence: a significant proportion of patients are completely cured, whilst a further proportion may have their symptoms eased for a significant time. Survival is a probability, not a slim possibility.[116]

If you need treatment, the specialists will generally recommend some combination of surgery, radiotherapy and hormone treatment, and they may recommend chemotherapy if the cancer is found to have spread.[117]

Let us look first at some of the treatment options for localised prostate cancer (confined to the prostate gland), which is generally managed in three different ways:

- Observation, with treatment at a later date if necessary ('watchful waiting').
- Radiotherapy: external-beam radiotherapy or brachytherapy (internal radiotherapy, involving the insertion of small needles carrying radioactive pellets).
- Surgery.

WATCHFUL WAITING

A good strategy for some patients with prostate cancer may be watchful waiting, with no immediate active treatment. This can be a good option for elderly men, although the Gleason score and PSA levels must be taken into account. The cancer is regularly and carefully observed and monitored. This approach may be recommended if a prostate cancer is not causing any symptoms, especially if it is very small and confined to one area of the prostate, if it is expected to grow very slowly, or if the patient is elderly or frail or has other serious health problems. Because prostate cancer often grows very slowly, many older men with the disease never need any treatment. Some men may decide that the side effects of treatment outweigh the benefits. Watchful waiting does not mean that more aggressive therapy cannot be used if the cancer begins to grow more quickly or causes symptoms.[118]

The following are Professor Waxman's criteria for patient selection for the watchful waiting option for those with localised prostate cancer:

- Good histology (low Gleason score).
- Minimal infiltration.
- Lack of symptoms.
- Older men.
- Patient preference.

One recent study[119] showed that men with prostate cancer who decided not to have surgery and instead opted only for treatment of their symptoms did as well as men who had surgery, at least in the first six or seven years after diagnosis. Men having surgery had only half the risk of dying from prostate cancer, but this was balanced by an increased risk of death from other causes. The researchers suggested that reasons might include a variety of complications such as blood clots following surgery.

SURGERY

In the case of prostate cancer, specialists generally prefer to go through the abdomen, often removing the entire prostate, the seminal vesicles and the pelvic lymph nodes. This route allows the specialist to see how far the disease has spread. This is major surgery, and as patients tend to be older it is risky, with the chances of complications increasing with age. After surgery, there is a 70 per cent risk of impotence and a 5 per cent risk of incontinence.[120]

Surgery for prostate cancer requires enormous skill – a skill that develops with practice. Radical prostatectomy has been refined over the last twenty years so that damage to nerves controlling sexual function can be limited. These will now not be removed, unless they are affected by the cancer. The name of the operation has been changed to reflect these advances and is now called a radical nerve-sparing prostatectomy.[121]

Admission to hospital is usually on the day before the operation. Prior to surgery, an anaesthetist will examine you, reviewing your overall medical state – in particular the state of your heart and lungs – to determine your fitness to undergo the procedure.

Try to talk to both your surgeon and your anaesthetist well ahead of the operation (standard practice at all good hospitals). Also at good hospitals it is standard practice for the surgeon to mark the area to be incised with a black felt-tip pen while you are fully awake. Although this is disturbing, just think how much more distressing it would be to come round from anaesthesia and find the wrong bit had been removed. If necessary, insist that this is carried out before you are given your 'pre-med' or tranquilliser.

There have also been reports of blood-transfusion-related problems, mostly caused by patients being transfused with the wrong type of blood. If you may need a blood transfusion, make sure that you know your own blood group and insist that the health professional checks that the blood is the correct one for you before allowing them to begin the transfusion or operation, if you are likely to be unconscious at the time of the transfusion.[122]

Several hours before the operation you will be given a pre-med injection to help you to relax. After the injection your throat may feel very dry and you will become sleepy. You will then be given a suppository to cause the bowel to empty, making surgery easier and reducing the risks of side effects such as infection. You will also be fitted with thigh-length support stockings to prevent blood clots forming in your leg veins. Patients are usually given an injection of Heparin, a drug that prevents blood clots forming (which happens more commonly in people undergoing operations). Antibiotics may also be given. Before the operation you will be wheeled into an anteroom and given an injection by an anaesthetist which will make you unconscious within seconds. Following removal of the prostate, the bladder neck must be reconstructed, which requires great skill because scarring can cause many of the side effects of such operations. A catheter is placed through the reconstructed bladder neck to drain urine before the abdomen is repaired. You are likely to spend two or three hours under observation in a recovery room before being sent back to the hospital ward.[123]

On waking back on the ward, you will find that you have a drip in your arm, a catheter in your penis and plastic tubes draining blood and serum from the surgical wounds in your abdomen. In most cases the drains are removed after five days and the catheter after one to two weeks. In a few cases problems due to scarring around the surgical join of the bladder and urethra can cause complete inability to urinate, requiring further minor surgery.

After the operation, it can take a minimum of three months to recover. Take it easy, gradually returning to a regular pattern of exercise.

Another type of operation, radical perineal prostatectomy, involves removing the prostate through an incision between the scrotum and anus. Nerve-sparing operations are more difficult by this approach, and lymph nodes cannot be removed.[124]

The following are Professor Waxman's criteria for patient selection for radical surgery:

- Age less than 70 years.
- Poorly differentiated tumours (high Gleason score).
- PSA less than 12–15.
- Sexual potency not at issue.
- No pre-existing radiation (not absolute).
- Informed consent.

- Patient desire.
- Patients without heart conditions or other serious illnesses.

There was a report in the *Lancet* about the possible spread of prostate cancer during surgical operations. Although it was considered that the jury was still out, the article noted that even a solid tumour such as prostate cancer may already have shed some cancer cells into the blood or lymph system, and that surgery could potentially worsen the situation. There is no doubt that anaesthesia damages the immune system and in China they frequently use acupuncture rather than anaesthesia for such operations for this reason.[125]

RADIOTHERAPY

Radiotherapy owes its origins to the first separation of the naturally occurring radioactive isotope radium-226 from a type of uranium ore by Marie Curie, who was a student of Henri Bequerel, the person who first discovered radioactivity.

Radiotherapy now relies on irradiating cancer with powerful X-rays (invisible but very powerful electromagnetic waves of energy) delivered using an externally applied beam, or in some cases by implanting radioactive sources which emit gamma rays (even higher energy rays). The machines most commonly used deliver powerful X-rays created by a machine called a linear accelerator. The exact method by which radiation destroys cancer cells is not known, but it is thought either to inflict genetic damage sufficient to kill cells directly, or to induce the cells to commit suicide by the process doctors call apoptosis. It relies on the fact that healthy tissues can repair the damage from radiation exposure more readily than cancer cells.

One of the main benefits of radiation therapy is that it can preserve the anatomical structure around the cancer, so it is less mutilating and disfiguring than surgery. Radiation can also destroy microscopic extensions of cancers that surgery can miss and is a safer option for older, frailer patients. Nevertheless, it sometimes fails to eradicate all the cancer cells in tumours and, like surgery, it is primarily a local treatment. It does not help in cases of metastastic cancer, except to relieve symptoms. Whole-body radiation exposure sufficient to kill all dispersed cancer cells would destroy tissues vital to life.

Many people are afraid of radioactivity, and rightly so. It is used a great deal in diagnostic medicine, including mammography, X-rays and bone scans, as well as in radiotherapy. It is worth remembering that in the UK, about 14 per cent of the average dose of ionising radiation to a UK citizen is from medical diagnostic procedures and treatment, compared with less than 1 per cent from industrial activity plus fallout from nuclear weapons; the remainder (about 85 per cent) comes from natural sources, including rocks, soils, buildings and food.[126]

In an investigation of hospital doctors' knowledge of radiation exposure,[127] it was found that few had any knowledge about the level of radiation that their patients were likely to be exposed to during investigations, despite all of them having taken the radiation protection course. This lack of awareness is particularly unfortunate considering the number of cancer patients who receive repeat investigations and treatments. This is unlikely to be a problem with radiotherapists, however, who, in my experience, are very knowledgeable about this subject.

There are two types of radiotherapy used to treat prostate cancer: external radiotherapy, which requires six weeks of treatment and kills all fast-reproducing cells in its line of fire, and brachytherapy, which involves implanting radioactive pellets into the prostate – this one-to-two-day treatment is more localised. It has growing support in the USA, but the UK still has relatively few centres. No long-term side effects of brachytherapy have yet been noted.[128]

External-beam radiotherapy

Radiotherapy involves sophisticated machinery and highly trained medical professionals. The first step in such treatment is planning. This involves determining precisely how to deliver the radiation to the area of the prostate to be treated and calculating the dose to be used, based on all the information obtained, especially from scanning. Planning should now routinely involve the use of computer imagery.[129]

Planning is a complex and highly skilled process, normally carried out by physicists to determine how to maximise the effects of radiation on malignant tissue while causing as little damage as possible to normal tissue.

A newer form of external-beam radiotherapy, known as three-dimensional conformal radiation therapy (3D-CRT), uses computers to map the cancer precisely and appears likely to increase the success rate and reduce the side effects of radiotherapy. Short-term results suggest that by aiming the radiation more accurately it is possible to reduce damage to tissues near the prostate and increase the radiation dose to the cancer.[130]

Recently intensity-modulated radiotherapy (IMRT) treatment for prostate cancer has been introduced. This is a refinement of conformal external-beam therapy, but employs a non-uniform beam to create greater conformity between the distribution of the radioactive dose and that of the cancerous tissue.[131]

Prior to radiotherapy you will be taken to the radiotherapy treatment centre to ensure that the plan is accurate. Be prepared for a room that looks like something from a science-fiction film. During this stage, one or more tiny permanent tattoo marks will be made on your skin to determine the positions of the radiotherapy delivery during the treatment process. I can still see the one above the top of my breastbone, but no one else seems to notice unless I point it out to them! The commonest treatment plans involve outpatient treatment five days a week for a period of six weeks, and many people continue to work daily (as I did during my treatment). It is entirely normal to be worried about radiotherapy, especially if there is a long wait for treatment, but once it begins most people adjust quickly.

Normally when you arrive for treatment you will be asked to wait in a waiting area with other patients.[132] Ensure that you talk only to patients with positive attitudes to calm any nerves. Always end conversations abruptly – rudely, if necessary – at the merest suggestion of a horror story.

When it is your turn for treatment you will be taken into the radiotherapy treatment room by a radiographer, who will position you and the radiotherapy machine correctly using laser beams and your tattoo or tattoos. The staff will then leave the room to reduce their exposure to radiation, but they will continue to observe you using a video camera. You should keep as still as possible throughout treatment. The radiotherapy treatment takes only a few moments, and you will be allowed to leave the hospital almost immediately afterwards. In most centres the time taken from arrival to completion of treatment is about 30 to 45 minutes.[133]

The following are Professor Waxman's criteria for patient selection for external-beam radiotherapy for patients with localised prostate cancer:

- Patient preference.
- Well-differentiated cancer.
- Small-volume tumours.
- Sexual potency not an issue.
- Age over 70 years.

- Any pre-existing history of colitis is a contra-indication to treatment, as colitis can be made worse.

Brachytherapy (internal radiation therapy)

Brachytherapy sounds very modern, but it is a method that has been around for decades. The procedure is relatively quick, requires short anaesthesia, and, after a few hours, you will usually be allowed to go home.[134]

The planning and administration of treatment is similar in many respects to external-beam radiotherapy, although it is initially more complex and involves an ultrasound probe being inserted into the rectum to take many measurements to assess the dimensions and configuration of the prostate and its relationship to other structures, such as the urethra. Up to forty needles may be used to insert radioactive pellets (each about the size of a grain of rice) of particular isotopes, such as iodine-125. These will keep their radioactivity long enough to treat the tumour, but the radioactivity will then gradually die away. A urinary catheter is frequently inserted into the prostate while the procedure is being carried out.[135]

Needles containing more radioactive material, high-dose-rate (HDR) brachytherapy, are generally used for less than a day and in combination with low-dose external-beam radiation. For about a week following insertion of the needles, patients may experience some pain and may have discoloration of their urine.[136]

The following are Professor Waxman's criteria for patient selection for brachytherapy for patients with localised prostate cancer:

- Younger men.
- All tumour grades.
- Tumour stage less than T2.
- PSA less than 10.

These highly selected patients would also be likely to have a very good prospect for cure by standard radiotherapy or surgery, or indeed a very low chance of progression of their tumour without any invasive treatment.

Effects of radiotherapy on the skin

Initially, the treatment has little or no effect, but gradually the skin looks and feels as if it has been very badly sunburned. Indeed, it is wise to be careful about ever sunbathing after having radiotherapy. Wash the burned area only with plain water using a low-power shower and never use soap or shower gels on the affected area. There are many different recommendations for treating the soreness caused by radiotherapy, including Aloe vera cream, but even herbal remedies contain preservatives which can aggravate symptoms. It is best to buy an Aloe vera plant and use a segment of a fresh leaf to rub on the affected area. Aloe vera has been used for centuries by desert Arabs against sunburn.

Some foods contain chemicals similar to those used in anti-radiation pills given to astronauts (more about this later).

Radiotherapy and chemotherapy have different side effects. In my own case, apart from the burn in the immediate irradiated area, I had no other problems. I know of no one treated by radiotherapy for prostate cancer who has lost his hair or felt nauseated (although irradiation of the head or digestive tract for other types of cancer can cause such symptoms). Throughout the radiotherapy you will be given blood tests to ensure that you can continue with the treatment. Also ask about the regularity with which the equipment is serviced and checked. This is very important, because poorly maintained radiotherapy equipment can be extremely dangerous. At the end of the treatment you should be given a thorough physical check-up, repeated after six weeks.

SOME OTHER SIDE EFFECTS OF RADIOTHERAPY AND SURGERY

Incontinence[137]

Incontinence is the inability to control the urine stream, resulting in leakage or dribbling of urine. There are three types: stress, overflow and urge incontinence.

- Stress incontinence, which is the commonest type after prostate surgery, occurs when coughing, laughing, sneezing or exercising and is usually caused by problems with the muscle valve, or sphincter, that keeps urine in the bladder. Prostate-cancer treatments may damage the valve or the nerves that keep it working.
- Overflow incontinence is associated with a dribbling stream of urine with little force, usually due to blockage or narrowing of the bladder outlet, by cancer or scar tissue.
- Men with urge incontinence often have a sudden need to pass urine, because the bladder is over-sensitive to stretching caused by urine build-up.

Depending on your situation, there are several ways to improve this condition, including surgery, medicine, and exercises, so do not be afraid to ask your doctor for help. They will have dealt with this problem many times before.

Cystitis (inflamed or sore bladder)

Cranberry juice is often recommended for cystitis, but it is useless where there is no infection and the problem simply reflects irritation. The patent medical cure Mist Pot Cit, which contains potassium citrate, should be avoided because it can increase the risk of cardiac problems.[138] It is best to drink lots of boiled, filtered (but certainly not fizzy) water.

Impotence[139]

Impotence, the inability to achieve an erection of the penis, can occur because of damage as a result of radiation therapy or radical prostatectomy. It is considered less likely after brachytherapy. Several solutions are available:

- Prostheses (penile implants) can restore the ability to have erections.
- Mechanical pumps, placed around the entire penis before intercourse.
- Certain drugs, such as sildenafil (Viagra), prostageandin E (administered as a urethral suppository (MUSE)), or injection of prostaglandin directly into the penis.[140] According to the orthodox doctors, the earlier that Viagra, or more modern alternatives, are tried, the more likely they are to work – and the later, the less likely.[141]

Do discuss such problems with your doctor and with your sexual partner.

Rectal damage and diarrhoea

Both external beam and brachytherapy can damage bowel and rectal tissue (proctitis), causing diarrhoea and colitis, and burning pain and diarrhoea, respectively. The doctors can treat this with drugs, but it should stop soon after the completion of treatment – though in some patients the radiation causes permanent scarring, leading to longer-term diarrhoea and sometimes rectal bleeding. In severe cases, surgery is required. Steroid enemas may be offered, but see my comments on steroid use in cancer treatment (see pp. 54–5).[142]

DEALING WITH PAIN

Do not hesitate to discuss pain with your doctors. Enduring unnecessary pain has no benefit, and pain medication does not interfere with cancer treatments. In fact getting effective pain relief can help some patients to be more active and may indirectly help them to live longer.[143]

I was lucky to have suffered very little pain after surgery. If I had I would have tried acupuncture rather than chemical painkillers, especially morphine. Acupuncture is said to have originated in China over 4,000 years ago, when it was realised that arrow-wounded soldiers often made surprising recoveries from long-standing illnesses.

Acupuncture for pain relief is one of the most widely accepted of all complementary medical disciplines. Indeed, the British Medical Association published a report on 'Alternative Therapy' in 1986, in which it accepted that there is a scientific basis for claims that acupuncture is effective as an analgesic (pain-reliever).[144] Some veterinary surgeons routinely use it for chronic pain relief for animals.[145] Overall, evidence from randomised controlled trials supports the use of acupuncture in pain conditions including post-operative pain. Such trials also provide evidence of an effect on nausea, hence acupuncture is a potentially valuable method of contributing to relieving some of the effects of cancer and cancer treatments and it does not add to the chemical burden of the body or cause other side effects.[146]

Acupuncture needles are extremely fine and do not hurt in the same way as, say, an injection; patients may even be unaware that a needle has been inserted. Many patients say they find acupuncture relaxing and sedating, though the method does not work well on everybody. If you use acupuncture it is essential to use only a fully qualified member of the British Acupuncture Council (or equivalent).

Variations include acupressure, where pressure is applied using studs on elasticated bands to the points traditionally used for acupuncture, and electroacupuncture (EAP), which uses an electrical pulse instead of inserting a needle in the acupuncture point. Lasers are sometimes used now instead of needles. Transcutaneous nerve stimulation or TENS does not use acupuncture points but stimulates nerves which block pain messages and it can be used at home. Hypnosis is another option for pain relief which is also thought to work by increasing endorphin production in the brain.

I refused, and continue to refuse as far as possible, to take medication prescribed by doctors or available over the counter from pharmacists. Steroids are sometimes given to suppress various types of discomfort associated with cancer or its treatment, but since they depress immune function I have always refused them. I also try to minimise my use of antibiotics and I cannot remember when I last used painkillers. None of these types of drugs is known to cause cancer, but I just do not like taking man-made chemicals if I can avoid doing so.

HORMONE OR DRUG TREATMENT*
This method is often used as prostate cancer is frequently hormonally driven. All hormonal treatments aim to negate the effects of androgens (more specifically testosterone) on prostate tissue, which they do in a variety of ways. They are given to patients with localised cancers or if the cancer is advanced and spreading to other tissues. Some types may be prescribed indefinitely. Injections may be given to block testosterone production, or tablets to neutralise the hormone; an operation may be recommended to remove the testes; or oestrogen tablets may be recommended to balance the testosterone. Lowering testosterone levels can make prostate cancers shrink or grow more slowly, but the therapy alone does not cure the cancer. Moreover, some prostate cancers are androgen-independent and some become androgen-independent after a few years of treatment. All forms of hormone treatment can have such side effects as impotence, loss of sex drive, hot flushes, breast swelling and osteoporosis.[147] Adjuvant hormonal therapy refers to treatment used in addition and prior to the start of surgery or radiotherapy, and it is claimed that it improves outcomes, especially for aggressive prostate cancers.

Orchiectomy   This is the medical name for surgical removal of the testes (castration). It is a relatively quick operation carried out under general or spinal anaesthetic. Some medical practitioners argue in favour of this treatment on the basis that it can be forgotten relatively quickly(!). Another argument of advocates of orchiectomy is that it is cost-effective – i.e. cheap – although this is disputed. It continues to be used if, having been fully informed about all of the options available, patients prefer this treatment.[148]

---

* The interaction of hormones with prostate tissue is described more fully in Chapter 2 and only abbreviations are used here, for example LHRH is used for luteinising hormone-releasing hormone.

Oestrogen therapy Oestrogens have been used to treat prostate cancer for more than 60 years. The main drug used is diethylstilboestrol (DES), a synthetic version of a female hormone oestrogen, generally taken in tablet form up to three times a day. This works by blocking the release of LHRH (*see* Chapter 2, p. 80), leading to the shutting off of testosterone production. Research has shown an increase in deaths from cardiovascular disease from this treatment, dating back to the mid-1960s.[149] Other symptoms include gastrointestinal problems and mood changes, and all patients suffer from swelling of the breasts, which can become very tender and profoundly enlarged. The argument for treatment with oestrogens in the UK is again that they are cheap. Although I refuse ever to advise individuals about their orthodox medical treatment I am aware that men on treatments that cause swollen breasts (called gynaecomastia by doctors) find this distressing and embarrassing. Waxman concludes that, because of all the serious side effects, oestrogens should not be prescribed as a treatment for prostate cancer.

Anti-androgens These work by blocking the binding of testosterone and DHT to androgen receptors in prostate tissue. The first drug of this type, Flutamide, was introduced for prostate-cancer treatment in the 1970s. Side effects can include severe depression, diarrhoea and, in rare cases, liver damage which is sometimes fatal.

In the late 1980s, another drug of this type called Bicalutamide was introduced for prostate-cancer treatment and is without major known side effects other than nipple tenderness – which may require radiotherapy. Approximately 40–60 per cent of all patients treated with this drug alone retain sexual potency.

Cyproterone acetate may cause fluid retention, strokes and heart attacks, and is so toxic to the liver that it can be used only for a very short period of time.

Gonadotrophin-releasing hormone (GnRH) agonists These treatments began in the early 1980s. They work by causing a decrease in LH and FSH levels produced by the pituitary. Subcutaneous implants requiring three-monthly replacement have been developed – a method regarded by Waxman as a humane and effective treatment of prostate cancer. Side effects include hot flushes (treated with yet more drugs) and, less commonly, anaemia and osteoporosis (on average about 2 per cent bone loss for every year of treatment). Any osteoporosis is treated with drugs called bisphosphonates (*see* overleaf).

Other hormone drugs   Megestrol acetate is sometimes used if first-line hormone treatments lose effectiveness. Ketoconazole, initially used for treating fungal infections and later found to also work as an anti-androgen, is another drug used for second-line hormone therapy.[150]

Other methods   These include combinations, for example of LHRH agonists with anti-androgens. Intermittent hormonal therapy may also be used in an attempt to allow the return of sexual potency, but the efficacy of this for treating prostate cancer remains unproven. Drugs that can prevent the adrenal glands from making androgens are sometimes used with other methods of hormone treatment for total androgen blockade, but once again doctors do not know whether this is more effective than treatments with single drugs.

Other drugs called bisphosphonates, used principally for treating osteoporosis, may also prolong the life of patients with prostate cancer whose cancer has spread to the bone. There has been debate for some years as to whether bisphosphonates have an anti-carcinogenic effect on malignant tumour cells, or whether they merely alter the bone so that the tumour doesn't spread as easily or grow so fast.[151] A systematic review of the role of bisphosphonates on damage to the skeleton (e.g. fracture, nerve-root compression and reduced mobility) in patients affected by metastatic cancer also found that bisphosphonates reduced these problems and extended the time to their onset.[152] In a personal communication Waxman points out that bisphosphonates do not improve survival.

As in the case of most prostate-cancer treatments, opinions as to the best methods are divided.[153]

One recent report suggested that 'hormone drugs attack a man in every department where he feels he is a man' – impotence, mood, lack of energy, inability to work. Patients may not be warned about these possible effects, and by the time they have had the treatment it is too late.[154] I have to say that I know many men on these types of treatment who appear to be coping very well.

CHEMOTHERAPY

The first chemotherapeutic drugs were developed during the 1940s and were a spin-off of the work carried out by the Nazis to develop methods of chemical warfare. Unfortunately, solid tumours such as prostate cancer are only rarely curable with chemotherapy alone.[155]

Chemotherapy involves the administration of anti-cancer drugs that travel throughout the whole body via the blood circulation system. Hence it is a systemic anti-cancer treatment. Many chemical compounds are currently in use, and new ones are constantly being screened and tested.

Chemotherapeutic drugs act by preventing cells from multiplying by interfering with their ability to replicate their DNA. In at least some cases, anti-cancer drugs (as in the case of radiotherapy) are thought to induce suicide of cancer cells. Unfortunately, while the chemotherapeutic agents are in the body they attack all cells undergoing cell division (mitosis). This is why they particularly affect tissues which have a fast turnover of cells such as the lining of the digestive tract, hair follicles and bone marrow. This is the reason for the common side effects of the treatment, which include nausea and vomiting, mouth sores, loss of hair, anaemia and increased risk of infection.

Damage to the rapidly replicating cells of the bone marrow can be particularly problematic because, as well as causing anaemia, it can damage the immune system. This reduces the ability to fight infections and can increase the potential for internal bleeding because too few red and white blood cells and platelets (the cells responsible for clotting) are produced.

One new study[156] claims that doctors should be wary of starting their patients on newly approved drugs because of the high rate of adverse side effects which can be undetected until late in the post-marketing surveillance period. Also, new anti-cancer drugs reaching the European market between 1995 and 2000 offered few or no substantial advantages over existing preparations, yet cost several times – in one case 350 times – as much.[157]

I find the following statement, from the ACS's website, particularly interesting since some of the prostate sufferers I have communicated with have been in remission following treatment with chemotherapy while keeping to my diet and lifestyle. The website states that chemotherapy is an option for patients whose prostate cancer has spread outside the prostate gland and for whom hormone therapy has failed. It is not expected to destroy all of the cancer cells, but it can slow tumour growth and reduce pain.[158] Also, chemotherapy, combined with my diet and lifestyle, saved my life when I had been given at best a few months to live. (I refused to take steroids, however, because they suppress the body's immune system. They are designed to relieve symptoms and I understand why they are prescribed in cases of advanced cancer. My doctors insisted but fortunately they were administered as pills, which I hid under my tongue and then spat them out. This was my decision, and you should discuss their use thoroughly with your doctor and agree what to do.)

Some of the chemotherapy drugs used in treating prostate cancer that has returned or continued to grow and spread after treatment with hormone therapy include doxorubicin, estramustine, etoposide, mitoxantrone, vinblastine, paclitaxel, and docetaxel. Two or more drugs are often given together to reduce the likelihood of the cancer cells becoming resistant to chemotherapy. Small-cell carcinoma is a rare type of prostate cancer that is more likely to respond to chemotherapy than to hormone therapy. Cisplatin and etoposide are the drugs recommended for treating such cancers.[159]

Do maintain an active interest in what is going on. Some years ago, I accompanied a friend for her chemotherapy treatment and she was almost accidentally given chemotherapy of twice the strength it should have been – and this had not been picked up by the doctor prescribing it, the computer system, the pharmacy or the senior nurse in charge of the ward. Had I not helped her collect her drugs and read the labels she could have had serious liver or kidney failure.

Some tips for coping with chemotherapy

If you are worried about losing your hair, treat yourself to a really good wig from a reputable company. A simple tip that many people facing chemotherapy find helpful is to involve your normal hairdresser, who can help you to choose a wig of the right colour and texture and trim it so that it looks almost identical to your normal hairstyle.

Ensure that you are given good anti-sickness pills such as those that actually block the receptors in the brain that tell you to feel sick. Also, some people develop horrendous haemorrhoids as a result of constipation caused by their anti-sickness pills. These can be dealt with easily by eating Linusit, which is organically grown linseed (also called flaxseed) and is widely available in health-food shops and has other benefits in combating cancer (*see* Chapter 5).

Additional advice from the National Cancer Institute (NCI) of America[160] includes telling your doctor about any side effects of the treatment, asking before you take any other medicine or supplement, and talking about your feelings (to counsellor, friends or family). Some further tips for eating if your appetite is badly affected by your treatment include:[161]

- Eat frequent, small meals or snacks whenever you want, perhaps four to six times a day, rather than three regular meals.
- Keep snacks (such as seeds, nuts, and fresh and dried fruits) within easy reach, so you can eat something when you feel like it.
- If you do not want to eat solid foods, try to drink soup, juice and herbal or green tea.
- When possible, take a walk before meals to stimulate your appetite.
- Eat with friends or family members, or, when eating alone, listen to the radio or watch TV.

Also, you can vary your diet by trying the new foods from this book and the recipes from *The Plant Programme*. One of the most common observations of patients following the diet recommended in this and my previous books when undergoing chemotherapy is how well they are able to withstand treatment, and this is often noted by their health-care professionals.

NEW TREATMENTS

A recent NIH (National Institutes of Health) Workshop on Selective Receptor Modulators (SRMS) focused on their potential use for treating hormonal-dependent cancers, including those of the prostate. Some SRMS, such as finasteride, are already being used for the clinical treatment of BPH and prostate cancer.[162]

A cancer treatment that encourages cancer cells to commit suicide by using biocatalysts that single out diseased cells is being developed by scientists at Exeter University.[163]

The US Food and Drug Administration (FDA) and the UK National Institute for Clinical Excellence (NICE) have approved a new drug, Gleevec, for patients with a rare but life-threatening form of leukaemia, and this is about to be tested on prostate cancer.[164]

Other new drugs with mechanisms of action that are not fully understood include Genasense, which is designed to work against a protein called Bcl-2 which allows cancer cells to ignore signals to commit suicide. When given to patients over several days before standard chemotherapy, Genasense is thought to help the other drugs kill the cancer cells. Bcl-2 over-expression plays a role in many types of cancer, including that of the prostate.[165]

Another drug that could prove a success story is Kahalalide F, which is based on a protein produced by tiny Hawaiian sea snails.

The drug has proved effective in tests on patients with prostate cancer. Molecules harvested from sea urchins, clams, algae, snails and sea cucumbers found off the coast of Venezuela are also under investigation as potential cancer cures. Laboratory tests showed that minute quantities of substances they produce can kill 50 per cent of cancer cells. One researcher is quoted as saying, 'Some outstanding growth inhibition was observed, suggesting that these organisms could be very promising sources of novel compounds.'[166]

TREATMENTS OF RECURRENT PROSTATE CANCER

Unfortunately, for some patients, prostate cancer can and does come back. Having repeated occurrences of cancer can be very distressing. I remember feeling suicidal the fifth time my cancer returned, and thinking that whatever I did to fight my cancer there was no escape. But try to remember that it is possible to recover from even advanced cancer. I did it, and I am aware of many men who have had recurrences of prostate cancer and are now in remission.

Recurrence frequently requires chemotherapy and, in advanced cases, radiotherapy or radioisotope treatment to control pain.

The use of chemotherapy agents depends on many factors, including the type and stage of prostate cancer, the medical history of the patient and, in some patients, their state of mind. The oncologist prescribing treatment will consider all of these factors and many others – including their own experience of clinical successes and failures – and I would always follow their recommendations as to which chemotherapeutic agents to use. The drugs in use in the past were highly toxic and more suited to treating younger men who could withstand their toxicity and side effects better than the elderly. Improved chemotherapy agents are available, including Mitozantrone, which is often given with steroids to limit its side effects (but see pp. 54–5). The side effects of this treatment are reported to be minimal, with a very few cases of nausea, vomiting or infection, and no hair loss.[167]

Systemic radiation therapy involving radioactive isotopes such as strontium-89, are used to treat bone pain caused by metastatic prostate cancer. This is usually more successful than external-beam radiation, but in the UK its high cost is an issue in treatment under the NHS where half-body (upper or lower half) radiotherapy is more commonly used. The latter treatment can have significant side effects, including anaemia, sickness and infection.[168]

I believe that prostate cancer has the same root cause as breast cancer, however, and in my own case I have survived for more than ten years cancer-free after five occurrences of breast cancer. I shall spend no more time therefore on the grim advice of orthodox medicine.

SUMMARY OF TIPS FOR COPING WITH ANTI-CANCER TREATMENT

General

1. Insist you are treated at a hospital with a specialist prostate-cancer team, which includes a urologist (not just a general surgeon), a radiotherapist and a chemotherapist.
2. Try to take a partner or discreet friend when you go for consultations with your doctors. Ensure that they are equipped with a notebook and pen to take notes to minimise confusion and additional stress.
3. If you know you are panicking or feeling emotional, ask your doctors for more time before making irrevocable choices about treatment options. Ensure that you are as calm as possible when you make important decisions or choices.

Diagnosis

4. Listen and read instructions carefully and follow them closely to minimise the need for repeat tests and hence to minimise your exposure to radioactivity and other impacts of diagnostic medicine.
5. If you have a bone scan, drink cola containing phosphoric acid afterwards, to try to flush the radioactive agent used for testing from your body as soon as possible. (This agent is usually attached to a phosphate compound so it will attach to your bones during testing.)

Surgery

6. Before surgery, while you are awake and fully conscious, ensure that the area to be operated on is clearly marked with a felt-tip pen by the surgeon who will be operating on you and that your blood type has been recorded correctly.

Radiotherapy

7. Wash the affected area with water only – using a low-power shower. Do not use soap. Use olive oil or the leaves

of Aloe vera plants on the skin but no creams – even herbal ones – that could contain irritating preservatives.

8. Eat seaweed, an organic egg a day and lots of garlic to give your body cysteine-like chemicals used, for instance, by astronauts to repair DNA (*see* Chapter 5).

Chemotherapy

9. Buy a wig with guidance from your normal hairdresser and have him/her style it to your usual hairdo. Drink juices to minimise or prevent the hair loss associated with some types of chemotherapy (*see* Chapter 5).

10. Drink only filtered water which has been boiled to kill organisms that can cause sickness and diarrhoea in immunosuppressed patients (*see* Chapter 5).

HERBAL THERAPIES

Natural substances have been used in Chinese medicine and Indian Ayurvedic medicine for about 3,500 years, and, as the WHO has pointed out, most of the people on Earth still rely on herbal treatments. Until the nineteenth century, drugs in western Europe, too, came mainly from plants – and botanic gardens were first established so that Renaisssance medical students could be trained to identify medicinal plants.

The international market for complementary and alternative medicine was worth an estimated $21.2 billion in the United States in 1997, more than half of which was paid directly by patients, and £450 million in Britain in 1998, with 90 per cent purchased privately.[169]

Complementary medicine is marginalised in many health-care systems, but calls for an integrated approach are growing louder. Basic courses in various complementary therapies are now available in many medical schools in Britain and the United States, albeit on an optional basis.

Complementary therapies are often seen by patients as more 'natural' and having fewer side effects than conventional treatments. The enthusiasm for them shows people's desire to help themselves, as well as their frustration with the limitations of conventional medicine. The holistic and patient-centred approach of many complementary therapists appeals, as does the sense of empowerment gained from their philosophies of care. One of the great benefits of complementary medicine is that users appreciate the greater amount of time devoted to the consultation.[170] Here I shall look only at herbal therapies. Other complementary therapies, including hypnosis, will be considered in Chapter 6.

The potential benefits of herbal medicines have been reviewed in an article by Ernst,[171] who suggests that a potential benefit could lie in their high acceptance by patients, their efficacy, their relative safety and their relatively low cost. He nevertheless points out the relatively small number of clinical trials in relation to the several thousand different plants being used for medicinal purposes worldwide. He attributes the paucity of such trials to the small size of the sector compared with that of pharmaceuticals. He also points out, however, that records of adverse effects associated with herbal medicine from 55 countries represent only a tiny fraction of the adverse effects associated with conventional drugs held on the WHO monitoring-centre database for the period 1968–1997.

It is worth remembering that the pharmaceutical industry sources several of its chemotherapeutic drugs from plants, including Pacific yew pine needles, Japanese marine algae and the periwinkle plant.[172]

Aspirin, which originally was a herbal medicine and one of the first to be commonly accepted by orthodox medicine, has been found to reduce the incidence of several types of cancer.[173] Its beneficial effects have been attributed to its content of salicylic acid.[174] I can find no specific studies of its use against prostate cancer, however. Remember to keep aspirin-based products – and indeed all medicines – away from children.[175]

In herbal medicine, Saw Palmetto has been used as a treatment for BPH. It may be that it might also be of use in cancer prevention, but again it has yet to be subjected to randomised clinical trials. If you plan to take Saw Palmetto, have your doctor monitor the concentration of dihydrotestosterone (DHT) (*see* Chapter 2), which is known to stimulate growth of the prostate, before you start and after you have taken the preparation, to see if the substance is helping to reduce DHT levels, and adjust the dose up or down.[176]

Astralagus, a traditional Chinese herbal medicine used for two thousand years or so for the treatment of cancer, has recently been studied extensively in the West. Cancer patients receiving Astralagus have been reported to have twice the survival rate of those receiving placebos. In the West, some herbalists routinely provide chemotherapy and radiotherapy patients with Astralagus, and, apart from boosting the immune system (which is damaged by such treatments), it is also claimed that it stops the spread of cancer cells. The EU is apparently planning to ban it on the pretext that, although it is a herb, it has not been on sale or in use in Europe for 30 years or more.[177] What a waste of time when such products are easily available over the Internet!

At a recent meeting of the British Society of Integrated Medicine in London, Dr Rosy Daniel, famous for her previous work with the Bristol Cancer Help Centre, described an Indian herbal formula from Ayurvedic medicine called Carctol that she had used with remarkable success to treat a range of cancers. Carctol, it is claimed, is distinguished from other conventional anti-cancer drugs in that it does not cause any side effects and is non-toxic. It also neutralises toxicity produced by chemotherapeutic agents. Carctol includes the following Ayurvedic ingredients: *Hemidesmus Indicus*, *Tribulus Terrestris*, *Piper Cubeba Linn*, *Ammani Vesicatoria*, *Lepidium Sativum Linn*, *Blepharis Edulis*, *Smilax China Linn* and *Rheumemodi Wall*.[178] Before using it, I strongly advise that you seek supervision from a doctor trained in integrated medicine, such as Dr Daniel.

Another combination of ingredients has been reported to help. Several prostate-cancer books variously recommend that sufferers of enlarged prostates take: Saw Palmetto oil (about 350mg); Panax ginseng (about 3 to 5mg); or Pygeum bark (about 100mg).[179]

PC-SPES, yet another herbal formula, contains *Chrysanthemum morifolium*, *Gandoderma lucidium*, *Glycyrrhiza glabra*, *Isatis indigotica*, *Panax pseudoginseng*, *Robdosia rubesceus*, *Scutellaria baicalensis* and *Serenoa repens*. The mixture has been shown to lower PSA in patients with prostate cancer and to inhibit the growth of prostate cancer cells *in vitro*.[180] These results are encouraging but require confirmation in clinical trials.[181] PC-SPES contains plant equivalents of DES (*see* p. 52) and has the same drawbacks.[182]

One of the most authoritative reference books on herbal medicine[183] recommends the following treatments for prostatitis and BPH, some of which might be helpful with the symptoms of prostate cancer:

Teas: Horsetail, Pulsatilla, Goldenrod.
Tablets or capsules: Echinacea, Pulsatilla.
Formula: Black Willow, Saw Palmetto, hydrangea, poke root, Thuja.

An extract of stinging nettles is also claimed to help against prostate cancer.

If you are going to use any of these treatments, inform your doctor and ideally ensure that your herbal treatment is supervised by a suitably qualified doctor, for example from the British Society for Integrated Medicine. Also check that they have an MB Ch B or equivalent basic medical qualification. I am wary of some herbalists and herbs which can come from unreputable sources. A few years ago, an importer in California brought in a Chinese herb mix, which he named PC-SPES. Word-of-mouth reports said that it relieved pain and symptoms of those with prostate cancer, especially advanced cancer. Researchers recently found, however, that apart from the eight natural herbal ingredients, the mix also contained DES (the synthetic oestrogen used in hormone treatment), indomethacin (an anti-inflammatory drug) and warfarin (an anticoagulant). Apparently, pre-1999, the Chinese had been adding the three compounds to the formula before shipment, and latterly just the warfarin. Doctors had been using PC-SPES with great success but noticed side effects like breast enlargement (typical of taking DES). When some people had blood clots and bleeding problems, investigations started. One wonders why they can't ask the Chinese to provide pure PC-SPES and test whether it works without the addition of Western drugs. In Europe, there is a herbal product called Protasol with many of the same ingredients but no trial results to date.[184]

Other treatments such as shark-fin extract are not only ineffective but their production involves cruelty.

PREVENTION ACCORDING TO CONVENTION[185]
The drug finasteride is being studied in the Prostate Cancer Prevention Trial, which involves thousands of men across the US who are participating for seven years, until 2004.

Scientists are also looking at ways to prevent recurrence among men who have been treated for prostate cancer. These approaches involve the use of drugs such as finasteride, flutamide, and LHRH agonists. Some studies have shown that hormonal therapy after radiation therapy or after radical prostatectomy can benefit certain men whose cancer has spread to nearby tissues.

The US-NCI-supported Prostate, Lung, Colorectal, and Ovarian Cancer Screening Trial is designed to show whether certain detection tests can reduce the number of deaths from these cancers. This trial is looking at the usefulness of prostate-cancer screening by performing a DRE and checking the PSA level in the blood in men ages 55 to 74. The results of this trial may change the way men are screened for prostate cancer.

Researchers are also (at last!) investigating whether diets that are low in fat and high in soya, fruit, vegetables, and other food products might prevent a recurrence.

THREE STORIES

Let me look briefly at what has happened to some close colleagues and friends who were diagnosed with prostate cancer shortly before *Your Life in Your Hands* was published and who followed my advice and are now alive and well. They are relatively free of symptoms, apart from one who is on a hormone-related treatment, and their initially very high PSA results have fallen to very low values – in one case below detection limit.

Take the case of Alec (a combination of several case studies), an engineer who I have worked with for many years. I remember on one occasion when we were driving together to work being surprised when he stopped the car at a motorway service centre and I saw his food choices – a meat-and-cheese burger, fries, peas and milky tea – but I said nothing at the time.

I still remember the day when I was told grimly by another male colleague that Alec wanted to speak to me – but he would not say what this was about. Anyway, almost immediately I returned to my office. Alec telephoned and asked if there was anyone else in the room. Having been reassured that I was alone and had closed the door to my secretary's office he began to tell me about his problem. He had just been diagnosed with advanced prostate cancer and had been given a fairly poor prognosis. He sounded depressed and anxious. My first reaction was to say that I would do everything I could to help and to try to reassure him as much as I could by pointing to my own survival against the odds. He was so sure that he would soon die that he gave up many of the positions he held on committees of learned societies and other organisations, despite my advice not to do so – and he still regrets this. Anyway, he went on my diet and followed it to the letter. He is still so evangelical about it that many of our mutual friends complain to me about how he nags at them if they do not follow my line – and of course this is all my fault (although I always refuse to behave like the food police). In discussions with his doctor (and I always refuse to be involved in orthodox medical choices, because I am not qualified to give such advice), Alec opted for external-beam radiotherapy, combined with my diet and lifestyle. He takes no ongoing medication. He now looks a picture of health and spends hours of enjoyment playing golf with his friends or taking his grandchildren out – but no longer for burgers, chips and milkshakes!

There is also Paul, a professor who lives a whirlwind lifestyle travelling around the world. His prostate cancer was detected by a very high PSA score (around 70) when his university first offered free health screening. He chose to have brachytherapy and went to a hospital in America for treatment. He also follows my diet and lifestyle closely and is on no other drug treatment. When I last saw him he told me delightedly that his latest PSA result had been less than 1.

Finally, a former senior executive from a leading UK company who loved his French cheeses and red wine. Again, he was found to have prostate cancer, with a PSA test result of about 15. He has followed my diet since he was first shown it in the *Daily Mail*. He chose to have radical surgery and continues to have hormone therapy of a type that has caused his breasts to develop – though he is always very smartly dressed and his breasts are not apparent.

The three examples I have chosen are all aged between about 46 and 75 years. I cannot tell you whether any of them have had other side effects. I am not medically trained and feel that I cannot question men – especially old and dear friends – about their sexual potency or their ability to urinate! All I know is that all three, and many, many other friends and colleagues who I am in contact with look well and healthy and tell me how well they are doing, frequently against the odds (with initially bad prognoses or recurrences of prostate cancer).

CONCLUSION

If you have read this far, you will have realised that, where prostate cancer is concerned, prevention is far, far better than cure. Shyness is a big problem. If a woman finds a lump in her breast she doesn't hesitate to go to the doctor, but men feel that talking about the prostate is embarrassing and so tend to avoid a visit to the doctor until it may be too late. Under-funding is perceived as another result of this shyness (but *see* Chapter 7). Men should be shouting about prostate cancer as much as women do about breast cancer. Although the UK government has increased funding for prostate-cancer research, it still falls short of that devoted to breast-cancer research from the government and via breast-cancer charities. The biggest UK prostate-cancer charity was founded only in 1996. The increased budget is, however, starting to work. Already new treatments like cryosurgery (freezing the prostate to kill cancer cells) or building viruses that attack the cancer cells and leave the healthy ones alone, are being developed. But the fact is we have one of the worst survival rates in Europe. Unless new and successful treatments are developed, the poor diagnostic techniques, the horrid nature of the current treatments with their side effects and the lack of an understanding of the real cause make having no treatment a real option.[186]

Meanwhile, the word is **PREVENT**. And in the following chapters I shall try to help you to do just that.

A FINAL QUOTE

The biomedical community needs to recognise and advocate approaches to prevent cancer with the same enthusiasm that it currently directs towards treating it.

Peter Greenwald,
Division of Cancer Prevention, National Cancer Institute,
National Institutes of Health, Bethesda, Maryland, USA.[187]

2 Cells Behaving Badly

In this chapter I explain what cancer is, in a way I wish I had been told when I was first diagnosed with the disease. The material is drawn from medical textbooks and recently published scientific papers, but it is explained in unscary, everyday language. The evidence shows that, with a few exceptions, prostate cancer is not caused by inherited faulty genes.

The chapter also deals with the roles of two groups of powerful biochemicals – hormones and growth factors – which act as chemical messengers in the body. They do this by docking with specific receptors within cells or on cell membranes to initiate processes in the cell such as growth, differentiation and proliferation. Growth factors and hormones are important in regulating these processes in normal cells, but disturbance of their activity and expression can promote cancer and help it to proliferate.

When I first told my mother of my illness, she said: 'But we've never had anything like *that* in our family!'

At first, I was startled by her reaction. Then I remembered that people used to look upon cancer as something almost shameful: a family secret to be concealed at all costs, as mental illness once was. Instead of saying someone had died of cancer, obituaries often euphemistically said the person had died 'after a long illness'. Perhaps the reason for this was fear, an emotion that the word cancer still invokes in most people to this day.

I think a lot of this fear stems from a basic lack of understanding of what cancer is, and when people have a rational understanding they can cope with the disease more effectively. As a scientist confronted with my own cancer, I had to find out as much as possible about what I was dealing with. I found that getting to grips with the most up-to-date facts enabled me to clear my mind of unhelpful old wives' tales, and having a modern understanding of cancer and its treatment helped me to feel less frightened. On one level, cancer is very easy to understand: it is a certain way in which some cells in the body begin to behave badly. What is 'bad' or odd or unusual about the behaviour of cancerous cells? Well, normally, parts of your body do not start to grow out of control, do not attack or consume other parts of your body and do not take off and start up a new colony elsewhere in your body. But cancer cells *do* act in these ways.

In order to understand why cancer is so hard to treat and cure, we need to look at it in a bit more detail and to acquire some basic information. If you're tempted to skip this short chapter, let me beg you not to – this isn't *Mastermind* and you're not going to be tested on it afterwards! Knowledge is power: if you understand the basic science of cancer, you're in a powerful position to protect yourself, to get involved in your treatment if you ever become a patient, and to play an important role in the increasingly public debate about threats to men's health.

WHEN BAD THINGS HAPPEN TO GOOD CELLS

As you probably know, your body is made up of millions and millions of cells living in complex interrelationships with each other. Normally, your cells do not grow out of control, they do not invade each other's territory, and cells from, say, the lining of your intestines or parts of your prostate gland do not take off and start growing in other organs such as your bones or liver, a process called metastasis. But, as indicated above, it is the property of cancer cells to do precisely these three things that makes them so dangerous.

Even when cancer cells are removed from the human body and grown in a laboratory culture, they behave very differently from normal cells. For example, normal cells are fussy about the nutrients they consume, but cancer cells are not. Also, normal cells reproduce only until they just touch each other, and then they stop (a phenomenon known as contact inhibition). By contrast, cancer cells keep on propagating and will pile up in mounds because they produce a substance called telomerase which stops them from counting how many times they have reproduced themselves.

Telomerase is an enzyme that regulates the length of chromosomes in higher organisms, known as telomeres. In most human cells, the activity of telomerase is suppressed, and telomeres shorten progressively with each cell division. By contrast, 80–90 per cent of human cancers have been found to have active telomerase, resulting in continued cell proliferation.[1]

So *why* do cancer cells start behaving badly? Why do they grow out of control and eventually, if unchecked, start migrating across the body, establishing secondary tumours? To understand why, you need first to be aware of the simple fact that your body must make new cells when necessary – and in some tissues 'necessary' is, in fact, almost constantly. As your body 'wears out', new cells are created to replace older, dead or damaged ones. This process is called cell division or, more technically, mitosis.

When cells reach a certain critical size and metabolic state, they divide and create new daughter cells. The daughter cell inherits an *exact* replica of the heredity information (an exact replica of the types of genes in an exact sequence) of the parent cell. Not all cells divide at the same rate. For example, liver cells in the adult do not normally divide, but they can be stimulated to do so if part of the liver is removed surgically. On the other hand, the stem cells in human bone marrow are a good example of cells that divide rapidly and almost constantly. The average red blood cell lives only about 120 days. There are about 2.5 trillion of them in an adult body. To maintain this number, about 2.5 million new red blood cells must be produced every second. In total, about 2 trillion cell divisions occur in an adult human every 24 hours; that's about 25 million a second!

Normally, the cells in your body reproduce only when instructed or allowed to do so by the cells around them, according to a complex and highly evolved system, which maintains the size and shape of your body throughout your life. Hence your ears and eyes, feet and legs stay in proportion to the rest of your body.

Now you can begin to imagine what would happen if this process goes wrong. If something happens to increase the rate at which one group of cells reproduce, the result will be an ever-increasing number of cells that have no beneficial function to the body, yet are absorbing nutrition at an increasing rate. And that's what a tumour is. If the cells remain in their place of origin and do not directly invade surrounding tissues, the tumour is said to be benign (or non-cancerous). If the cells invade neighbouring tissue and cause distant secondary growths (metastases), the tumour is known as malignant. Hippocrates called this abnormal cell process 'karkinos', literally meaning 'crab', from which the modern word 'cancer' is derived.

THE WRONG KNITTING PATTERN

How can this process go wrong? Well, it's all a matter of control. Cell division (mitosis) happens according to a well-established cycle. First, the cells increase in size and make new proteins before a resting phase; then they make two *exact* copies of the cell chromosomes. (Chromosomes are the strings of DNA that contain our gene sequence and they carry all the instructions about how to make us: blue eyes, curly hair, and so on.) Next, the chromosomes line up and finally they divide into two. The whole process is designed to make new cells that are *exact* copies of the ones they are replacing. This sequence of events is controlled by the cell's genes.

Each cell in the human body contains tens of thousands of genes which provide detailed instructions that determine not only the colour of our eyes or hair, but also instructions about cell division, growth and death. Genes can be thought of as knitting patterns or computer programs which, in the case of cancer cells, have somehow had a few mistakes introduced. Just think how a sweater would turn out of it was made from a pattern with a mistake in it. It's the same idea.

Most cells, no matter what their shape or function, have an outer surface – the cell membrane – inside which is a thick fluid called cytoplasm. Then, with the exception of red blood cells, all cells have a 'control centre', called a cell nucleus. In the cell nucleus are the chromosomes, made of strands of a special substance called DNA that contains our genes. The genes specify how to make particular proteins that carry out their work. When a gene is activated it causes such proteins to be made. Mutations (mistakes in genes) can cause the wrong amounts or types of the protein to be produced, thus sending the wrong message. Then, when the cell begins its cycle of mitosis, there are errors – just like the misshapen sweater made from the misprinted knitting pattern.

All cells, including prostate cells, have receptors for chemical messengers such as hormones and immunity and growth factors. Receptors are special parts of the cell designed to allow chemical messengers such as particular hormones or growth factors to 'dock' and deliver their messages. In the case of growth factors, for example, one end of each receptor protrudes into the fluid between the cells, the other end projects into the cell's cytoplasm and in this way creates a conduit along which the message starts to be transmitted. So, for example, when a growth factor docks on to an appropriate receptor its message is passed directly into the cytoplasm. There it begins the relay of a message that is carried from one protein to the next until it reaches the cell nucleus. This relay occurs along what is sometimes called a pathway. Once in the cell nucleus, the message activates genes to initiate their instructions – in this case, for the cell to begin its growth cycle. But cells can receive other messages as well.

There are basically three types of genes in normal cells that can go wrong to produce cancer: those that say 'grow', called proto-oncogenes by doctors and researchers; those that say 'don't grow', called tumour-suppressor genes; and those that say 'fix it', instructing the cell to repair damage or, in extreme situations, self-destruct, called apoptotic genes.[2]

Currently, most doctors think that the cells in a cancer are descended from a common ancestral cell that at some point in time – probably years before any tumour is detected – initiated a programme of inappropriate reproduction. Somehow one or more of the knitting patterns for the 'grow', 'don't grow' and 'fix it' genes crucial to cell mitosis accumulated a series of mistakes resulting in the ancestral cancer cell. Normally, the body has a complex 'quality control' system to ensure that such errors are detected and eliminated – to the extent of causing damaged cells to self-destruct (the cell's ability to commit suicide, 'apoptosis'). But somehow, the ancestral cancer cell avoided the body's quality-control safeguards and began to grow out of control. Normal DNA repair mechanisms didn't work and, for some reason, the body's immune system didn't recognise the cancer cells as abnormal and so failed to kill them off. Even the 'final solution' of cell suicide failed to work. You can see from this sequence of events that cancer is actually the result of a series of failures, starting from mistakes in the cell's genes – the knitting patterns.

These mistakes in the genes are called mutations, and most cancers possess mutations in one or more of the three main gene categories. The progression of cancers from an individual damaged cell to a cluster of damaged cells, then to non-aggressive cancer and finally to highly aggressive cancer is generally considered to result from the continued accumulation of muta-tions. Cells from advanced cancer typically have many genetic changes and chromosome rearrangements, although these are considered to be the result rather than the cause of malignancy. The number of mutations required for the development of cancer varies with the cancer type.

The first genes that can go wrong are the 'grow' genes, the genes which produce normal growth proteins in our cells, which relay signals to the nucleus (the control centre of the cell), stimulating growth in response to proteins and other substances in the intercellular fluid. The signalling process involves a series of steps which begin at receptors on the cell membrane (or within the cell, in the case of steroid hormones), then involve a host of intermediary proteins in the cell cytoplasm and end with the activation of factors in the cell nucleus which help to move it

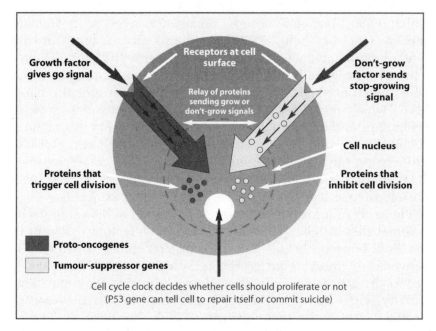

Figure 2.1: 'Grow' and 'don't-grow' signalling in normal cells.

through its cycle of growth and replication (Figure 2.1). The abnormal degree of proliferation in cancer-cell populations generally results from over-activity in one or more of these steps.[3] Interestingly, one of the diagrams in Woolf's book, *Pathology, Basic and Systemic*, illustrating how cancer cells behave, shows a marked increase in growth factors in the intercellular fluid, followed by an increase in growth-factor receptors and in signal transmission, followed by an increased response to their signalling. There is no indication that the increased levels of growth factors could be because of factors outside the body. This is despite the fact that nutritional intake has been shown to be a strong determinant of levels of circulating growth factors such as insulin-like growth factor I (IGF-I).[4] The role of IGF-I in promoting cancer has been investigated for many years, but recently, as discussed in Chapter 4, the quality and quantity of evidence of its role in promoting prostate cancer, including the role of diet, has increased greatly.[5]

The activation of a normal 'grow' or proto-oncogene to become a cancer-causing 'oncogene' can occur in several ways: by altering DNA at a particular point on the chromosome, by rearranging chromosomes or by increasing the numbers of normal proto-oncogenes in a cell.[6] There are several such genes which, when damaged, become oncogenes involved in prostate cancer. One of them, ERBB2, contains instructions for the production of or codes for an epidermal-growth-factor-like protein; this oncogene is also involved in ovarian and other cancers. Others include: FGF3, which codes for fibroblast growth factor; MYC, which codes for a factor involved in activating growth-promotion in the cell nucleus and is also involved in ovarian and colon cancer; and ROS1, which codes for insulin-receptor-like proteins on the cell membrane. The location of proto-oncogenes at particular sites on particular chromosomes is now well documented as a result of the Human Genome Project.

The relay of information between a receptor and a cell nucleus is sometimes called a pathway. When growth factors – present in the fluid between cells – attach to cell receptors, a pathway is activated or 'fired'. That is, the relay of the 'grow' message is begun. In cancerous cells, the relaying proteins maintain their activity when they should have 'switched off'. In the case of prostate cancer, the proto-oncogenes with the mistakes – those that keep telling the cell to fire when it should have stopped – are thought to be those that control how the receptors for growth factors behave.

Pharmaceutical companies are currently working on drugs intended to shut down growth-factor receptors that have gone wrong, as a way to treat the cancer. Shut-down methods have been shown to work in cultures of cancer cells, but they have not yet been shown to work in the human body. Research is in progress to formulate a substance that will increase the activity of IGF-binding protein 3 (IGFBP-3)[7] in prostate-cancer patients, either directly or by stimulating its production in the body.

The second class of genes which can go wrong to produce cancer are called tumour-suppressor genes. In normal cells these genes encode for a sequence of proteins to restrict cell growth, including by cell-to-cell signalling via the fluid between cells – the intercellular fluid. So, if a cell is growing out of control, these genes can make a set of proteins to send a different relay of signals to the nucleus. This time it is to say 'don't grow'. It is the inheritance of mutated forms of the BRCA1 gene and the BRCA2 gene (both tumour-suppressor genes) that is thought to cause an estimated 5–10 per cent of all inherited or familial breast-cancer cases. There is also evidence that the same genes are involved in inherited prostate cancer. For example, work by a team at Cambridge University, UK, has shown that men who carry the mutated BRCA2 gene are four to five times more likely to get prostate cancer.[8]

In recent years, much more has become known about the behaviour of the BRCA genes. More than two thousand papers have been published in peer-reviewed journals on the BRCA1 gene alone. From this work, scientists have learned that this gene, in its normal, unmutated form, helps to guard DNA against damage. The BRCA1 protein seems to act like a plumber, fixing breaks in the genome as they occur. The BRCA1 protein physically binds to damaged DNA and then recruits other molecules to assemble the equivalent of a DNA repair kit. Scientists have further demonstrated that the absence of the BRCA1 protein does not directly cause cancer but makes cells more susceptible to changes that can lead to cancer.[9] It has been suggested that the BRCA1 protein works via the intercellular fluid, from where it interacts with surrounding cells to keep them cancer-free.[10]

Within affected families, the BRCA1 or BRCA2 gene can be passed directly from generation to generation, through either the male or the female line. However, not everyone who carries the mutated genes goes on to develop cancer. Furthermore, just because a close relative has had prostate cancer it does not mean that there is genetic cancer in your family.

Several studies have looked into the family history of patients with prostate cancer. One study carried out in Canada and published in 1995 showed that, out of a sample of over 7,000 men with prostate cancer, only 159 had a positive family history – unlike the situation for many other cancers. These results suggest that for most patients genes have relatively little to do with the development of their prostate cancer.[11]

It has been suggested that true hereditary prostate cancer occurs in a very small number of men and tends to develop at a very early age (less than 55 years old).[12]

Some researchers have suggested that faults in the BRCA genes are involved in types of prostate cancer other than familial. So presumably the genes can be damaged during an individual's lifetime. Unlike some other cancer genes, which produce proteins that are more unreachable because they are located deep within the cell near the cell nucleus, the proteins that the BRCA genes encode for are secreted into the fluid between cells. In healthy cells, these proteins are thought to be the method by which the prostate protects itself against unruly cell division and, hence, cancer.

It may be important for people to know if they have inherited the mutated forms of the tumour-suppressor genes involved in predisposing them to prostate cancer.

If you wish to find out whether or not you have inherited faulty genes, you will need to consult an appropriate medical specialist. However, I believe that since the inherited mutated genes implicated in prostate cancer are tumour-suppressor genes, they are simply failing to 'close the door after the horse has bolted'. I believe that changing certain aspects of your diet and lifestyle could help to reduce your individual risk by reducing your exposure to growth factors, as discussed under proto-oncogenes, above, and hormone and hormone-mimicking substances.

The third group of genes involved in cancer are those controlling the replication and repair of DNA – the 'fix it' genes. An example of this type of gene, which is defective in many human cancers, is the p53 gene.

The p53 gene, although often grouped with tumour-suppressor genes, actually operates within the cell nucleus, by inducing repair or cell suicide. Damage to the p53 gene, which can produce a protein capable of halting the whole cell cycle and hence cell division until DNA damage is repaired or cell suicide is triggered, continues to be regarded as a key factor in human cancers. More than half of all human cancers have mutations in the p53 gene and hence no functioning p53 (messenger) protein. It has been suggested that a virus called SV40, which knocks out the p53 gene, was a contaminant in polio vaccines administered in the USA and possibly other countries between 1955 and 1963.[13]

In several types of cancer the genes that have gone wrong encode for proteins deep within the cell. In the case of prostate cancer, recent research is hopeful and suggests that the problems are related to proteins responsible for transmitting messages to stimulate or slow down growth, between the cells and intercellular fluid, rather than deep in the cell as in the case of some other cancers. This suggests that changes in body chemistry such as those achieved through changes in diet or lifestyle, can help to prevent and treat the disease. This is discussed further in Chapters 4, 5 and 6.

ALL IN THE GENES?

One of the first things patients do when they receive a diagnosis of cancer is to look to their lives to try to establish what it is that has caused their illness. They often ask themselves, 'Is it me, or is it something I've done?'[14] In other words, 'Have I got cancer because of my genes or because of my particular lifestyle?'

According to Professor Waxman, all the evidence seems to point to predominantly environmental causes for prostate cancer. I agree with him entirely.

Following the Human Genome Project, we have all been encouraged to believe that we are simply a collection of genes in a hermetically sealed bag and that developing a disease is the result of a faulty gene switching in.

Because there is clear genetic damage in the causation of cancer, many scientists and lay people seem to take it for granted that cancer is, by definition, a genetic disease. Let me explain the way this reasoning runs:

1. Cancer results from genetic errors.
2. Cancer is therefore a genetic disease.
3. There's nothing you can do about your genes, so there's nothing you can do about your risk of getting cancer.
4. The cure for cancer will therefore be a genetic one: spend a few more billion on researching gene therapy and one day we'll find the answer.

This is faulty logic. Unfortunately, many people who ought to know better seem to believe this mistaken line of reasoning. I do not.

Even the term 'proto-oncogenes', which literally means 'first cancer genes' (it is quite a mouthful!) implies that we have genes in our body whose only purpose is to lurk in hiding just waiting for their opportunity to malfunction and cause cancer. In fact, these genes are *essential* for the growth cycle of normal cells. Only *mutated* or *damaged* forms of these genes lead to cancer. But you wouldn't think so from the name.

The simplistic genetic model totally fails to take account of our interface with our environment – such as exposure to toxic chemicals like those in tobacco smoke, which are known to trigger lung cancer. I do not believe that most of those suffering from tobacco- or asbestos-induced lung cancer would be affected if they had not been exposed to cancer-causing agents. And neither do I believe that most men have genes that will lead them to suffer from prostate cancer without being exposed to something that promotes it. As we shall see, damage to the DNA, the material that makes up our genes, is critical to the initiation of cancer,[15] and both this damage and the promotion and progression of prostate cancer are critically linked to factors in our lifestyle and environment. There are various repair mechanisms, and it is only when damage persists that cancer becomes established as a disease.

So why does all the research, including that arising from the much-vaunted genome project, not lead to cures? Probably because all the 'new' methods face the same problems and must overcome many of the same obstacles faced by standard chemotherapy. Hence, for any method to be effective, it must find, penetrate and then change or destroy cancer cells without irreparably damaging normal, healthy cells.

One of the main results of all the recent scientific research activity has been to show that there are only minimal differences between cancer and normal cells.[16] Only a minute fraction of the tens of thousands of genes in individual cancer cells are damaged and altered. Hence it is extremely difficult to devise treatments against cancer that will not damage normal tissue as much as cancerous tissue.

Cancer treatments may work well in cultures of cancer cells or sometimes in laboratory animals. In the human body however, not only must the anti-cancer agent, whether chemical or biological, find the cancer, but it must also find a way to penetrate tumours sufficiently to be effective *without* causing such serious side effects that it cannot be used on human patients. Solid tumours, such as those of the prostate typically, have many barriers to drug delivery; not much blood flows within them, and some agents do not easily diffuse out of the blood vessels into the cancer itself.[17] Also, there are the problems of toxicity, side effects and the emergence of drug resistance in the tumour cells and immune resistance to foreign proteins in the body generally. Moreover, cancer cells are genetically unstable and can mutate or change so rapidly that they can readily evade recognition by immunology-based treatments and/or rapidly become resistant to many different methods of treatment, including those based on chemicals or gene therapy. Finally, as discussed in Chapter 1, the cost of researching the 'new' methods of treatment is extremely high and any drugs developed are likely to be so expensive that they are unlikely to be widely available to prostate-cancer patients – even if they could be made to work in human beings with active cancer.

Many new methods of cancer treatment are being developed. They include methods based on gene therapy to correct defective genes (though current procedures fail to deliver genes to a high-enough proportion of cells in cancers); molecular medicine aimed at correcting the proteins produced by faulty genes; methods to make cancer cells commit suicide; methods of blocking the formation of small blood vessels to choke off the blood supply that cancers need to grow (angiogenesis inhibitors); and methods to prevent cancer cells metastasising. New immunological methods designed to stimulate the body's own immune system into recognising and destroying cancer cells are also under development. Such methods presently increase time to disease progression by only a few months, however – hardly a triumph compared with my survival of eleven years due to a simple, low-tech, low-cost approach based on science and common sense!

Recent work[18] provides a scientific basis for the success of my approach. The authors of this research point out that, while much recent attention has focused on the human genome project, the genes that have been identified as causing cancer so far account for only a small proportion of major cancers. The rapid increase in the incidence of cancers that have accompanied economic development, together with the findings of twin studies – which compare cancer risk in identical and non-identical twins to determine the relative influence of genetic and environmental factors – both point to the importance of non-genomic factors[19] – in other words, to the importance of environmental factors.

FROM DNA DAMAGE TO DISEASE

There are now considered to be three main stages in the development of cancer (Figure 2.2). The initiation stage, which is characterised by the conversion of an initial ancestral cell to a

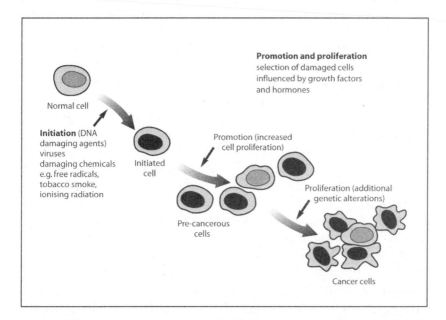

Figure 2.2: Initiation, promotion and proliferation of cancer cells (modified from Greenwald, Peter, 2002. Cancer chemoprevention, *BMJ*, 324, 714–718).

pre-cancerous condition in response to agents that damage DNA. As discussed above, some cancers are caused by inherited cells which have already been damaged, but in most cases the damage is caused by something in our lifestyle or environment.

The initiation stage is followed by the promotion stage, in which the initiated cell is transformed into a population of pre-cancerous cells, associated with further DNA damage. Thirdly, there is the proliferation stage, involving further transformation of pre-cancerous cells to a population of cancer cells and helping their spread.[20]

The body has many mechanisms and checks and balances for eliminating damaged cells. The fact that cancer cells not only survive but proliferate faster than normal cells suggests that some agent is preferentially fostering their growth relative to normal cells. The promotion and progression stages are thus extremely important in understanding, preventing and treating cancer.

INITIATION, OR BAD BEGINNINGS

Of the factors that damage DNA, environmental contaminants and chemicals such as tobacco smoke are considered further in Chapter 6, Lifestyle Factor 6. Viruses are also able to change DNA in human cells, by many different mechanisms. They can convert normal 'grow' genes into cancer genes, which stimulate uncontrolled cell growth and division by various means. Ionising radiation, including that from radiotherapy and other medical X-rays, can change the nature of chemicals in the body, including DNA, and cause genetic mutations that can be passed to offspring. Some of the principal sources of ionising radiation were discussed in the previous chapter.

There is increasing emphasis on the role of free radicals in causing damage to DNA. Free radicals are highly reactive molecules that typically have very short lifetimes. The best way to think of the effect of free radicals in the body is to imagine a pat of butter or a piece of meat or some nuts going rancid. This occurs because of a chemical process called oxidation caused by free radicals. More technically, free radicals are defined as chemical species that possess an unpaired electron in the outer (valence) shell.[21] This means, in practice, that they are very short-lived, because they generally attack any nearby molecules, including proteins, fats, carbohydrates and DNA, to 'steal' their missing electrons. The attacked molecule that loses its electrons then becomes a free radical itself, beginning a chain reaction that, once started, can become a cascade that results in cell disruption.

Free radicals are produced continuously in cells, including as by-products of normal metabolism.[22]

The best-known defence against the generation of free radicals and the damage that they cause is the activity of antioxidants. Sources of antioxidants are discussed further in Chapter 5, where I examine the role of diet in the chemoprevention of cancer.

It is worth re-emphasising that of the tens of thousands of genes in the normal cell the principal genes that are altered in cancer cells are the 'grow', 'don't-grow' and 'fix-it' genes. What we are looking for, therefore, are factors which preferentially encourage the growth of cancer cells, in which these types of genes are damaged, so that we can eliminate such factors from our lives.

PROMOTION AND PROGRESSION OF CANCER, OR SURVIVAL OF THE UNFIT

Since reliable cancer registers began to be kept in the 1950s and 1960s, the age-standardised incidence of hormone-dependent cancers (breast, prostate, endometrial (lining of the womb), testicular and ovarian) have increased in most industrialised countries, over and above that which can be attributed to the introduction of screening.

Cancers of the prostate have generally been considered to be sex-hormone dependent.[23] The strongest link has been a positive association with androgen status, especially with testosterone.[24]

The use of hormone levels to identify individuals or groups of people at risk of developing reproductive cancer has so far proved unsuccessful, and several reasons have been used to explain these negative findings.[28] There is, however, much more compelling evidence of links between hormones and the progression of established cancers. For example, some prostate cancers may regress following hormone-deprivation therapy, including removal or ablation of the testicles, or as a result of the use of anti-androgens (see Chapter 1). Conversely, there is evidence that administration of steroid hormones increases the growth of reproductive tumours. In the case of prostate cancer, the most important seems to be testosterone (see p. 124). As discussed in Chapter 1, many drug treatments for prostate cancer are aimed at reducing tumour levels of testosterone. The main benefits of such therapy are for testosterone-receptor-positive cancers.[29]

Hormonal and other influences on the prostate
The male hormone system is orchestrated by the hypothalamus gland at the base of the brain, which sends signals to the body's master gland, the pituitary gland, immediately beneath it. The whole process is controlled by gonadotrophin-releasing hormone, also called luteinising hormone-releasing hormone (LHRH), produced by the hypothalamus. The most significant hormones produced by the pituitary for male reproductive and sexual function are luteinising hormone (LH) and folical-stimulating hormone (FSH), which, respectively, control male hormone and sperm production in the testes. When LH and FSH are released from the pituitary into the bloodstream, they induce the production of testosterone and sperm in the testes. Approximately 95 per cent of testosterone in the blood derives from the testes, and a lesser amount from the adrenal gland. Testosterone is a relatively inactive hormone, which becomes activated by a special enzyme to form dihydrotestosterone (DHT).[25] Androgens such as testosterone represent the primary steroid hormone affecting gene expression in the prostate.[26]

Although the prostate is clearly a sex-steroid-(androgen)-dependent tissue, there is much evidence to indicate the involvement of numerous other hormones, as well as growth factors and substances called cytokines (a unique group of growth factors normally involved in the body's immune response) in the development and progression of tumours affecting it. Factors such as IGF-I, fibroblast growth factor (FGF), members of the erbB family, and others, as well as their receptors and binding proteins, and other small bioactive hormones, are now also implicated in the development, growth and differentiation of the prostate.[27]

The evidence that the two groups of biochemically powerful chemicals, hormones and growth factors, promote and progress prostate cancer is considered further below.

CHEMICAL MESSENGERS

As discussed above, hormones are secreted in special endocrine glands which contain a rich network of blood capillaries through which the hormones are released into the bloodstream. They circulate in the blood, usually in tiny amounts, until they interact with the target cell by way of highly specific receptors, located either on the cell surface or within the cell cytoplasm. This docking activates a series of intracellular reactions, including gene activation. By this means, hormones and growth factors enable the organism to exert control over a host of metabolic functions and to alter these functions in response to changes in conditions. The sex hormones, testosterone and oestrogen, for example, are involved in the onset of puberty in males and females.

Hormones can be divided into two classes, peptides (proteins), which interact with receptors on cell membranes, and steroids (fatty or fat-soluble substances), which also interact with receptors but within the cell cytoplasm, through which they can directly affect the proteins released from a large number of target genes.

There is increasing concern now about man-made chemicals. The most important for cancers of the reproductive system, such as prostate cancer, are thought to be chemicals which can disrupt the hormone system, in some cases because of their hormone-like behaviour.

The second class of chemical messengers – growth factors – also interact with cells by way of specific receptors and are increasingly strongly implicated in the promotion of prostate cancer.[30] Essentially, growth factors are proteins that bind to receptors on the cell surfaces to activate cell proliferation and differentiation. Some growth factors stimulate numerous different cell types while others are specific to a particular cell type. They are generally less well understood, including by many medical professionals.

The discovery of growth factors dates back to the early 1950s, when the Italian biochemist and 1986 Nobel laureate, Rita Levi-Montalcini, was working with tissue cultures of peripheral nerve cells. She found that, while the cultures would maintain themselves in a medium containing the right combination of nutrients, they did not grow much. However, when they were supplied with an extract derived from mouse salivary glands, they grew dramatically, extending towards the highest concentration of the extract. The substance was finally purified and characterised as a low-molecular-weight protein with chemical properties similar to that of insulin, which was called nerve-growth factor (NGF). NGF is now known to be just one of a large number of such small protein growth factors derived from a variety of tissues generally named according to the tissue from which they have been purified rather than that on which they act. They include, for instance, brain-derived neurotrophic factor (BDNF),[31] as well as the insulin-derived growth factors IGF-I and IGF-II. The authoritative textbook, *Biochemistry* by Donald and

Judith Voet,[32] states that EGF (epidermal growth factor), which, like the IGFs, is implicated in reproductive cancers such as prostate cancer (see p. 113), is a hormonally active polypeptide which stimulates cell proliferation. IGF-I is very powerful and has profound effects on tissue such as that of the prostate, even when it is present in only tiny amounts in the blood (0.2 millionth of a gram per millilitre).[33]

Let's look at some of the suspect chemicals, starting with the one most strongly implicated in prostate cancer, IGF-I. There is now little doubt about the role of the IGFs in increasing the risk of prostate cancer. At a one-day meeting of the Royal Society of Medicine in London in October 2003, entitled 'Biology of IGF-I: its interaction with insulin in health and malignant states', eight papers were devoted to the topic of IGF-I and cancer. For example, one paper by Grimberg, a distinguished endocrinologist from Philadelphia in the USA, illustrated how IGF-I signalling may contribute to each stage of cancer progression, including enhancing the survival and proliferation of cancer cells. She also presented evidence that IGF-I may promote cancer in-directly by interaction with other hormones, especially testosterone and oestrogen, the sex steroids long implicated in prostate and breast cancer. Other authors have also suggested that there is a direct effect of IGF-I on cancer incidence because it is critical for maintaining cell survival, particularly of transformed cells.[34]

Initial mutations can result in fragility of the DNA within damaged cells that inappropriately survive; they may then accrue further mutations to progress into a tumour.[35] Both growth hormones (GH) and IGF-I have been reported to increase chromosome fragility, in vitro[36] and in vivo[37].

The IGFs, IGF-I and IGF-II, have a similar structure to that of insulin, but their concentrations in the blood are much higher because they are bound by specific binding proteins (e.g. IGFBP-1 to -6). These binding proteins prevent the IGFs from docking with their receptors and stimulating cancer cells. The main carrier protein, IGFBP-3, is particularly important in determining the extent to which IGF-I is free to dock with its receptors on prostate-cancer cells.[38] Most (90 per cent) of the circulating IGF-I is bound to IGFBP-3, and associations of IGFs with prostate cancer are generally strongest where the ratio of IGF-I to IGFBP-3 is highest – in other words, where there is more free IGF-I to lock onto receptors on the prostate.[39]

Recent evidence indicates that IGFBP-3 also promotes suicide of prostate-cancer cells.[40] High ratios of IGFs to IGFBP-3 show a consistent association with prostate-cancer risk.[41] Professor Yu of Yale University and his colleague Professor Rohan have also reported that high circulating levels of IGFs and low levels of IGFBP-3 are associated with increased risk of several common cancers, including those of the prostate, breast, colorectum and lung.[42]

In their review of more than three hundred publications on the role of IGFs in cancer progression, Yu and Rohan[43] state that the evidence consistently shows that the IGFs strongly stimulate cancer cells and prevent their suicide. They also act together with other growth factors and steroid hormones in promoting cancer growth.

Experiments involving cancer-causing viruses in experimental mice indicate that IGF-II is also involved in tumour development[44] and has been reported to reduce suicide of cancer cells five-fold.[45]

As discussed earlier in this chapter, most human tumours develop by a multi-step process in which cells accumulate mutations. Spontaneous gene mutations undoubtedly occur frequently and naturally throughout life, and such events may be increased by viruses or chemicals in the environment.[46] It is increasingly recognised that the sophisticated defence mechanisms to eliminate such damaged cells in the body, including cell suicide, can be overridden by external 'survival' signals. The most potent survival factor for many such cell types appears to be IGF-I.[47] New work also concludes that the recent findings about IGF-I provide a potential mechanism through which an array of previously identified risk factors (see Chapter 1, pp. 10–11) may act.[48]

Interestingly, Oliver and others[49] have examined the relationship between serum IGF-I and PSA in 367 healthy men with no evidence of prostate cancer and found a positive association between the two chemicals. In other words those with high IGF-I levels have correspondingly high PSA levels and those with low IGF-I levels have low PSA levels. They observed that the association between IGF-I and PSA was stronger in older men, which they suggest reflects the induction of cell proliferation in the prostate gland; the association was clear, even at very low PSA levels (less than 2). Serum PSA was also found to be closely related to prostate size, suggesting that IGF-I may induce proliferation of prostatic epithelium (the thin tissue forming the outer layer of the body's surface and lining the alimentary canal and other hollow structures). Hence the authors suggest that high circulating levels of IGF-I may increase the risk of both prostate cancer and BPH, as a result of inducing increased cell proliferation. The findings are consistent with a recent study conducted in Shanghai, China,[50] which also observed high circulating IGF-I levels and symptomatic BPH.

Another study[51] showed that both IGF-I and IGF-II are associated with increased risk of prostate cancer detected using PSA tests. The strength of the association was found to be stronger in advanced cases. As discussed in Chapter 1, over-diagnosis and over-treatment are major problems associated with prostate-cancer screening based on the PSA test.[52] Oliver and others[53] suggest that if measurement of the IGFs can distinguish aggressive prostate tumours from other, less aggressive types, unnecessary invasive medical interventions could be restricted.

Holly and others also suggest that the strong association between circulating IGF-I and subsequent clinical presentation with prostate cancer suggests that measuring IGF-I as part of a screening profile may indicate the men more likely to benefit from invasive medical intervention. Measuring IGF-I may also be of value in monitoring risk-reduction strategies.[54] (Interestingly, two American professors have had their IGF-I levels monitored before and after following my dietary regime, and found that they dropped markedly.)

There is no doubt that an enormous amount of scientific effort continues to be spent on research into growth factors such as IGF-I and IGF-II to prevent them stimulating the growth and proliferation of breast (and other) cancer cells. There are now major textbooks aimed at cancer scientists and doctors such as the reference book entitled *Growth Factors and their Receptors in Cancer Metastasis*,[55] which aims to provide state-of-the-art knowledge of the role of growth factors and their receptors in cancer metastasis. The importance of growth factors in promoting breast cancer is no longer in dispute.

The new evidence on IGF-I suggests a simple model for prostate-cancer promotion. Levels of IGFs and their binding proteins are produced in the body and show little variation with gender, but vary substantially with age. Serum IGF-I and IGF-II levels increase until puberty. IGF-I levels then decline with age, while IGF-II levels remain stable.[56] This evidence suggests that the IGFs instruct cells to proliferate markedly during puberty, but of course such instructions are inappropriate later in life. Such a model would explain how prostate-cancer risk increases with increasing age in those with high circulating concentrations of IGFs.

Holly and others[57] conclude that the new understanding of cell biology, together with the new epidemiology, suggests that circulating IGF-I levels are as strongly associated with risk of cancers (such as those of the prostate) as any other factors yet described. They suggest increased emphasis on prevention.

The problem in persuading some medical professionals that dietary changes can help to prevent and treat prostate cancer seems to be that many research workers appear to assume that the development of cancer reflects abnormal over-expression of growth factors such as the IGFs[58] or their receptors because of processes entirely within the body. In fact, dietary factors, especially the consumption of certain types of animal produce and over-refined carbohydrates, can increase circulating levels of the hormones and growth factors that have receptors in prostate and breast tissue. Yu and Rohan, following their recent comprehensive literature review of the actions of IGF-I and all the evidence incriminating elevated levels of this circulating growth factor with high risks of breast, prostate and other cancers, emphasised 'the feasibility and validity of implementing dietary interventions to reduce IGF levels with the goal of preventing cancer'.[59] They find that nutritional status is critical to circulating levels of IGFs and that studies of normal adults demonstrate that, as protein levels in the diet increase, so do those of circulating IGF-I. A 50 per cent reduction in calorie intake or a 30 per cent reduction in protein intake significantly reduced levels of circulating IGF-I. Although the work of Yu and Rohan in linking circulating levels of IGF-I to an increased risk of breast, prostate and other cancers has been praised by Professor Epstein of Illinois University, he is critical of their apparent lack of awareness of the significance of milk – especially that treated with rBGH – as a source of IGF-I.[60]

Professor Epstein's conclusion follows the similar conclusions of an extensive review of the scientific literature of IGF-I by Outwater and others,[61] and the EU Scientific Committee on Veterinary Measures Relating to Public Health (see p. 125), and more recently those of Gunnell and others.[62]

We have always used euphemisms for cancer: it is now 'neoplasms', but in my younger days it was 'growths' – and what a clue that was, given all the new findings on the role of growth factors! Indeed, the emerging evidence suggests that growth factors are to an initiated cancer cell what oxygen is to a spark.

Additional information on the role of diet, including limiting exposure to foods with high levels of hormones and/or growth factors likely to promote prostate-cancer cells, is considered in Chapter 5, together with food and drinks protective against the disease. Reducing risks from exposure to hormone-disrupting chemicals is considered further in Chapter 6 on lifestyle factors.

3 The Third Strawberry

In this chapter, I explain how I used my science, knowledge and experience of working in China and Korea, and with scientific colleagues from Thailand and Japan – as well as a large dollop of good luck – to identify what I believe to be the main factor that promotes prostate and breast cancer. I compare recent information on the incidence and death rates for prostate cancer between low-risk oriental and high-risk Western countries. Such comparisons, together with migration and twin studies, support the evidence that prostate cancer is closely associated with the Western diet and lifestyle. Despite this association, the conventional medical advice continues to be based on the same old risk factors such as age and family association. This may be because so many more studies have been carried out within countries than between countries, although the latter comparison shows much more significant differences in prostate-cancer rates.

In my own case, once the panic and fear had subsided after my cancer returned for the fifth time, I began to realise that the only thing that could save me was my scientific knowledge and approach.

It was all too clear from what my doctors said, and from reading medical textbooks, that chemotherapy treatment alone was unlikely to cure me. For five years, I had done everything my doctors had advised and undergone all the treatments that they had prescribed. Also, I had followed to the letter the anti-cancer diet and lifestyle then recommended in the famous Bristol diet.[1] Nevertheless, I now had a hard, cancerous lump in my neck that looked like half a small boiled egg sticking out above my collar bone, and this had grown in only ten days. Clearly, my lymph system was badly affected by breast cancer cells. It is important to realise that, when cancer spreads from its original location to another part of the body, the new tumour has the same kind of abnormal cells and therefore the same name as the primary tumour. For example, if prostate cancer spreads to the bones, the cancer cells in the new tumour are prostate-cancer cells. The disease is metastatic prostate cancer; it is not bone cancer.[2] This is very important because it means that reducing risk factors for prostate cancer can help even when the disease has spread to other organs.

Years before I had cancer, I had worked with an American doctor who specialised in multiple sclerosis (MS). At that time, he had described the disease to me as a 'slot machine disease'. It was a strange expression, and the first time I heard it, I asked him what he meant.

'Think Las Vegas,' he replied. 'You're playing the slot machines. You get one strawberry – no big deal. You get two strawberries in a row – still nothing special. But if you get three strawberries, then you've hit the jackpot big-time.'

What he was saying is this: if a person had two out of the three factors that he thought were implicated in MS (or as he put it more graphically, two strawberries and a lemon) they would not develop any symptoms. But in the comparatively rare event of three strawberries coming up, then you would have problems – you would develop the disease. In the case of MS, my colleague had suggested that the three factors were a genetic predisposition, an infection – and at the time slow viruses were the fashionable scientific interpretation – and an environmental or lifestyle factor. (My involvement in his work had been an attempt to identify potential environmental factors, particularly in the Orkney Islands and other parts of northern Scotland where the incidence of MS is unusually high.)

Cancer, like MS, can be seen as a multifactorial disease. This thought gave me my first real glimmer of hope: although there was nothing I could do about whatever might originally have *initiated* my own cancer (probably many years previously), there might be a lot I could do to eliminate whatever might be *promoting* it right now.

Since cancer develops at different rates over different periods of time in different people, it seemed likely that something in the body maintains an environment that promotes the cancer cells, enabling them to multiply out of control and eventually allowing them to invade other organs in the body. Such a model could explain why, in some individuals, cancer goes into remission for long periods of time, or even fails to recur. On that basis, I had to identify and eliminate that something, that one 'strawberry', in order to overcome my disease.

So here I was – a scientist about to embark upon the most vital piece of research I had ever faced. Like a plot straight out of a nightmare, the deal was starkly, exquisitely terrible: if I got it right, I could have my life back; if not, then it would be the last piece of research I would ever do.

THE SCIENTIST WITHIN

Now, I want to tell you something about myself which greatly benefited me at the time. As an earth and environmental scientist

I am trained to observe natural phenomena such as rocks, fossils, volcanoes and earthquakes and to piece together observations to develop theories to try to understand how the Earth and its systems have developed.

Natural scientists like me work in a very different way to biological and medical scientists. If you think about it, we have to: the time scales of earth processes are so vast (up to thousands of millions of years) that it is impossible to carry out experiments in test tubes or under controlled laboratory conditions.

Instead, natural scientists work by piecing together fragments of, often very sparse, information; producing, synthesising and refining their theories from observations, observations and yet more observations.

This approach has been astonishingly successful. In less than a century and a half, such methods have allowed the amazing story of the Earth and the evolution of its life forms to be pieced together. We now know, for example, that the Earth was formed about 4,500 million years ago. It has been transformed by a complex interplay of physico-chemical and biological processes from a hot ball of dust spinning through space into a planet with a cool and varied surface environment where abundant water and an oxygenated atmosphere are capable of supporting complex and diverse life forms. We also know that the outer layer of the Earth is divided into huge plates. These move on million-year time scales in a complex interrelationship with convection currents deep in the Earth; with volcanoes and earthquakes concentrated along the plate margins. Life began more than 3,500 million years ago, since when various diverse life forms have evolved and become extinct, or survived, in response to changes in environmental conditions.

The findings of natural scientists have often been opposed by the orthodox scientific establishment. For example, in the second half of the nineteenth century, the famous natural scientist Charles Darwin suggested, on the basis of careful and extensive observations of rocks and fossils in relation to the modern world, that the Earth and its life forms had required more than 3,000 million years to evolve. At the time Darwin's views were vehemently opposed by many other scientists. Lord Kelvin, in dismissing Darwin's findings, used physical calculations to show that the Earth was only 20 million years old. Kelvin was wrong by a factor of approximately one hundred and fifty in his calculation – an enormous error for a physicist to make! He made this mistake because he had failed to take account of the heat generated within the Earth by its own natural radioactivity. Darwin, the careful observer, was eventually proved right and the orthodox physical scientist was proved wrong.

Later, the earth scientist Alfred Wegener proposed the then heretical theory that the continents had once formed one large land mass that had split apart to form the present-day oceans and continents. Despite being founded upon careful observation, Wegener's theory was vehemently rubbished by orthodox scientists, who said there could be no mechanism for such a process. Again, as evidence mounted and Wegener's ideas became irrefutable, the theory of plate tectonics finally became widely accepted by the entire scientific community.

So, having no alternative but to die or find a way out myself, I determined to take control of my situation using my training as a natural scientist. I would work in the way that had taken me to the top of my career.

I reminded myself that, despite the billions of dollars spent on cancer research worldwide, little had been achieved in combating the global upward trend in the cancer death rate. Despite the dedication of doctors working to treat patients with cancer, the tools that they had at their disposal were essentially the same as those of twenty years ago. If any other area of scientific research had produced so little benefit for such a high cost, it would have been closed down long ago. I would reject the orthodoxy that predicted – on the basis of a classification of the type of cancer I had and the stage that it had reached – that I would die in, at most, three to six months. I decided that, instead, I would look at my cancer in a detached way as a natural scientist, and try to understand the disease as a type of natural phenomenon. I would try to look at it in a holistic way in the tradition of Darwin. This, therefore, was to be my initial approach: look at the facts, the figures, the statistics, the data and observe, observe, observe.

THE GAME'S AFOOT

'Come, Watson, come!' Sherlock Holmes used to cry when he was on the trail of a particularly exciting case. 'The game is afoot. Not a word! Into your clothes and come!'

There's a certain kick you get when you're doing scientific detective work, even when it's a rather grim race against time. Even though I was, at that time, undergoing chemotherapy and so from time to time feeling desperately sick, I still felt the thrill of the chase as I started to use my brain for my own survival. But I still wasn't sure where to start looking.

Scientists are supposed to be logical, dispassionate types who labour long and hard for their results, but you'd be surprised how many real scientific breakthroughs would never have happened without a healthy dollop of good, old-fashioned luck. And that's what happened to me.

The first clue to understanding what was promoting my breast cancer came when my husband arrived back from working in China while I was being 'plugged in' for a chemotherapy session. He had brought with him cards and letters as well as some amazing herbal suppositories sent by my friends and colleagues in China as a cure. I do not know what they contained but they looked like firework rockets. I gave them to Charing Cross Hospital for their research, but I was never able to obtain the results. Despite the awfulness of the situation, we both had a good belly-laugh and I remember saying that if this was the treatment for breast cancer in China, then it was little wonder that Chinese women do not get the disease!

Those words echoed in my mind. *Why* didn't Chinese women get breast cancer? My mind flashed up the image of an atlas called *The Atlas of Cancer Mortality in the People's Republic of China*, which I had been given by Chinese colleagues when I had been working with them a few years earlier. I had been helping to develop a collaborative project between Britain and China, aimed at examining the links between soil chemistry and disease. Specifically, we were examining how low levels of the chemical element selenium might be related to the occurrence of a type of heart disorder called Keshan disease, and also a crippling condition characterised by enlargement and deformity as a result of the degeneration of cartilage called Kashin-Beck disease (nicknamed 'big-bone' disease).

Keshan disease is now accepted to be a selenium-responsive endemic condition that mainly affects children and women of child-bearing age and which, untreated, results in heart failure and death. Subsequent field trials of selenium supplementation involving thousands of children proved that selenium could effectively prevent Keshan disease.[3]

Initially, Western doctors and scientists had been highly sceptical of the findings of the Chinese scientists. It was not until organisations such as the famous Rowett Research Institute of Animal Health in Aberdeen, Scotland, replicated Keshan disease in laboratory animals by feeding them selenium-deficient diets, that the findings of the Chinese scientists were accepted. The scientific community, just like the wider community, can often be very chauvinistic when it comes to accepting the results of 'foreign' scientists from certain countries.

More recently, the British Geological Survey (BGS), where I work as Chief Scientist, has worked with Chinese colleagues to develop methods to mitigate the problem of selenium deficiency caused by crops grown on certain soils, and the incidence and death rates of Keshan disease in China are now greatly reduced. It is perhaps worth emphasising again that without an understanding of the fundamental causes of such problems – which lay in the environment – there would have been little or nothing that conventional Western medicine could have done.

THE NEWS FROM CHINA

The Atlas of Cancer Mortality in the People's Republic of China had always intrigued me. It shows the markedly different distributions of the various types of cancer over the country. The distribution of lung cancer, for example, shows the disease to be concentrated mainly in urban areas (consistent with research in the West, which indicates that lung cancer rates in polluted cities exceed those in rural areas, especially among smokers); and locally in areas of tin or uranium mining where inhalation of radioactive aerosols is likely to be a factor. Overall, the mortality rate for stomach cancer in China is high; but the atlas shows that it occurs almost entirely in the cooler, wetter and mountainous areas of the north while levels are extremely low in the southern tropical areas of the country. This is consistent with the idea that this type of cancer is caused by carcinogens, including aflatoxins produced by micro-organisms that grow in food stored for winter in poor and unhygienic conditions. In contrast, cancer of the nose and mouth is concentrated in south China in a well-defined region north of Hong Kong and Hainan Island. The data in the atlas underlines the view that cancer is not one disease but many different diseases with different distributions and causes.

What struck me the first time I looked through the atlas was the amazingly low rate of breast cancer shown *throughout* China. The background rate on the map is 1 cancer death in 100,000 women, which is very much lower than rates in the West which are about 1 in 10 women in many Western countries. I knew, however, that data from different countries could not be compared this simply. They must first be converted to fit a model age distribution for the population using a method developed by Professor Sir Richard Doll of Oxford University (the man who first demonstrated the link between smoking and lung cancer).

Otherwise, false assumptions might be made. For example, if a type of cancer affects mainly middle-aged and elderly people, as prostate and breast cancer do, and population A has many more young people than population B, then the overall cancer rate would appear to be much lower in population A than in population B – an erroneous impression. Therefore, statisticians have developed a simple method for adjusting data that takes these age differences into account. Data adjusted this way are termed 'age-standardised'.

Nevertheless, even using the age-standardised rates of incidence for prostate and breast cancer for China and Japan, compiled by the International Agency for Research on Cancer (IARC) (part of the World Health Organization, WHO) the rates are *extremely* low compared to Western countries (*see* below).[4]

The difference between the incidence of prostate cancer in the West and in oriental countries is spectacular. Cancer is now the biggest killer of men in the UK overtaking heart disease (not including stroke) for the first time, according to new figures released by Cancer Research UK,[5] and a recent report by the WHO (World Cancer Report) predicts that world cancer rates will double by 2020. The report calls for increased efforts to promote a healthy diet and persuade people to stop smoking.[6]

The current official figure for 'lifetime risk' of prostate cancer among men in the UK is one in thirteen. Last year there were approximately 20,000 cases. However, the figures are confused by the issue of BPH. Men in their 70s and 80s will almost certainly have an enlarged prostate, and it has been estimated that at least one in three of these will be cancerous. Ninety-five per cent of prostate cancers diagnosed are in men over sixty. One study in the USA of men over the age of 50 who had died of other causes reported that 40 per cent were found to have prostate cancer in autopsies[7] (though others suggest a figure of 50 per cent, *see* box overleaf).

Prostate cancer is the second most common life-threatening (non-skin) cancer in men in most Western countries[8], and is rapidly overtaking the first – lung cancer; it accounted for over 31,000 deaths in the USA alone in 2000.[9] It was estimated that by 2002 about 180,000 men would be diagnosed with prostate cancer, and about 32,000 would die from the disease. The National Cancer Institute confirms that prostate cancer is now the most frequently diagnosed non-skin cancer in American men.[10] As discussed in Chapter 1, the only risk factors widely accepted by the orthodox medical profession continue to be age, family history and ethnicity.

TWELVE FACTS ABOUT PROSTATE CANCER IN THE USA

- Prostate cancer is the most common form of cancer in men.
- Prostate cancer is the second leading cause of cancer death after lung cancer.
- The risk of developing prostate cancer increases with age.
- 80 per cent of men over the age of 65 who have cancer have prostate cancer (American Cancer Society Data).
- One in five men will develop prostate cancer in their lifetime.
- Approximately 335,000 men will be diagnosed with prostate cancer each year.
- Nearly 42,000 men will lose their lives to prostate cancer each year.
- African-American men have the highest prostate cancer incidence in the world.
- African-American men are twice as likely to die from prostate cancer as other men.
- Approximately 71 per cent of men diagnosed with prostate cancer and treated will live more than five years.
- For every man diagnosed with prostate cancer, there are two men with prostate cancer who are not diagnosed.
- Autopsies performed on men over the age of 50 who died from other causes showed approximately 50 per cent had undiagnosed prostate cancer.

From http://www.fgcu.edu/chp/deadlytomen/info.html

Prostate cancer does run in families, and men who have a father or brother with the disease have a five- to twenty-fold increased risk, depending upon which study you read. According to the University of Michigan Health System Comprehensive Cancer Center,[11] the risk increases in men of any age who have a first-degree relative (father, brother) with prostate cancer. These, it is claimed, have approximately a two-fold increased risk of developing prostate cancer during their lifetime, and an individual who has two first-degree relatives with prostate cancer has five times the chance.

In America, African-American men, more especially those of a Sub-Saharan African descent have an incidence of prostate cancer that is 1.5 times that of whites. It has been suggested that there are complex differences between the DNA on the Y chromosome of Afro-Caribbeans and Caucasians which could explain why Afro-Caribbean Americans would be more susceptible to prostate cancer, but the low incidence of prostate cancer in rural areas of Africa throws doubt on this hypothesis. Interestingly, although

Japanese immigrants to the United States have a higher incidence of prostate cancer than Japanese living in Japan, their rate is still about half that of US whites[12] (which could be understood if some of the men maintain their traditional diet and lifestyle while others adopt, partly or wholly, that of their adopted country).

By far the greatest differences in risk of prostate cancer are between men living a Western lifestyle and men in the Far East (Japan, China, Thailand, Korea and south-east Asia generally) (Tables 3.1 and 3.2 on pages 97 and 98), who have the lowest incidence (though this changes if they move to the West).[13] The incidence of prostate cancer is generally agreed to be lowest in these parts of Asia (5 per 100,000 men).[14]

Interestingly, even in Japan, long one of the most Westernised oriental countries, prostate cancer detected at autopsy is only about 1 in 2,800, which contrasts with about 1 in 570 in white men in the USA.[15]

As discussed in Chapters 2 and 4, there is increasing evidence that the IGFs and their ratios to their binding proteins may increase the risk of prostate and breast cancer.[16]

Prostate-cancer incidence has been rising over the past 40 years throughout the West. Deaths had increased in the 1970s and 1980s, according to researchers from Oxford University, but have since fallen by 20 per cent in the European Union, and by 30 per cent in America in men aged 50 to 74, attributed to earlier detection and hormonal treatments.[17]

The higher survival rates in the United States have been attributed to the use of more aggressive treatment with radical prostatectomy (which is associated with serious side effects) rather than with the more conservative treatment based on radiotherapy plus endocrine therapy that tends to be used in Britain,[18] but comparison is difficult because incidence rates are higher in the US (Tables 3.1 and 3.2), possibly reflecting the greater use of the PSA screening test there (*see* Chapter 1).

The data I used to look at the incidence and mortality rates of prostate cancer for *Your Life in Your Hands* – which are also the data that I use now – are those of the WHO. The age-standardised data on the incidence of prostate cancer (Tables 3.1 and 3.2) that I used in both editions of the book show that the lowest age-standardised prostate-cancer rate was only 0.5 and has risen to 1.7 per 100,000 males in rural China (Qidong county). This rate approximately quadruples in Chinese cities (such as Shanghai and Tianjin, Table 3.1) and at the time I was initially looking into the different rates of breast and prostate cancer I thought this was probably because of the serious urban pollution problem, the severity of which is rapidly overtaking anything the West can produce.

In highly urbanised Hong Kong, the rate for prostate cancer was approximately 4 times that in the rest of China – but still affects only approximately 8 men in 100,000. The Japanese cities of Hiroshima and Nagasaki have rates of prostate cancer similar to those of Hong Kong (Table 3.1): and remember, both cities were attacked with nuclear weapons so, in addition to the usual pollution-related cancers, one would also expect to find some radiation-related cases of cancer.

The conclusion I drew from the data at the time struck me with some force. If a Western woman were living a Japanese lifestyle in industrialised, irradiated Hiroshima, *she would slash her risk of contracting breast cancer by half.* If an American man were to do the same, *he would slash his risk of contracting prostate cancer by a staggering factor of between 9 and 12!*

The conclusion is inescapable. Clearly, some lifestyle factor not related to urbanisation or pollution is seriously increasing the chance of contracting breast or prostate cancer in those living a Western lifestyle.

The latest data from the WHO (Table 3.2) show that the crude background rate for prostate cancer in China remains so low that it is not mapped.[19] The latest age-standardised rates (ASR) of the incidence of prostate cancer in China and other oriental countries, with their distinctive diets and lifestyles, are compared with those of several Western countries in Table 3.2. The countries presented are all countries I have worked in and where I have been able to discuss the data with local doctors. I have talked to doctors in China, for example, who hardly remember treating a case of prostate (or breast) cancer in their entire careers (though this is changing now, as the Western diet becomes fashionable). I have also selected the countries where data are available for migrant communities (e.g. Chinese or Japanese migrants to America or Australia). These studies show that within a generation or so such communities acquire rates of prostate cancer approaching those of their host populations – indicating the importance of dietary and lifestyle factors rather than genes as the key factor. These are the strawberries that can be eliminated.

Migration studies such as those published recently by Kolonel into cancer incidence in different ethnic populations of first- and second-generation migrants to Hawaii[20] add considerable weight to the evidence of earlier migration studies that most

Table 3.1: Age-standardised rates (ASR) of incidence (per 100,000)	Prostate cancer in males
China, Qidong county (rural)	0.5
China, Shanghai (urban)	2.3
China, Tianjin (urban)	1.9
Hong Kong	7.9
Japan, Hiroshima	10.9
Japan, Miyagi	9.0
Japan, Nagasaki	9.1
Japan, Osaka	6.8
Japan, Saka	6.7
Japan, Yamagata	7.9
England and Wales	28.0
Scotland	31.2
USA (whites)	100.8
USA (blacks)	137.0

Data from *Cancer Incidence in Five Continents*, 1997. Vol. VII, published by the IARC (International Agency for Research on Cancer)

cancers are environmentally determined. Professor Kolonel's research is now focusing on the interaction of diet with genetic susceptibility in determining cancer risk because the potential for understanding cancer through studies of ethnic and migrant populations has, he states, never been greater.[21] Migration studies of cancer incidence in migrants between different continents indicate large dietary influences on the incidence of epithelial cancers generally, including prostate cancer.[22]

It is difficult to compare the data in Table 3.1 with those in Table 3.2 directly because of changes in the groupings and methods used by the WHO IARC. Nevertheless, the more recent age-standardised data from the WHO (Table 3.2) still clearly show that incidence rates of prostate cancer and breast cancer are much higher in Western countries than in oriental countries. It is worth emphasising that many oriental countries, such as South Korea and Japan, are densely populated and have been highly industrialised and urbanised for many years, yet their rates of prostate and breast cancer remain extremely low. Compare this with the USA, where, as indicated above, prostate cancer was the most frequently diagnosed non-skin

Table 3.2: Age-standardised rates (ASR) of incidence
(per 100,000), year 2000

	Prostate cancer in males
China	1.7
China (Hong Kong)	7.6
Japan	11.0
Thailand	4.4
Korea	4.2
New Zealand	101.1
Australia	76.0
Canada	83.9
UK	40.2
USA	104.3

Data from WHO International Agency for Research on Cancer (IARC), IARC Cancer Epidemiology Database. GLOBOCAN 2000. Cancer incidence, mortality and prevalence worldwide. Ferlay, J., Bray, F., Piesci, P. and Parkin, D.M. (eds). www.dep.iarc.fr/globocan/database.pdf

cancer by 2002. Such evidence continues to indicate strongly that it is an environmental or lifestyle factor that promotes the disease.

The death rate from prostate cancer (Figure 3.1 opposite) shows two quite distinct groupings: Western countries, such as Germany, the UK and the USA, with high mortality rates; and oriental countries, such as Thailand and China, with very low rates. The death rate in Japan is rising, however, as the Japanese become more and more Westernised, while that in some Western countries, including the UK, is falling. In the USA, it has been suggested that the difference in the likelihood of surviving cancer between black and white men may stem from the difference in access to chemotherapy, or even to the doctors who prescribe it.

Interpretation of the data is complicated, however, by the extent to which some prostate cancers are slow growing and cause no problems during a normal lifetime while others are potentially life-threatening – metastatic cancers. From autopsies performed on men who have died of other causes, it is known that small amounts of cancer can be found within the prostates of many men. These lesions can first be detected shortly after the onset of puberty, with the frequency increasing steadily with age.

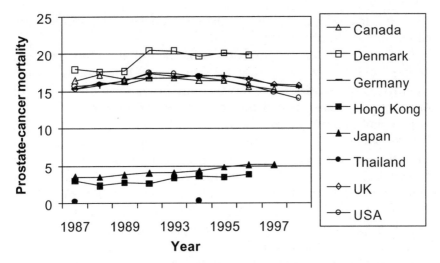

Figure 3.1: prostate-cancer mortality (annual, per 100,00), age-standardised rates (worldwide), 1987 to 1998, by country. Data from WHO/IARC Worldwide Cancer Mortality Statistics, ASR(W) for Annual Mortality per 100,000 by sex and age group. http://www.depd.iarc.fr/who/menu.htm

By the time men reach the age of 70 and above, 80–100 per cent will have such lesions. While these numbers are high, only approximately 1/3 per cent of these patients will develop metastatic prostate cancer in any given year. Because it is only metastatic prostate cancer that is potentially lethal, it is important to understand what stimulates the cancer to spread beyond the confines of the gland.[23]

One clue to the puzzle of why some cancers metastasise comes from studies done in Japan and other Asian countries. There, localised prostate cancer increases with age, just as it does in the United States and Europe. However, the occurrence of metastatic disease in Japan is approximately 1/10th that in the United States. The incidence of prostate cancer varies by 120-fold when third-world countries are compared with the United States and Europe. As discussed previously, migration studies strongly suggest a dietary or lifestyle rather than a genetic cause to explain the large variation in the incidence of metastatic prostate cancer. For example, when Japanese men move to America, their risk of developing metastatic prostate cancer increases in proportion to the number of years they have lived there, and the risk continues to rise with each succeeding generation born there. The implications of this finding are profound: it suggests, for example, that if Americans could adopt aspects of the

Japanese lifestyle, they might reduce the death rate from prostate cancer by as much as 90 per cent.[24]

This evidence is supported by the fact that, when oriental people adopt a Western lifestyle in Hong Kong or as some wealthy Chinese do in Malaysia and Singapore, the rates of prostate and breast cancer approach those of the West.

The slang name for breast cancer in China translates as 'Rich Woman's Disease'. This is because, in China, only the better-off can afford to eat what is termed 'Hong Kong food'. The Chinese describe all Western food, including everything from ice cream and chocolate bars to spaghetti and feta cheese, as 'Hong Kong food' because of the availability of Western food in the former British colony and its scarcity, in the past, in mainland China.

Finally, let me just remind you that the statistics we have been examining aren't simply the abstract results of some obscure laboratory experiment. They are real-world, real-life body counts. The knowledge that these studies give us has been obtained at an extraordinarily high price: for example, the neat little graph in Figure 3.1 reflects the loss of hundreds of thousands of individual lives. The least we can do, as scientists, is to study these figures very carefully and to learn everything we can from them. From all the data, it seemed a fair bet that the factor – the 'third strawberry' – that I was looking for when I had cancer is probably related to a long-standing cultural difference between oriental and Western countries.

I remember saying to my husband: 'Come on Peter, you have just come back from China. What is it about the Chinese way of life that is so different? Why don't they get breast cancer?'

Over the next couple of weeks Peter and I examined the results of the China study (*see* p. 136).

So the Chinese ate a low-fat diet: but so did I. The diet I had been living on for years before I contracted breast cancer was very low in fat and high in fibre.

Peter and I persevered and discussed the suggestions made by some scientists that it was the high levels of soya consumption in oriental countries such as China that gave the female population protection against breast cancer. The protective value of soya is discussed further in Chapter 5.

Soya, provided it is organically grown and not genetically modified, is an excellent source of protein and it has many other benefits, especially for menopausal women.[25] However, at that time I had been consuming so much soya in various forms that I did not believe that this could be the factor that I was looking for.

A BELL RINGS

Then one day a couple of weeks later something rather special happened.

Peter and I have worked together so closely over the years that I am not sure which one of us first said: 'The Chinese don't eat dairy produce!'

It is hard to explain to a non-scientist the sudden emotional and mental buzz you get when you know you have had an important insight. It's as if you have had a lot of pieces of a jigsaw in your mind and suddenly, in a second, they all fall into place and the whole picture is clear. Whenever that has happened to me in the past, I have always been proved right – even if, initially, my suggestions were regarded as controversial.

This is precisely the feeling I experienced. I felt the same buzz or to use the German-derived word which sums up the feeling so well: *gestalt*. Suddenly, I recalled how many Chinese people were lactose-intolerant, how the Chinese people I had worked with had always said that milk was only for babies, and how one of my close friends, who is of Chinese origin, always politely turned down the cheese course at dinner parties. I knew then of no Chinese people who lived a traditional Chinese life who ever used cow or other dairy food to feed their babies. The tradition was to use a wet nurse but never, ever dairy products.

Culturally, the Chinese used to find our Western preoccupation with milk and milk products very strange. I remember entertaining a large delegation of Chinese scientists shortly after the ending of the Cultural Revolution in the 1980s. On advice from the Foreign Office, we had asked the caterer to provide a pudding that contained a lot of ice cream. After enquiring what the pudding consisted of, all of the Chinese including their interpreter, politely but firmly refused to eat it. At the time we were all delighted and ate extra large portions!

In 1996, I attended an international conference in Beijing and was having lunch with two senior Chinese women scientists. A man smelling strongly of spices and garlic walked past, and I suppose my reaction showed. One of my companions giggled, and shyly asked me, 'What do Chinese people smell of to you?'

I thought about it carefully and replied honestly, 'Nothing in particular.' Then, deciding that I could legitimately ask the question in reverse, I said: 'And what do we Westerners smell of to you?'

There was considerable laughter – usually reflecting embarrassment in Chinese people – but after encouragement on my

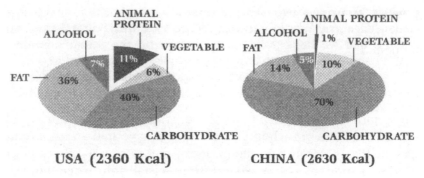

Figure 3.2: Comparison of American and Chinese diets

part, they finally said: 'Westerners smell to us of sour milk!' – 'But', they added reassuringly, 'you don't.'

Recently I checked several Oriental (Chinese, Japanese, Korean and Thai) cookbooks. None mentioned dairy produce at all.

Since I wrote the first edition of *Your Life in Your Hands*, the evidence has continued to indicate strongly that the distinctive difference in rates of prostate and breast cancer between Western and oriental countries relates to diet.

The differences between the Chinese and American diets were thoroughly investigated and documented in 1994 by Campbell and Junshi,[26] and are shown as pie charts in Figure 3.2. The advantages of the Chinese diet include the following factors:

- It is low in fat. Only 14 per cent of calories in the average Chinese diet were from fat, compared with almost 36 per cent in America.
- It is high in fibre, which helps to eliminate excess hormones and toxins from the body. Animal protein was found to make up only 1 per cent of an average Chinese diet, compared with 11 per cent of the average American diet. Vegetables are the main source of protein in China, giving an average fibre intake of 34g per day, compared with the average US fibre intake of only 10–12g per day.
- It is high in phyto-oestrogens, which are protective against prostate and breast cancer. Vegetables rich in phyto-oestrogens, such as soya, are the main source of protein in China.
- Traditionally Chinese people did not eat dairy produce, whereas in the West this can account for up to 40 per cent of the diet.[27]

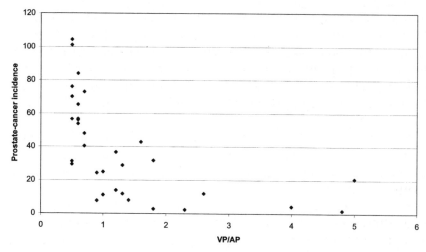

Figure 3.3: Relationship between prostate-cancer incidence and the ratio of vegetable protein (VP) to animal protein (AP) in the diet. Age-standardised cancer data from WHO/IARC, IARC Cancer Epidemiology Database. GLOBOCAN 2000, Cancer incidence, mortality and prevalence worldwide. Ferlay, J., Bray, F., Piesci, P. and Parkin, D.M. (eds). http://www.dep.iarc.fr/globocan/database.pdf. Diet data from Frassetto, L.A., Todd, K.M., Morris, R.C., Jr and Sebastian, A., 2000. Worldwide incidence of hip fracture in elderly women: relation to consumption of animal and vegetable foods. *J Geront: Med Sci*, 55A, (10), M585–M592.

Interestingly, the study by Campbell and Junshi showed that the Chinese took in more calories than Americans, but were much less obese, strongly suggesting that it is the type of food and not the calorie intake that is important. The data in Figure 3.3 also clearly show the importance of a diet high in vegetable, rather than animal, protein.

Unfortunately, the traditional oriental diet is being replaced by the typical Western diet, high in dairy and junk food. According to Chinese colleagues, just as in the West, dairy is being marketed as being essential for strong bones – an idea completely refuted by informed and distinguished doctors and scientists,[28] and more recently by my book *Understanding, Preventing and Overcoming Osteoporosis*, written with Gill Tidey, which is based on an in-depth analysis of the peer-reviewed medical and scientific literature.[29]

Figure 3.3 shows the proportion of vegetable to animal protein in the diet of 33 countries (compiled from the Food and Agriculture Organisation of the United Nations (FAO) food fact sheets[30]) plotted against prostate-cancer incidence. There is a clear relationship between diets with a high ratio of vegetable to animal protein and low prostate-cancer risk. The critical ratio of vegetable to animal protein is between 1 to 1 and 2 to 1. Put more simply, the data suggest that you can decrease your risk of developing prostate cancer by eating larger amounts of vegetable than animal protein. But note that this refers only to protein, and I recommend eating masses of vegetables and fruits as well (*see* Chapter 5).

Nevertheless, despite the mounting evidence of the links between the Western diet and prostate cancer, most conventional medicine continues to promulgate the same old risk factors (*see* Chapter 1).

Much of the information on conventional risk factors may be relevant within countries such as the USA or the UK, but it completely ignores all the epidemiological evidence of the much lower rates in China and other oriental countries, evidence which strongly implicates the Western diet and lifestyle as the main causative factor.

One of the problems, it seems to me, is that researchers tend to look at their own populations. Using Figure 3.1 as an example, they are frequently looking at minor perturbations in the lines at the top of the graph (i.e. rates within individual Western countries), while ignoring the much more significant differences between prostate- and breast-cancer rates in different countries. These differences between Western and oriental countries have been clear and sustained ever since reliable standardised cancer registers were first kept. The data strongly indicate that the difference in diet and lifestyle, especially exposure to hormones and growth factors in food and drink and to hormone-mimicking chemicals in food, drink and the environment, are at the root of the problem of the increasing incidence of prostate, breast and other reproductive cancers in the West – a trend now being followed in the East as they strive to become more and more Westernised.

A very high proportion of non-Caucasian human populations, as well as some Caucasians, become lactose intolerant after weaning, when the child's body stops producing lactase, the enzyme needed to metabolise lactose. This is a clear signal from nature that, as the Chinese used to say, 'milk is for babies' – and they meant human milk. Five thousand years of milk drinking has masked some of the most obvious ill effects of dairy consumption in Western countries.

Another clue that milk drinking by adults is unnatural is that no other mammal drinks the milk of another species. Wildlife programmes show animals eating the flesh and eggs of other species, and living on vegetable matter, but I have yet to see an example of an adult mammal suckling an adult mammal of another species for food.

We all know the old maxim 'you are what you eat'. In the West, the idea of using diet to treat illness goes back to the Hippocratic School of Medicine that originated in Greece in about 400 BC. Hippocrates scorned the belief that disease is caused by magical or supernatural forces, and said that everything had a rational origin. He also noted the body's ability to heal itself, given the right conditions.

THE FINGER POINTS

In my years of exploring alternative health systems – since I first had breast cancer – I have learned that many naturopaths believe that the part of the body that is diseased provides a clue as to the cause of the illness. This seems to be particularly the case for cancers for which we know the cause. For example, lung cancers reflect inhalation of cancer-causing cigarette smoke, radioactive aerosols such as the naturally occurring radioactive gas radon, or asbestos dust. Skin cancers frequently reflect excessive exposure to sunlight whilst cervical cancer is associated with infection by the sexually transmitted human wart (or papilloma) virus. It seemed highly likely that consuming a powerful biochemical solution from the mammary gland of one species of animal (milk) could be sending the wrong signals to my own mammary glands – my breasts.

And I'd certainly been a big milk drinker. Before I had breast cancer the first time, I had consumed a lot of dairy produce as skimmed milk and particularly as low-fat cheeses and yoghurt, which I had used as my main source of protein. I also ate some cheap but lean minced beef (which I have since realised was probably ground up *dairy* cow) as hamburgers with my children, especially when we went out for treats, or made it into spaghetti bolognese or other low-cost meat dishes.

At the time of my last recurrence of cancer in the lymph nodes in my neck, I had been eating yoghurt and some skimmed organic milk which I boiled before drinking, as allowed in the Gerson and Bristol diets. The original Bristol diet by Forbes[31] recommended Indian-style ghee (clarified butter) for cooking and one of the salad dressings for which a recipe is given is based entirely on yoghurt. A detailed case history describing a breast cancer cure in the Bristol diet book also refers to the extensive use of yoghurt. I had been careful to choose only those brands of yoghurt labelled as 'live' and 'organic' or I had often made my own yoghurt using milk labelled as 'organic'. In order to cope with the chemotherapy, I had initially been eating organic yoghurts as a way of helping my digestive tract to recover and repopulate my gut with 'good' bacteria.

However, following Peter's and my insight into the Chinese diet, I decided to give up all dairy produce immediately. Cheese, butter, milk and yoghurt and anything else that contained dairy produce – it all went into the rubbish bin. It is surprising how many products, including commercial soups, biscuits and cakes, contain some form of dairy produce. Even many brands of margarine marketed as soya, sunflower or olive oil spreads can contain significant quantities of dairy produce. Many prescription and herbal drugs are in a lactose base. I therefore became an avid reader of the small print on food and drug labels.

I discovered that as far back as 1989 yoghurt had been implicated in ovarian cancer.[32] Dr Daniel Cramer of Harvard University studied the diet of hundreds of women with ovarian cancer and compared the data with that for a group of women similar in age and other factors, but who had not developed cancer. There was one thing that distinguished the two groups: the women with cancer had eaten much more dairy produce, especially supposedly 'healthy' yoghurt, than women without cancer.

Dr Cramer suggested that the problem was the milk sugar, not the fat, so yoghurt and cottage cheese produced using bacteria, which increase the production of galactose from lactose (milk sugar) were of most concern. Although I am not sure that I agree with the underlying explanation proposed by Dr Cramer or with the chemical he implicated, the link he so clearly demonstrated certainly explained my situation and my observations and hypothesis. How I wish Dr Cramer's information had been more widely publicised at the time. If it had been, I believe I could have avoided any recurrence of my cancer.

I BECOME A HUMAN GUINEA PIG

Up to this point, I had been steadfastly measuring the progress of my latest and greatest lump with callipers and plotting the results. Despite all the encouraging comments and positive feedback from my doctors and nurses, my own precise observations told me the bitter truth: the first chemotherapy session had produced no effect – the lump was still the same size.

Then I eliminated dairy products.

Within days, the lump started to shrink. About two weeks after my second chemotherapy session and one week after I gave up dairy produce the lump in my neck started to itch, and then it began to reduce in size. The line on the graph, which had shown no change, was now pointing downwards as the tumour got smaller and smaller. And, very significantly, I noted that instead of declining exponentially (a graceful curve) as cancer is meant to do, the tumour's decrease in size plotted on a straight line heading off the bottom of the graph, indicating a cure: not suppression or remission of the tumour.

One Saturday afternoon after about six weeks of excluding all dairy produce from my diet, I practised an hour of meditation (more of that later) then felt for what was left of the lump. I could not find it. I went downstairs and asked my husband to feel my neck. He could not find any trace of the lump either. On the following Thursday, my cancer specialist examined me thoroughly, especially my neck where the tumour had been. He was initially bemused and then delighted as he said, 'but I cannot find it'. He was as overjoyed as I was. When I saw the same specialist for my annual check-up in 2001, he told me that my chemotherapy treatment had been only the same basic type that has been used for breast cancer for the past twenty years. None of my doctors, it appeared, had expected someone with my type and stage of cancer (which had clearly spread to the lymph system) to have survived, let alone be so hale and hearty.

When I first discussed my ideas with my cancer specialist he was understandably sceptical. But I understand that he now uses maps from *The Atlas of Cancer Mortality in the People's Republic of China* in his lectures and recommends that his other patients read my books.

I now believe that the link between dairy produce and breast and prostate cancer is fast becoming as well established as that between smoking and lung cancer, as discussed further in Chapters 2 and 4.

I believe that identifying the link between breast cancer and dairy produce, and then developing a diet based on my findings, cured me. Initially, it was difficult for me, as it may be difficult for you, to accept that a substance supposedly as 'natural' and wholesome as milk might have such ominous health implications. In the next chapter, I want to show you some of the particular factors in dairy products that I believe to be to blame.

At the beginning of this chapter I used the idea of a slot machine and its combination of lemons and strawberries to communicate the idea that prostate cancer and breast cancer are what scientists call multifactorial diseases, involving several different risk factors. I explained that, while there is little that we can do about some of our risk factors – or strawberries – such as our genes, eliminating some controllable risks, and changing at least one strawberry to a lemon, can prevent prostate cancer or breast cancer (*see* pp. 87–8). Indeed, even when we have one of these cancers, we can put the disease into remission by eliminating one of the strawberries – as I have done for the last eleven years.

4 Milk is a Four-Letter Word

In this chapter, I explain much of the compelling scientific evidence that has accumulated over the years, even since I wrote the first book in 2000, suggesting that prostate cancer and breast cancer are associated with the Western diet and its high proportion of dairy produce. Milk contains hormones, such as prolactin and oestrogen, and growth factors, such as IGF-I and IGF-II, substances which, according to leading international experts, promote prostate cancer and other types of cancer. The chapter also explains why giving up dairy is unlikely to cause health problems, but, on the contrary, is likely to cut your risk of suffering not only from cancer of the prostate and other reproductive organs but from many other diseases as well.

Just as oriental people used to be astonished when they saw Westerners consuming so much dairy produce, many of us have found it difficult to understand how anyone could possibly live healthily without it. Certainly I was one of those who had bought into the message, pushed by the industry, that dairy produce, especially yoghurt, was essential for good health.

It is all a matter of perception. One person's milk is another person's bowl of cockroaches. The reaction of both groups is 'yuk'.

In most of Western society, milk is promoted as a healthy, natural food: vital for babies, full of protein for active adults, and essential for older women, at risk of osteoporosis. Yoghurt continues to be promoted as being essential for keeping the gut flora in balance. In short, dairy continues to be marketed as all things to all people.

But this carefully crafted marketing image is just that – an image. There is no scientific evidence that we need to consume milk after weaning – in fact, we're the only species that intentionally does so. Even stranger is our obsession with the milk of other species: the cow or goat. Can you imagine drinking dogs' milk, pigs' milk, or rats' milk? Just the thought fills us with disgust – maybe that's how we ought to feel about cows' or goat's milk, too.

One best-selling supposedly anti-cancer diet I read recently recommended consuming meat and dairy produce to protect against cancer (advice I strongly refuted in *Your Life in Your Hands* and *The Plant Programme*), and another book still available in the UK continues to recommend yoghurt as part of an anti-breast-cancer diet. Anything good in dairy produce, whether calcium or the now highly promoted conjugated linoleic acids (CLAs), comes from plants or the action on them of microbes in the gut. Surely it is better to eat salads and vegetables, which are not unlike the grasses that are eaten by cows in the first place – after all, they are the real source of the immensely strong bones of animals designed to be totally vegan, such as cows and hippopotamuses!

Cows' milk isn't intended by nature for consumption by any species other than baby cows. If we compare its profile of nutrients with that of human breast milk, you'll see some major differences.[1] The vertical line on Figure 4.1 represents the nutritional profile of human milk; the horizontal bars show how cows' milk compares. It is clear that cows' milk contains about three times as much protein as human milk, and far more calcium – both of which can place an excessive burden on the human kidney. The high calcium in dairy also causes other problems.

Many scientists believe that the amount of dairy produce in our diet is now far too high. Recently the Royal Society,[2] Britain's most authoritative scientific organisation, has suggested that routes of human exposure to oestrogen that changed in the latter half of the twentieth century included increased consumption of dairy produce. They went on to point out that dairy practices have changed such that pregnant cows continue to be milked. The US Department of Agriculture has estimated that the average American's diet comprises more than 40 per cent dairy produce, more than double most official guidelines.[3] The American diet is certainly not a healthy one. It is estimated that a staggering 60 per cent of Americans are now overweight enough to begin experiencing health problems as a result. About 25 per cent of all Americans under 19 are overweight or obese, a figure that has doubled in 30 years.[4]

In Bill Bryson's book *The Lost Continent* he repeatedly refers to the obesity of the American population:

Iowa women are almost always sensationally overweight – you see them at Merle Hay Mall in Des Moines on Saturdays, clammy and meaty in their shorts and halter tops, looking a little like elephants dressed in children's clothes, yelling at their kids, calling out names like Dwayne and Shauna.

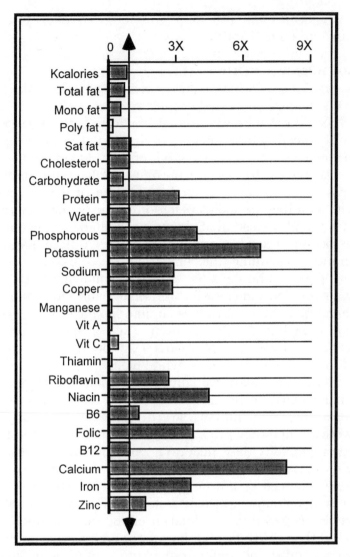

Figure 4.1: Comparison of the composition of typical cows' and human milk. The vertical line represents the composition of typical human milk.

Several recently published books such as *Fat Land: How Americans Became the Fattest People in the World* and *Fast Food Nation* raise concerns about the American diet. According to a review of the former in the *BMJ*,[5] the book is a well-written report on the obese American, and how they got that way. 'And if America is out in front,' the reviewer asks, 'can the United Kingdom be far behind?'

The eight food factors and the eight lifestyle factors, set out in the following two chapters to help you to prevent and treat prostate cancer, will also help you to avoid obesity and its associated diseases.

MILK – WHAT A COCKTAIL!

Let us first look at a list of the incredibly biochemically active chemicals that are contained in milk.

Why should dairy be so strongly implicated? Mammals developed fairly recently in the history of the Earth (they have existed for only about 200 million years, out of the 4,500 million years of the age of the Earth) and are the most evolved and intelligent creatures on the planet. Their high degree of development is achieved by a long period of gestation in the womb, where they are fed a complex cocktail of chemicals, including hormones and growth factors, which bring about cell growth, differentiation and proliferation, including the migration of embryonic cells to different parts of the developing foetus. Following birth, infant mammals are suckled (ideally, in humans, for about one and a half years) because milk carries similar chemical messengers to maintain growth and differentiation. The transport medium for the chemical messengers – plasma – simply changes from red blood to white milk, known as 'white blood' in some cultures.

Milk from every mammal contains hormones, growth factors and other biochemically active substances. The reason why all mammals, other than humans, stop drinking milk at a certain age is because by then they produce all the hormones, growth factors and other peptides they need. The production, secretion and levels of these substances are regulated through a complex, delicately balanced system of interaction. This can be impaired by absorbing extra quantities of such substances from cows' milk, goats' milk or the meat of animals used for dairy production.

Some of the growth factors, hormones and peptides in human milk, cows' milk and milk from other mammals include the following[6] [my bold]:

- bombesine (a neuropeptide).[7] Milk contains both bombesine and GRP (bombesine-like peptide).[8] Bombesine levels in milk are three times higher than in blood,[9] and GRP and bombesine have been implicated in prostate cancer[10] and breast cancer.[11]
- GRP (Gastrin-releasing peptide).[12]
- substance P (a neurotransmitter),[13] which increases vascular permeability[14] and stimulates histamine secretion,[15] causing allergic reactions.

- CGRP (calcitonin-gene-related peptide, also a neurotransmitter).[16]
- **IGF-I and IGF-II[17] (insulin-like growth factors)**. IGF-I and IGF-II are quite resistant to decomposition by enzymes.[18] They promote both prostate[19] and breast cancer.[20] See also the work of He[21] and Perks and Holly.[22]
- **EGF (Epidermal growth factor)**.[23] Like IGF, EGF is quite resistant to decomposition by enzymes.[24] EGF enhances prostate cancer[25] and breast cancer,[26] and was the first growth factor to be shown to be absorbed by the blood through the gut wall.[27] It is to be strongly avoided by those with tumours over-expressing the HER-2 protein. EGF has been implicated in androgen-independent prostate cancer.[28]
- NGF (Nerve growth factor).[29]
- **Prolactin**. To be able to breastfeed, the female body is better equipped to cope with temporarily increased prolactin production. Males are not, and prolactin-producing tumours in men are therefore larger, more active and resistant to treatment.[30] Prolactin enhances prostate cancer[31] and breast cancer.[32]
- PRP (Prolactin-releasing peptide).[33]
- **LHRH** (or: GnRH, stimulates secretion of LH and FSH).[34]
- **progesterone**.[35]
- peptide YY.[36]
- peptide histidine methionine.[37]
- neuropeptide Y (stimulating appetite).[38]
- T3 (Triiodothyronine).[39] T3 increases the number of oestrogen receptors, increasing oestrogen-influence.[40]
- TSH (stimulating T3 and T4 secretion).[41]
- TRH (stimulating TSH secretion).[42] TRH stimulates prolactin[43] and growth-hormone (GH) secretion,[44] through T3.[45]
- GHRF (Growth-hormone-releasing factor).[46] GHRF stimulates GH and hence **IGF-I and IGF-II** secretion.[47]
- ACTH (regulating cortisol secretion).[48]
- neurotensine.[49]
- cortisol.[50]
- insulin (regulating blood-glucose level).[51]
- beta-endorphin (opioid peptide).[52]

Since many of the powerful chemicals contained in milk are known to have an important role in the development of young mammals, including cell division, and milk is designed for this purpose, it is worth asking the question: what happens if the chemicals which are intended by nature to stimulate cell growth in newly born animals such as cows and goats send similar signals to adult tissue?

Many of the growth factors, hormones and other biochemicals contained in dairy milk are implicated in the production and development of other cancers.[53] It has been suggested that different growth factors increase the cancer-risk in different tissues. Excessive LHRH (*see* p. 80), which is concentrated in milk, stimulates secretion of LH and/or FSH, which, in turn, have been implicated in prostate,[54] ovarian[55] and testicular cancer.[56] It has also been suggested that different growth factors promote types of cancer not associated with the reproductive system. There is evidence for the role of milk in promoting lung cancer. For example, in Japan, in 1996 people consumed more than three times as many cigarettes as in Norway,[57] but in Norway lung-cancer mortality in men was higher.[58] Also in countries such as Russia, UK, France, Canada, USA and Australia fewer cigarettes are smoked,[59] but lung-cancer mortality in men is higher than in Japan.[60] In all these countries more milk, containing cancer-promoting substances, is consumed,[61] again suggesting that dairy contains substances that select for damaged or initiated cancer cells.

THE INSULIN-LIKE GROWTH FACTORS (IGF-I AND IGF-II) AND PROSTATE CANCER

Let us look at the role of the insulin-like growth factors, especially IGF-I, for which evidence of its role in prostate and breast cancers continues to mount.

Why should such substances cause prostate or breast cancer?

In humans, free, or circulating IGF-I levels decline with age, consistent with their role in growth. IGF-I levels are higher in teenage girls than boys and the difference extends into adulthood. Levels are elevated in pregnant women. Although IGF-I is essential for growth, its levels do not correlate closely with growth rates; supporting other evidence that some IGF-I may be of dietary origin. It was suggested some years ago by distinguished biochemists that IGF-I levels may be affected by nutritional status.[62]

The levels of IGF-I in the blood are highest during the years of puberty which is, of course, a time of rapid growth. Indeed, at the onset of puberty, IGF-I signals to prostate and breast cells to begin dividing so that the prostate and breasts will grow in adolescent boys and girls.

Both insulin and the IGFs cause cells to increase in size. Insulin has a simple short-term action of cleaning excess nutrients from the circulation and storing them in cells. In contrast, the IGFs are involved in cell proliferation and differentiation, and a complex set of factors have evolved to ensure that IGF activity occurs only when conditions are optimal for growth. Zinc levels are particularly important in the case of the prostate,[63] which seems to store zinc.[64] See Chapter 5 and Lifestyle Factor 1 in Chapter 6 for healthy and unhealthy sources of zinc.

In 1990 researchers at Stanford University reported that IGF-I promotes the growth of prostate cancer cells. In 1995 researchers at the National Institutes of Health reported that IGF-I plays a central role in the progression of many cancers, including that of the prostate. According to Hans R Larsen, the evidence of a strong link between cancer risk and a high level of IGF-I is now indisputable.[65]

Pollack[66] has recently suggested that the relation of IGF physiology to carcinogenesis will become relevant in cancer-risk assessment and chemoprevention, although he continues to emphasise the potential value of drugs that target the IGF-I receptor and indicate that several candidate pharmaceuticals are awaiting clinical trials. Lonning also recommends that future therapeutic strategies in treating breast cancer should consider total blockade of the IGF-I receptor.[67] Yee and Sachdev also state that there are abundant data from human, animal and in vitro studies supporting a role for the IGFs in cancer and that interactions with their receptors have been shown to stimulate cancer proliferation, prevent cell suicide and enhance metastasis. Again, their research centres on targeting the IGF-I receptor.[68] Pollack raises particular concern about the use of IGF-I levels and GH to prevent ageing in humans.[69]

Several prospective studies, using stored blood collected up to fourteen years before the onset of disease, have shown associations between IGF-I and prostate cancer.[70] The associations remain when people whose blood samples were taken soon before diagnosis are excluded from statistical analysis, suggesting that the observed relationships do not reflect release of the growth factor by pre-clinical cancers.[71] The effects are sizable and stronger than the effects of most previously reported risk factors.[72]

This study and that of Chan and others, published in 1998,[73] into IGF-I levels and prostate cancer, discussed below, are both prospective studies whereby symptomless groups of patients are followed for years and data for those developing disease are compared with data for those who do not. Such studies are generally considered most convincing for indicating causal relationships, rather than retrospective studies carried out after the disease has developed, in which case there is a chance the disease could be causing the high measured levels of IGF-I.

Researchers from Canada's McGill University and the Harvard School of Public Health in the United States have also found increased levels of IGF-I circulating in the blood to be a strong predictor of prostate cancer.[74] Men with the highest levels of circulating IGF-I had a 4.3-fold increased risk of developing prostate cancer compared with those with the lowest IGF-I levels. In the article in the magazine *Science*, Professor Pollack writes that 'until now, researchers interested in prostate cancer have focussed on male hormones such as testosterone, but these (IGF-I) results open up a whole new direction of research. This is of the same order of magnitude as the relationship between cholesterol levels and the risk of heart disease'. Also according to Pollack, most recent population studies and laboratory investigations support initial prospective studies linking risk of future diagnosis of prostate or premenopausal breast cancer with levels of circulating IGF-I.[75] Significantly, one of the ways in which the drug Tamoxifen is thought to work is by reducing circulating IGF-I levels.[76] Yet another recent study from 1998 confirms that increased IGF-I levels in blood are associated with large relative risks for common cancers.[77]

Another recent study, based on an eighteen-year follow-up of policemen, reports that circulating GH concentrations are significantly associated with increased risk of malignancy;[78] again, this was a prospective study in which GH measurements were undertaken in a healthy male population and related to subsequent cancers detected in a long-term follow-up (an average eighteen years). Such long-term studies are limited in number by the relatively recent introduction of reliable assays for GH and IGF-I. The prospective study of GH in the police was based on results from an early GH assay, the imprecision of which may have resulted in underestimating the association with malignancy.[79]

Much recent scientific evidence supports the link between dairy consumption and prostate cancer. IGF-I is exactly the same chemical whether it is in the milk of goats, sheep, cows, humans or other mammalian species. Levels of IGF-I are naturally higher in cows' milk (and in that of sheep and goats) than human milk because these animals grow more rapidly. As pointed out by John

Robbins in his book *A Diet for a New America*,[80] while a human normally takes 180 days to double its birth weight, a cow takes only 47 days and a goat even less – just 19 days – so such milk is likely to be particularly bad for us because it will contain more growth factors than human milk.

The fact that dairy products are rich in growth factors is illustrated by the normal practice of isolating growth factors for research studies from milk or cheese whey.[81]

The average concentration of IGF-I in milk from cows treated with a genetically modified hormone-recombinant bovine growth hormone (rBGH; also known as bovine somatotropin or BST) is *even higher* than in untreated milk (estimates vary from two to five times higher concentration in treated milk) and there is about two times more IGF-I in the meat of treated cows than in that of untreated cows.[82] In the US, the rBGH is available without veterinary prescription. Its use is banned in the EU, although under the GATT (General Agreement on Tariffs and Trade) it has not been possible to ban imported milk products from the US.[83]

One of the most important effects of rBGH, as far as prostate and breast cancer studies are concerned, is that it releases extra quantities of IGF-I and IGF-II. The conventional medical view is that the highest proportion of IGF-I is made by the liver. It would also be true to say that we manufacture our own cholesterol, but cholesterol-related disease (e.g. heart disease) is caused by consuming *extra* amounts of the substance from dairy and other animal products. Could a similar situation not apply in the case of IGF-I? Specifically that, yes, we manufacture our own IGF-I but could not *disease* be caused by consuming extra quantities of IGF-I from dairy produce and the meat of animals used for dairying?

Independent studies show that substances contained in milk closely similar to IGF-I are not destroyed by the digestive system because of the protective effect of casein (the principal protein in milk).[84] The 1999 report of the EU Scientific Committee states 'there is clear evidence that orally ingested IGF-I reaches the receptor sites in the gut in its biologically active form'.[85] Moreover, research published by the Cancer Epidemiology Unit at Oxford University[86] has shown that serum IGF-I was 9 per cent lower in vegan men than in meat eaters (also thought to consume dairy produce) and milk-consuming vegetarians.

Different breeds of cows have different levels of IGF-I. For example, the Brahman breed generally has higher blood levels of IGF-I than the Angus breed of cattle.[87]

Over the years, the dairy industry has chosen to increase the average milk yield by selectively breeding from cattle which are better milk producers. This has resulted in the selection of cows which have higher levels of naturally occurring BGH, so that even before the era of rBGH, levels of IGF-I in milk were increasing. Also, the long-term treatment of cows with the hormone implant oestradiol as a growth promoter increases secretion of IGF-I. IGF-I is not destroyed during pasteurisation of milk. In experiments, after being treated at 175°C for 45 seconds (longer than the US Department of Agriculture Pasteurization Protocol), the concentration of IGF-I was not reduced.[88]

IGF-I has growth-promoting effects in response to concentrations as low as 1ng/ml. Milk contains approximately 30ng/ml so that 2, 8oz glasses of milk a day would contain 200ng of IGF-I per kilogram of body weight per day for a person weighing 70kg.[89] Also, milk secretions of mammals contain special forms of IGF-I which is ten times more potent than normal IGF-I. In normal cows' milk 3 per cent of the IGF-I is reported to be in this form.[90]

Because IGF-I is known to be so biologically active in humans, the increased levels in milk raise the question: is it the increase in ingestion of IGFs from milk or the meat of dairy animals (which is known to be closely associated with prostate cancer) that has been a key factor in the increased incidence in this and other reproductive cancers noted, for example, by Miller and Sharpe?

The evidence of such a dietary link continues to mount. In one recent study, Dr Chan and her colleagues investigated the relationship between dairy calcium and prostate cancer in 20,885 men in the Physicians' Health Study.[91] The results clearly showed that men consuming more than 600mg a day of dairy calcium had a 32 per cent higher risk of prostate cancer than men consuming less than or equal to 150mg of dairy calcium a day, even after adjusting for other risk factors such as age, smoking, exercise levels and body mass index. Chan concluded that the results support the hypothesis that dairy products and calcium are associated with a greater risk of prostate cancer.[92] The study also found that those who ate the most dairy produce had 17 per cent less vitamin D in their bloodstream than those who consumed the least. This vitamin is known to play a protective role against prostate cancer.[93]

Evidence of a dose-response relationship between dairy consumption and prostate cancer has also been noted by Barnard,[94] who goes on to say that mechanisms that may explain the association include the deleterious effect of high-calcium foods on vitamin D balance, increased serum IGF-I concentrations and the effect of dairy products on testosterone concentration or activity.

Studies of breast-cancer cell lines demonstrate that vitamin D compounds block the cancer-promoting activity of IGF-I.[95] It is therefore likely that the anti-cancer effect of vitamin D involves interfering with the IGF-I/IGF-II signalling pathway. A recent study of the treatment of rats with a vitamin D analogue found that it caused a marked regression in prostate cancer, accompanied by an increase in the expression of IGFBP-2, -3, -4 and -5. In addition, a significant increase in the number of apoptotic cells was observed from the vitamin D-treated animals compared with control animals. The results suggest that vitamin D exerts its growth-inhibiting effects on prostate cells by interfering with the IGF-I signalling pathway, which eventually leads to induction of cell suicide.[96] Studies of Vitamin D on EGF and its receptor show a similar relationship, but most of the studies relate to breast cancer.[97]

Remember, however, that too much vitamin D is toxic, and I strongly recommend against either pills or dairy as a source of this vitamin in most cases (see further in Chapters 5 and 6).

Colleen Doyle, director of nutrition and physical activity for the American Cancer Society in Atlanta, explains: 'Calcium, especially when it is taken as a supplement, has the ability to temporarily suppress the amount of vitamin D that circulates in the blood. Vitamin D is thought to be important in suppressing the growth of prostate cells.'[98]

Research directed at understanding the mechanism of vitamin D action on normal and malignant prostate cells is being carried out with the goal of developing prevention and treatment strategies to improve prostate-cancer therapy. Its main actions were reported to be to help resistant prostate-cancer cells to become more treatable. Vitamin D was reported to be anti-proliferative and to promote differentiation.[99] It has been suggested that vitamin D compounds help to normalise telomerase activity (*see* Chapter 2).[100]

One type of vitamin D has been shown to delay the rate of increase of serum PSA in a pilot trial involving men with early recurrent prostate cancer after primary therapy with radiation or surgery.[101] Harvard Medical School has shown that men who eat dairy products regularly have a 30 per cent greater chance of suffering prostate cancer than those who eat less than half a serving per day.[102] This study is the largest to date, by arguably one of the most respected epidemiology teams in the world. Milk is loaded with calcium, and taking large amounts of calcium lowers blood levels of a particular type of the body's form of vitamin D which prevents cancers.[103] This study shows that men who have more than six glasses per week of milk fortified with vitamin D have lower levels of vitamin D than those who have fewer than two glasses.[104] These studies imply that you don't need to drink milk and that taking calcium supplements may harm you.[105]

There now seems to be an emerging consensus. Vitamin D is present in small quantities in our food and it has been proved to reduce the incidence of prostate cancer significantly, but its ability to do this is limited by the effects of protein and calcium in the diet. Perhaps this is one of the connections to the Western diet with its high levels of protein and dairy.[106]

Another researcher, E Giovannucci, concludes:

> For prostate cancer, epidemiologic studies consistently show a positive association with high consumption of milk, dairy products and meats.[107]

and

> Diets high in dairy products and meats are related to higher risk of prostate cancer incidence or mortality in most ecologic, case-control and prospective studies.[108]

A recent Scandinavian report also links the volume of dairy consumption to the level of risk of prostate cancer. High dairy consumption was reported to increase risk by 50 per cent.[109]

Other studies have also linked high circulating levels of bioavailable/bioactive IGF-I with an increased risk of developing prostate[110] and other[111] cancers.

These and other recent findings provide compelling evidence that dairy consumption is one of the key factors contributing to prostate cancer (and breast cancer) – though all of the other dietary factors in Chapter 5 are important too.

As indicated in Chapter 2, DNA can be damaged by many factors, although the body is well equipped to repair or eliminate damaged cells. The problem of cancer developing into a disease is more likely to reflect the influence of factors favouring the growth of damaged, relative to normal, cells over the longer term.

Absorbing growth factors and hormones through the diet will preferentially favour such damaged cells – those least able to deal with growth factors – and hence promote cancer. Eventually, tumours can start producing more growth factors, stimulating their own reproduction, but probably only in very advanced cases. Even so, some natural substances can help to block their activity (*see* Chapter 5).

Hence, many scientific investigations reveal that consuming dairy increases the risk of prostate cancer[112] and breast cancer.[113] There are a few studies that purport to show the opposite, but, as discussed in the final chapter, their validity has been questioned.

In *Your Life in Your Hands*, I quoted other studies that suggested such a link, including that of Outwater and others[114] which was based on a review of more than 130 peer-reviewed publications. I also quoted the findings of an EU scientific committee that concluded that excess levels of IGF-I in milk posed an increased risk of prostate and breast cancer.[115] Strong evidence of a causal association between higher levels of milk consumption and IGF also came from a comparison between people whose diets were supplemented with milk and a control sample of people whose diet was not supplemented.[116] Associations of calcium, milk and dairy products with IGF-I also suggest a link between diet and prostate cancer.[117]

Together, the evidence suggests that the association between IGF-I and cancer incidence complies with many of the accepted criteria for causality;[118] the association is strong and specific, it demonstrates the correct temporal sequence, it is dose responsive, it has biological plausibility, and it has coherence with other documented associations. More prospective studies with longer follow-up are required to confirm the link. The last remaining criterion of causality to be satisfied would then depend on interventions, showing that reducing circulating IGF-I levels reduces cancer incidence.[119]

Holly and others[120] point out that the strong dependence of circulating IGF-I concentrations on nutrition raises the prospect of being able to reduce cancer risk by less aggressive interventions. Investigation of nutritional interventions aimed at reducing serum IGF-I concentrations would be warranted if such reductions were confirmed to reduce the risk of cancer.

More recently, Gunnell and others, from a consortium of British universities including Bristol and Cambridge, examined the association of diet with the IGFs in healthy middle-aged men. They found that raised levels of IGF-I, relative to the binding protein that prevents it locking onto receptors, were associated with higher intakes of milk, dairy products, calcium, carbohydrate and polyunsaturated fats, while lower levels were correlated with high vegetable consumption, particularly tomatoes. They found no evidence of an association with red meat. Their findings that vegetable intake was weakly related to lower bioavailable/bioactive IGF-I is consistent with the observation that vegetable-rich diets protect against prostate, breast and colorectal cancer.[121] Their findings were not affected by socioeconomic status or other lifestyle factors such as smoking.[122] These associations, with the exception of carbohydrates, support all the factors I proposed as limiting levels of circulating IGF-I in *Your Life in Your Hands*. Unfortunately Gunnell and his co-workers looked at carbohydrates as a whole, whereas I advised against refined carbohydrates but not against others, basing this advice on scientific evidence that refined white bread increases circulating IGF-I levels whereas whole-grain cereals contain chemopreventive chemicals active against prostate and breast cancer (*see* further in Lifestyle Factor 1, Chapter 6). Other studies had previously reported reduced levels of IGF-I with increased tomato consumption[123] and in those on vegan diets.[124]

Prostate and breast cancers have existed in Western populations for a long time. A mid-seventeenth century painting by Rembrandt entitled *Bathsheeba at her Toilet* (1654), which hangs in the Louvre in Paris, clearly shows that the model had a large tumour in her right breast. Since the time Western man developed stable, farming communities they have consumed significant quantities of milk, and it is worth remembering that, even without the use of genetically engineered hormones and the practices of the modern industrialised dairy industry, milk contains quantities of IGF-I that have been steadily increasing over the centuries because of the selection of higher-yielding dairy cows.

IGF-I is only *one* of the powerful chemicals in milk which may have a significant role to play in the development of prostate and breast cancer. What about all of the others? Here are some of them.

IGF-II

According to Outwater and others,[125] IGF-II is also a potent mitogen (a substance that induces cell division) present in dairy milk. The US Food and Drug Administration (FDA) reported that IGF-I levels are approximately 30ng/ml. Those of IGF-II are approximately 350ng/ml – more than ten times greater. Most studies have concentrated on IGF-I because of the effects of rBGH on its concentration, and there is little about IGF-II in the literature. One experiment, however, which involved increasing IGF-II levels in transgenic mice 20–30 fold, indicated the development of a wide range of tumours after eighteen months.

PROLACTIN

Prolactin receptors have been demonstrated in the rat prostate. Expression of the receptor gene(s) appears to be controlled differently in different parts of the prostate, one form being regulated by prolactin, testosterone and oestrogen. The study may have implications for prostate-cancer progression since prolactin increases epithelial cell DNA synthesis. This research also concluded that prolactin may increase prostate-cancer progression because it increases synthesis of epithelial-cell DNA.[126]

The hormone prolactin is a key milk-supporting hormone and is found in all milk, although there are differences between human prolactin and that of other species. Prolactin has been linked to prostate and breast cancer by several research groups. For example, Clevenger and others[127] from the University of Pennsylvania writing in the *American Journal of Pathology* in 1995 concluded that their data suggested a role for prolactin in the pathogenesis of breast cancer. The ability of bovine prolactin to act as a mitogen in cultures of rodent breast cancer cells is undisputed. Struman and others in 1999[128] also showed that the human prolactin/GH family are angiogenic – that is they promote the development of microvascular structures – remember from Chapter 2 that cancers need to develop a blood-supply system and scientists are trying to develop anti-angiogenic substances to effectively starve cancers. The same molecules however, can have anti-angiogenic properties. These properties are thought to be important in the development of the vascular connections between the mother and developing foetus (stress and some drugs, including some for treating psychotic disorders, increase the body's circulating prolactin).

Most amazingly, in the lab prolactin is actually measured by adding milk to cultures of a type of cancer cell (rat lymphoma) and weighing the increase in the mass of the cancer to calculate the concentration of prolactin! This technique has been shown to be a sensitive bio-assay method (relies on biological rather than chemical reaction) for determining the levels of prolactin in milk, and it *depends upon* prolactin's ability to stimulate the growth of cancer cells. I actually first discovered this in a book entitled *Breastfeeding – A Guide to the Medical Profession*.[129] Genetically engineered prolactin is also marketed and sold for experiments on prolactin-dependent tumours.[130]

Prolactin in milk has been described as biologically potent and in new, suckling infant mammals it influences fluid, sodium, potassium and calcium transport. Again, we manufacture our own prolactin. Is it not likely that, as in the case of cholesterol, triglycerides and IGF-I, disease could be caused by consuming foods (especially in large quantities) in which *extra amounts* of this chemical are concentrated?

Hence, at least one hormone (prolactin) and a potent growth factor (IGF-I) contained in milk and the meat from slaughtered dairy cows have been shown to be cancer promoters. There is evidence that IGF-II is also a cancer promoter. And these are only three of the many powerful biologically active chemicals in milk designed to influence development of the newborn of the same species. EGF, which is also a mitogen (promoting cell division), also occurs in milk. It is well established that EGF stimulates the proliferation of epidermal and epithelial tissues generally.[131]

If prostate tissue is frequently bathed in fluid with elevated levels of growth factors used in nature to signal to young males to develop their prostate glands during puberty for the production of semen and a hormone for which the prostate has been shown to have receptors, is it surprising that prostate cells make mistakes that can lead to cancer?

TESTOSTERONE AND OESTROGEN

Officially, testosterone has been considered to be one of the main hormones to affect prostate cancer, and oestrogen to affect breast cancer.[132,133]

The association between prostate-cancer risk and IGF-I is stronger in men over 60 years of age, however, when androgens such as testosterone are likely to have less influence.[134] An alternative explanation might be that IGF-I enhances the production of steroids from the testis[135] and the ovary.[136] The proliferative effects of steroids on prostate and breast tissue can also be made worse by IGF-I[137] – indeed IGF-I has been reported to be able to activate the androgen receptor even in the absence of androgens in prostate cells.[138] Increased IGF-I, derived from the circulation, could therefore enhance and add to the effects of testosterone on the prostate. A combination of such potential interacting mechanisms involving IGF-I effects on steroids is a plausible explanation of the associations of testosterone with prostate cancer and oestrogen with breast cancer.[139]

The findings of the EU Scientific Committee on Veterinary Measures Relating to Public Health[140] state 'The physiological actions of IGF-I and IGF-II relate to growth and development of the embryo and foetus and to cellular differentiation, proliferation and cancer.' Is this not just a modern, high-technology way of saying what the Chinese have always known: that milk (and they meant human milk) is just for (human) babies?

IN SUMMARY

This chapter has presented you with a lot of scientific evidence drawn from peer-reviewed scientific papers published in reputable international scientific journals or from the findings of international panels of experts about the potential causes of prostate (and breast) cancer. Let me summarise what all this information means.

- A rational explanation of cause and effect has been found for many types of cancer, following Professor Richard Doll's breakthrough in the 1950s, which showed the link between smoking tobacco and lung cancer. For many types of cancer, we know that the disease is caused or triggered by something we are exposed to, including industrial chemicals and viral or bacterial infections. Some members of the exposed population may be more likely to be affected because of their genetic make-up, but many cancers for which there is now a well-established rational cause are related to dietary or lifestyle factors rather than genetic factors.
- The incidence of prostate cancer in some Western countries, especially the eastern seaboard of the USA, which includes many ethnic groups and hence a mixed gene pool, is similar to that of the incidence of lung cancer among heavy smokers.
- Oriental communities have traditionally had exceptionally low rates of prostate (and breast) cancer compared to Western countries. However, when oriental people move to live in the West their rates of prostate and breast cancer approach those of Western countries.
- The rates of prostate and breast cancer also increase when oriental people adopt a Western lifestyle in their own countries. Typically oriental diets have included most of the things eaten in the West, including meat such as pork,

chicken and duck (although in much smaller quantities), but traditionally oriental diets have *not* included any dairy products.

- The consumption of Western food including dairy products such as milk, ice cream and reprocessed dairy cow meat such as sausages and burgers, is increasing as countries such as Japan, Korea and, increasingly, China embrace 'development'. This process of Westernisation typically begins in urban centres, and, as we have seen from the data in Chapter 3, prostate- and breast-cancer rates in oriental countries are significantly higher in urban areas than in rural ones.

- Modern genetic research and molecular protein studies indicate that in the case of prostate and breast cancer the damage to the cell, which causes the wrong chain of protein signals to be relayed causing the uncontrolled growth that is cancer, is at a superficial level in the cell (between the receptors and intercellular fluid) – not deep inside the cell as is the case in some other types of cancers.

- Only a very small proportion of prostate cancers are the result of inherited mutated (damaged) genes, which are called tumour-suppressor genes. These genes normally produce proteins to slow down cell growth. However, the disease does not always develop, even in those carrying the mutated gene. This observation and the fact that they are tumour-suppressor genes suggests that even where people have inherited mutated genes their risk of cancer *can be reduced* if factors signalling to the cell to produce too much, or the wrong sorts of, growth factors are removed.

- Milk and the meat of dairy animals contain significant amounts of the growth factors IGF-I and IGF-II, and hormones such as prolactin.

- The levels of IGF-I in milk have probably increased due to selective stock breeding and the adoption of high-yielding species for dairying.

- The use of the genetically engineered hormone rBGH to increase milk yield is associated with the highest IGF-I levels in milk.

- IGF-I and prolactin are known to promote the growth of prostate- and breast-cancer cells in laboratory cultures. This strongly suggests that they can do the same in humans, too, if they enter the bloodstream. Prostate tissue has receptors for IGF-I, IGF-II and prolactin.

- Casein, the main milk protein, has been shown to protect such substances contained in milk from being broken down during digestion.
- Research on humans, including gold-standard prospective studies, shows that men with high levels of circulating IGF-I are at greater risk of suffering from prostate cancer than those with lower levels.
- Research also now shows convincingly that circulating levels of IGF-I reflect the diet, especially high dairy and calcium intakes[141] and other factors described in Chapter 5.

I RECOMMEND

Overall, the evidence of a connection between dairy consumption and prostate and breast cancer has become even more compelling since *Your Life in Your Hands* was first published in 2000. Such a connection would explain the increase in prostate- and breast-cancer incidence with increasing age if, by consuming dairy produce on a daily basis, we are exposing prostate and breast tissue, which should be turning off or turned off, to growth factors and hormones designed to cause the tissue to grow and proliferate as is the case naturally in adolescence. I therefore recommend that all men who wish to prevent or treat prostate cancer should *totally eliminate all forms of dairy produce from cows, goats or any animal source from their diet and make the other dietary and lifestyle changes indicated in Chapters 5 and 6*. Those with active cancer, particularly, should cut down their intake of foods of animal origin as much as possible.

THE RISK WE RUN

I know that there will be many people who will read this book and say that they have consumed dairy produce all their lives with no ill effect – just as there are people who point out that someone they know has smoked 40–60 cigarettes a day and lived to be 100. The problem is one of increasing risk to those in the population who, for genetic or other reasons, are more vulnerable. Risk is a difficult idea to explain. Many scientists who are specialists in risk (which is a concept based on statistical probabilities) point out that no one would buy lottery tickets if they understood the subject, but human behaviour is based more on personal experience and emotions than mathematical concepts.

The best way of explaining cancer risk is perhaps the aeroplane analogy, which I use to try to persuade people to stop smoking.

According to this example, you should think how you would feel if you were going to fly in an aeroplane and you knew with certainty that one out of every ten flights was going to crash. Would you fly? I don't think you would! Perhaps because they understand risk, very few scientists smoke.

I have never smoked, and, knowing that I am vulnerable to breast cancer, I will no longer eat any dairy produce (including meat from animals used for dairying) in any form, at any time. I have lived without any dairy produce whatsoever in my diet for more than ten years. Since then, a large cancer in my neck that was thought to be incurable, shrivelled and disappeared and has not returned. My previously brittle nails are now long and strong, my skin is in excellent condition and I have no signs of osteoporosis. I have few grey hairs and most people think I am younger than my 59 years. Similar advice to give up dairy is given by Dr RM Kradjian, MD, in his book, *Save Yourself from Breast Cancer*,[142] and in a letter entitled 'The Milk Letter: A Message to my Patients'.[143]

I believe that I, and all those who have suffered from prostate cancer or breast cancer but shared my advice, have avoided death by dairy.

However, don't think that this is the only benefit to be gained from eliminating dairy from your diet. There are many other diseases which are helped by avoiding dairy. Some of these are described below, and many of the beneficial effects of a dairy-free diet have been confirmed over and over again by communications from followers of the dietary and lifestyle factors outlined in this book.

SOME OTHER PROBLEMS WITH MILK AND HEALTH
Scientists have linked the consumption of cows' milk to a wide range of human health problems. Here are some of them.

Cows' milk and human infants
Babies who are fed cows' milk in the first year of life are at risk of developing iron deficiency. The iron in cows' milk isn't easy for babies to absorb, and such milk also appears to interfere with the body's absorption of iron from other foods. Even worse, cows' milk has been shown to cause iron loss by producing gastro-intestinal bleeding.[144] Many authorities, including the American Academy of Pediatrics Committee on Nutrition, recommend that whole cows' milk should be excluded from the diet in the first year of life.[145] The UK Department of Health has

recently endorsed the resolution passed at the World Health Assembly in May 2001 that babies should be exclusively breast fed for the first six months of life.[146] Paediatricians learned long ago that cows' milk was often a cause of colic in young infants, and even breast-feeding mothers consuming cows' milk can have colicky babies.[147] This is how one British consultant paediatrician describes allergy to cows' milk in infants: 'An infant receiving cows' milk protein (CMP) may be persistently restless, screaming at intervals and appearing in pain. His appetite may be excessively greedy, he may regurgitate freely and he may have loose, mucousy stools in which blood and sometimes sugars are detected. There may be impaired weight gain and anaemia is common. Infants, especially if their parents or siblings suffer from eczema/hay fever/asthma, may develop facial or generalised eczema, persistent nasal congestion and noisy wheezing when CMP is introduced, or these symptoms may be accentuated at that time, with or without gastrointestinal disturbance.'[148]

Milk and allergies

Milk is one of the most common causes of food allergies. It is the single most common cause of allergy in infants,[149] and CMP has frequently been implicated in causing eczema, asthma and migraine. It has been suggested that some of the thousands of cases of cot death that occur in the USA every year might be caused by cows' milk allergy.[150] Respiratory problems, canker sores, skin conditions, and other subtle and not-so-subtle allergies can all be caused by dairy products. Over 70 per cent of the world's adult population are unable to digest the milk sugar, lactose, suggesting that this is the normal condition for adults, not some sort of deficiency.[151] The symptoms, which include abdominal pain, flatulence and diarrhoea, are relieved by taking the enzyme that breaks down lactose, called lactase. Lactose intolerance would seem to be nature's early warning system!

According to an article in *FDA Consumer*,[152] a food allergy, or hypersensitivity, is an abnormal response to a food triggered by the immune system. Many people often have gas, bloating or other unpleasant reactions to something they eat, but this is not a true allergic response. Such a reaction is called 'food intolerance'. Lactose (milk sugar) intolerance is very common, especially among non-Caucasians. This is of particular concern since it is used as the matrix or filler for many orthodox and herbal tablets. The article continues:

The food protein fragments responsible for an allergic reaction are not broken down by cooking or by stomach acids or enzymes that digest food. These proteins can cross the gastrointestinal lining, travel through the bloodstream and cause allergic reactions throughout the body.

The timing and location of an allergic reaction to food is affected by digestion. For example, an allergic person may first experience a severe itching of the tongue or 'tingling lips'. Vomiting, cramps or diarrhoea may follow. Later, as allergens enter the bloodstream and travel throughout the body, they can cause a drop in blood pressure or eczema, or asthma when they reach the lungs. The onset of these symptoms may vary from a few minutes to an hour or two after the food is eaten.

Over 170 foods have been documented in the scientific literature as causing allergic reactions.[153] Most sufferers are affected by the so-called 'big eight': milk, eggs, soya, wheat, peanuts, shellfish, fruits and tree nuts, which between them account for the great majority of food allergies.[154]

Pending legislation on allergens in manufactured foods, the UK Institute of Food Science & Technology makes the following recommendations for label warnings (to take the example of dairy): 'where calcium caseinate is the MSA (major serious allergen) concerned, the warning should read "Contains MILK PROTEIN". It would be helpful to the purchaser to add to this category of warning the words "to which some people may be allergic" '.[155]

Let me quote from a recent article in the *Sunday Times*[156] on the role of milk in allergies.

> Hippocrates, the father of medicine, swore by milk-exclusion diets for curing all sorts: enfeebled babies, diarrhoea, skin complaints, wheezing, painful joints ... As Hippocrates suspected, the white stuff [milk] is the commonest cause of childhood allergies. Standard medical advice is that such allergies usually desist by the age of three. But in a recent Finnish study, two thirds of a group of 56 infants diagnosed with cows'-milk allergy were still allergic and highly symptomatic at the age of 10. Other studies show that many children are milk allergic but don't know it. Reactions include runny noses, wheezing, coughing, ear infections, rashes and stomach upsets. When milk

is withdrawn from their diet, symptoms improve or clear altogether, and reintroducing it leads to relapse in the majority. The chief culprits appear to be lactose and bovine protein.

Insulin-dependent diabetes (Type I or childhood-onset) is linked to dairy products. Epidemiological studies of various countries show a strong correlation between the use of dairy products and the incidence of insulin-dependent diabetes. This disease, which tends to strike in early teenage years and accounts for many deaths a year in the UK alone, starts with the immune system destroying the beta cells in the pancreas that produce insulin. It has been suggested that there may be a genetic predisposition, but mounting evidence suggests that the disease is linked to an allergy to bovine (cows') protein.[157]

'Dirty milk' and infectious illnesses

Milk is an excellent culture medium for the growth and transmission of many bacteria and micro-organisms. Pasteurisation was originally developed to destroy Coxiella burnetii (the organism responsible for Q-fever) and Mycobacterium tuberculosis (the organism responsible for tuberculosis), which were thought to be the most heat-resistant pathogens likely to be present in raw milk. However, new studies suggest that a microbe called Mycobacterium paratuberculosis may survive pasteurisation if it is present in high numbers prior to heat treatment.[158] In cows, the microbe causes Johne's disease, which is an incurable, chronic, infectious disease characterised by diarrhoea, weight loss and debilitation. It is one of the most widespread bacterial diseases of domestic animals throughout the world, and is believed to be associated with irritable bowel syndrome in humans[159] (which affects 20 per cent of the population in the USA[160]). This problem has made headlines in prestigious newspapers in Britain. For example, an article entitled 'TB bacteria found in treated milk' (*Sunday Times*, February 20, 2000) discussed links between mycobacterium paratuberculosis and Britain's 80,000 cases of Crohn's disease. The article goes on to describe serious outbreaks of food poisoning also involving pasteurised milk which, in one case, affected sixty people, killing one child and requiring a second child to have a kidney transplant. Hugh Pennington, Professor of Microbiology at Aberdeen University, who traced the outbreak to milk contaminated by faecal E-coli 0157 bacteria, is quoted as saying 'There have been enough problems with milk in recent years to show there is an issue here. Most of the time farmers will get away with dirty milk, but when things go wrong it can be disastrous.'

Also, drinking milk contaminated with bovine tuberculosis can affect tumours. By the end of 2003, 3,015 herds of cattle in Britain were under movement restrictions due to TB incidents extending from England (2,313 herds) to Scotland (78 herds).[161]

Listeria monocytogenes is a bacterium which can occur in soft cheeses and cause very serious illness, including meningitis and septicaemia; the mortality rate can be as high as 30 per cent in those affected by Listeriosis.[162] The most vulnerable people include those who are immunosuppressed, which of course includes those on chemotherapy. The incubation period before the development of the disease can be as long as ten weeks, causing considerable difficulty in identifying the source of infection.

The dairy industry also contributes to the spread of many other nasty infectious illnesses such as brucellosis, leptospirosis (Weil's disease) and cryptosporidium (a malaria-like parasite, which is resistant to normal water disinfection processes and is now affecting even some of our major groundwater sources), not to mention BSE and new-variant CJD.

As if these allergies and unpleasant infectious illnesses were not bad enough, a wide range of chemicals can be administered legally to dairy animals.[163] These chemicals include antibiotics to treat infection and for use as growth promoters, and anti-parasitic drugs including those active against worms. In the USA and some other countries, hormones, including oxytocin, are used as veterinary prescription drugs. It is claimed that their use in cows does not pose human food safety concerns, provided that they are used according to directions. They can, however, be misused – for example oxytocin can be used to increase milk production – and highly effective policing is needed to ensure milk does not contain excess residues of hormones administered by dairy farmers.[164]

The trend towards intensive farming means that fewer and fewer cows are being forced, unnaturally, to produce more and more milk. In the USA, for example, there has been an almost constant annual increase in milk yield per cow of 1.5–2 per cent. One of the consequences of this highly artificial, high-pressure environment is an increase in infections of cows' udders, which can cause pus to be present in milk. Even in the EU, milk for human consumption can be sold legally even when it contains up to 400,000 somatic pus cells/ml (EU directive 92/46/EEC), so one teaspoon of milk can contain 2 million pus cells. Because increased pus diminishes the value of milk, dairy farmers use antibiotics on their animals. In 1990, an FDA survey found antibiotics and other drugs in 51 per cent of 70 milk samples taken in 14 cities.[165] There is growing concern that residues such as these may increase the human allergic response to milk, as well as increasing the immunity of bacteria to antibiotics, making human diseases more difficult to treat. It is estimated by the EU that 3-10 per cent of the human population is allergic to penicillin and the other antibiotics most commonly used to treat mastitis in cows. Their report also states that increased use of anti-microbial substances in treating mastitis might lead to the selection of resistant bacteria.[166]

Milk is designed to be a concentrated source of chemicals which ensure the growth and well-being of newly born and young mammals. Unfortunately, many harmful man-made chemicals which the body cannot distinguish from natural substances also become concentrated in milk. See further in Chapter 6, Lifestyle Factor 6.

Dairy and osteoporosis

Dairy is strongly and wrongly promoted as protecting against osteoporosis. Indeed, the most commonly asked questions from those recommended to adopt a dairy-free diet are 'Won't I get osteoporosis?' or 'Where do I get my calcium from?' The marketing of dairy produce as an essential source of calcium has been so strong that even some medical professionals, who should know better, insist that eliminating dairy produce from the diet will lead to calcium deficiency and hence increase the risk of osteoporosis. For many people, cheese is likely to be part of the cause, not the cure, of osteoporosis. The widely publicised scientific evidence on the real causes of osteoporosis, presented in *Understanding, Preventing and Overcoming Osteoporosis*,[167] appears to have made no impact on conventional thinking. We were unable to find a single website from an orthodox medical source, national or international agency or charity that did not recommend dairy as a source of calcium and protection against osteoporosis. In our book, we present evidence, from the peer-reviewed scientific literature, which strongly and convincingly refutes this.

I shall quote here from John Robbins's bestselling book *Diet for a New America*:[168]

The [US] National Dairy Council has spent tens of millions of dollars to make us think that osteoporosis can be prevented by drinking more milk and eating more dairy products. **But the only research that even begins to suggest that the consumption of dairy products might be helpful has been paid for by the National Dairy Council itself [my bold].**

And finally
Let me finish with a statement from a review of *Your Life in Your Hands* posted on the Amazon.com website by a physician in the USA: 'In my practice I see so many patients with acid reflux disease, asthma, frequent migraine headaches, feeling tired all the time. As soon as we stop the milk and related products their improvement is remarkable. I think it does not make sense that millions of our citizens take medications for the above-mentioned disorders and do not follow a common sense approach by discontinuing milk products and giving themselves a chance to feel better naturally. I switch all my patients from milk to soy on their first visit and in one week they feel the difference.'

For further information on the problems of dairy foods you may wish to update yourself regularly using the website of the AntiDairy coalition, http://www.antidairycoalition.com.

5 The Food Factors

Let your food be your medicine and your medicine be your food.
Hippocrates

In this chapter, I explain the eight dietary factors to help you cut your risk of suffering from prostate cancer.

Let me begin by stating the potential for cancer prevention, which is presented by the major international report *Food, Nutrition and the Prevention of Cancer: a Global Perspective*, published in 1997.[1] The report reviewed more than 4,500 research studies and involved more than 120 contributors and peer-reviewers, including from the WHO, the FAO and the US National Cancer Institute.

The Potential of Prevention
- Eating right, plus staying physically active and maintaining a healthy weight, can cut cancer risk by 30 to 40 per cent.
- Recommended dietary choices coupled with not smoking have the potential to reduce cancer risk by 60 to 70 per cent.
- As many as 375,000 cases of cancer, at current cancer rates, could be prevented each year in the USA through healthy dietary choices.
- A simple change, such as eating the recommended five servings of fruit and vegetables each day, could by itself reduce cancer rates by more than 20 per cent.

All this advice agrees closely with that of the American-based Physicians Committee for Responsible Medicine,[2] and with most of the recommendations on diet and lifestyle in this and my previous books,[3] although these are considerably more detailed.

The evidence that a diet that includes lots of fruit and vegetables is preventive against cancer continues to increase. One review of more than 250 studies found that the data overwhelmingly supported an inverse association between consumption of fruit and vegetables and cancer risk, with associations more consistently observed for vegetables than for fruit.[4]

Considerable research in this field is currently focused on identifying biomarkers, such as the extent of DNA damage, rather than overt cancer, to allow smaller, less expensive trials of shorter duration to be carried out. An example of a useful biomarker for diet is the finding that a person's fruit and vegetable intake can be determined reliably by measuring the level of carotenoids in their blood.[5] Carotenoids are natural fat-soluble pigments found mainly in plants, algae, yeasts, moulds and some bacteria. They are antioxidants, helping protect organisms against damage by light, oxygen and free radicals generally. They are responsible for many of the red, orange and yellow hues of fruit and vegetables such as carrots. Recent findings include the observation that lycopene (*see* p. 153), which is a carotenoid, significantly reduces the extent of a type of diffuse, high-grade prostate cancer.[6]

Even the Beef USA factsheet,[7] aimed at promoting beef and dairy as sources of conjugated linoleic acid (CLA) as anti-carcinogens, states, 'Of the vast number of naturally occurring substances demonstrated to have anti-carcinogenic activity, all but a very few are of plant origin.'[8] Another source states that CLA is the *only* known antioxidant/anti-carcinogen primarily associated with animal foods.[9]

The numerous components in vegetables and fruit thought to contribute to the reduced risk of cancer include dietary fibre, vitamins, minerals and various phytochemicals (or plant chemicals) – which include antioxidants.

Table 5.1 shows the relationship between phytochemicals in foods and their suggested modes of action.

In the case of prostate cancer, it has been known for the last 20 years that the disease has a significant dietary basis. Indeed, there may be additional protection against cancer from *specific* diets. The China study[10] showed a reduction in risk in those consuming oriental diets, using data from impeccable sources. Moreover, it has been known for some time that people from the Mediterranean region are much less likely to develop prostate cancer than other Europeans. One reason for this may be that their diets are rich in cooked tomato products.[11] Another reason may be their use of olive oil in place of butter. Also, in Chapter 3 we showed the clear relationship between a high ratio of vegetable to animal protein in the diet and low risk of prostate cancer.

All of this evidence supports the case for a change to a predominantly plant-based diet to prevent and treat prostate cancer and breast cancer.

According to some conventional medicine, the evidence currently available suggests that prostate cancer could be prevented

Table 5.1: Food sources of phytochemicals and proposed mechanisms of action

Phytochemical	Food	Proposed mechanism(s) of action
Allicin Diallyl sulphide S-allyl-L-cysteine	Garlic Onions	Inhibits enzymes that activate cancer-causing chemicals (carcinogens) Stimulates enzymes that detoxify carcinogens
Catechins	Tea (green)	Antioxidant
Ellagic acid	Grapes Strawberries	Antioxidant
Flavonoids: *Citrus* – Diosmin and Hesperidin	Grapefruit juice Orange juice	Decreases levels of biochemicals that influence cell growth and proliferation
Noncitrus – Genistein and Daidzein (phyto-oestrogens)	Apples Grapes (red) Soya	Antioxidant Blocks oestrogen and androgen hormones from binding to their receptors (retarding cell proliferation)
Indoles	Cabbage Turnips	Increases conversion of oestrogens to inactive forms Stimulates enzymes that increase carcinogen detoxification

Table 5.1: *Continued*

Phytochemical	Food	Proposed mechanism(s) of action
Isothiocyanates	Cruciferous vegetables	Inhibits enzymes that activate carcinogens Stimulates enzymes that detoxify carcinogens
Lignans	Flaxseed and grains	Prevents oestrogen and prostaglandin hormones from binding to their receptors (retarding cell proliferation)
Lutein and Zeaxanthin	Kale Okra Romaine lettuce Spinach	Antioxidant
Lycopene	Tomatoes Watermelon	Antioxidant
Monoterpenes: Limonene	Lemon peel Orange peel	Decreases cell proliferation by decreasing activity of ornithine decarboxylase (ODC), an enzyme that helps trigger cancer Decreases activity of growth-promoting proteins Prevents expression of oncogenes Stimulates enzymes that detoxify carcinogens

Phenols	Berries Grapes Mustard Tea Turmeric Sesame seeds	Antioxidant Inhibits formation of carcinogens such as nitrosamines Stimulates enzymes that detoxify carcinogens
Phytate	Grains Nuts Seeds Soya beans	Inhibits cell proliferation and the spread of cancer cells (metastasis)
Polyphenols	Artichokes	Antioxidant Stimulates enzymes that detoxify carcinogens
Protease inhibitors	Dried beans Lentils Soya beans	Antioxidant Inhibits transformation of normal cells into cancerous ones Inhibits expression of certain genes and cellular processes that promote cancer
Sulphoraphane	Broccoli	Stimulates enzymes that detoxify carcinogens

Adapted from the MD Anderson Practice Guidelines on Nutrition and Cancer Risk Reduction http://www.mdanderson.org/departments/nutrition/display.cfm/id51175998-98b2-11d5-81330050b603a14&methoddisplayfull&pn

by simple healthy dietary measures. It is also maintained, however, that once cancer has developed there is little evidence to suggest that changing diet will treat the cancer or prolong survival, and that to do so in such circumstances can be detrimental.[12] I disagree with this advice, based on the correspondence I continue to receive from prostate-cancer sufferers. It also shows a failure to understand that removing the factors that favour the promotion and proliferation stages of cancer cells will help treatment. Nevertheless, the diet is meant to complement, not replace, conventional medical treatment.

BACKGROUND TO THE DIET

The eight food factors that follow from page 142 are based on the principles of the Chinese diet. The cookbook, *The Plant Programme*, is designed to accompany the food factors, with recipes adapted to suit Western tastes. All the recipes contain high levels of foods known to be protective against prostate cancer or breast cancer and to contain no foods known to promote these diseases. The recipes are delicious – and are also practical and easy to make for busy people.

Before discussing the eight food factors further, I want to tell you a little more about the Chinese diet. This has evolved over thousands of years of observation and practical experience and has been thoroughly documented and referenced.[13] It is not a new fad diet based on the latest single-issue biochemical theory, but has evolved over more than 5,000 years as a sustainable system of nutrition and agriculture by one of the most biologically successful people on Earth.

In Japan, where the traditional diet is similar to that of China, a healthy diet is believed to be based on eating at least thirty different ingredients a day. Compare this with the diet of the average American, for whom 40 per cent of all that they consume is from dairy.

THE CHINESE WAY

In some parts of China less than 3 per cent of the population under 65 years of age die from any form of cancer, and prostate and breast cancer are almost unknown. Stomach cancer is more prevalent in China, but it is attributed by most experts to unhygienic methods of storing and preserving food, so that it becomes contaminated with micro-organisms that generate carcinogens. The prevalence of the disease is declining as more people use refrigerators.

The Chinese diet has been handed down from generation to generation, using the pictogram system of writing, which was developed early in their history. Chinese writing has evolved progressively into the sophisticated system in use today (an educated person in China is expected to know at least 10,000 different pictograms) and, like the diet that is recommended here, continues to evolve.

Legend in China describes how Emperor Shen Nung, known as 'the divine farmer' and revered as the founder of Chinese agriculture, set out in 3494 BC to discover the healing properties of plants. Each day he would taste various plants to determine their properties – poisoning himself several times in the process, so that he also had to find many antidotes. This story of Emperor Shen Nung may well be a metaphor for the trial-and-error method of the discovery of the properties of plants, but there is little doubt that Chinese agriculture and medicine are derived from knowledge accumulated over the last three to five thousand years. It is worth recalling that China had reached a considerable level of sophistication while the British Isles were still emerging from the Stone Age.

To those used to modern Western science and medicine, some concepts basic to the Chinese approach to diet, such as balancing yin and yang foods, sound like mumbo-jumbo, but in reality it is a memorable way of capturing well-documented concepts! Let me give an example from my own subject, Earth sciences, to illustrate why I strongly believe that observation, which is the basis on which the Chinese diet has developed, is sound.

In Japan, people used to believe that their islands were situated on the back of a large turtle. When the turtle became angry, it shook itself, causing massive shock waves, which destroyed buildings and communications. We now know that there is no angry turtle, but that the Japanese Islands occur in a particularly unstable geological setting on the so-called 'ring of fire', which encircles the Pacific Ocean and is marked by volcanoes and earthquakes caused by deep geological forces. Despite the explanation of the angry turtle being seen now as just a quaint superstition, it was a metaphor which allowed the Japanese to develop an excellent and practical response to the earthquakes that frequently shattered their towns and villages. They lived in small houses of one or two stories, built of light wood with thin rice-paper walls and paper lampshades, and they slept in roll-up beds called futons that were easy to carry around. This minimalist lifestyle was far better protection to human life than the highly engineered structures developed today, even when we know so very much more about the Earth and earthquakes and earth-quake engineering. Just think of the terrible loss of life and destruction of property caused by the 1995 Kobe earthquake.

The Chinese diet and Chinese medicine should be viewed in a similar light. The basis may sound strange to modern scientists, but the observations provide excellent responses to nutritional and environmental problems.

Of course, it is not just Asian traditions that have messages for today's generation. Let us take just two examples of how folklore and customs have grown up and become part of a culture that works to protect people from environmental problems in Britain. In some parts of Scotland there are granites which are naturally radioactive, and consequently emit small amounts of the radioac-tive gas radon. Radon is colourless and odourless, but if people are exposed to it for long periods of time, then the incidence of a type of lung cancer increases. When I worked in northeast Scotland in the 1970s I noticed that local people are always keen to be in very well-ventilated rooms, ideally sleeping with the windows open, even on the coldest of nights. Good ventilation is, of course, the best defence against dangerous accumulations of radon gas.

Also while working in Scotland early in my career, I noticed that many locals would run the water for a long time before filling the kettle – especially in the morning. This is a custom that forms a very good defence against dissolved lead, leached from the plumbing systems in old houses by the naturally acid water there.

In each case, people were unable to give a scientific explana-tion for their behaviour. When questioned about the water, for example, they would say that 'it would have turned stale overnight'. Despite not understanding the real scientific basis of problems that could cause ill health, these communities had nevertheless developed protective behaviour that was passed down through the generations. It is this kind of well-tried, observation-based depth of tradition, particularly from China and other parts of Asia, that forms the principles of the food factors described here.

FOOD FACTOR 1: FROM DAIRY TO SOYA

Soya consumption has been shown to be inversely related to prostate-cancer risk.[14] As discussed below, it contains a wealth of anti-cancer agents and helps to prevent the spread of cancer generally. Phyto-oestrogens in soya are particularly helpful in all cases of hormone-dependent cancers, such as prostate cancer, by blocking receptor sites for hormones and growth factors in the cell or on the cell surface. One report stated that consuming two glasses of soya milk per day cut the risk of prostate cancer by 40 per cent.

Prostate cancer is hormonally driven, and, as discussed earlier, dairy influences natural hormone levels adversely.[15] One of the first and most essential things you can do to reduce your risk of prostate cancer is to substitute soya products for **ALL** dairy products (whether from cows, sheep, goats or any other animals) in your diet.

By doing this you will immediately and dramatically reduce your body's exposure to a powerful cocktail of hormones and growth factors increasingly shown in scientific paper after scientific paper (*see* Chapters 2 and 4) to promote prostate cancer. You will also be reducing your exposure to antibiotic residues and other powerful biologically active chemicals (including man-made endocrine-disrupting chemicals, which can become particularly concentrated in milk – *see* Chapter 6). You will reduce your cholesterol and triglyceride intake, with great benefits for your heart and circulatory system, thereby reducing the possibility of developing thrombosis, to which patients undergoing surgery, chemotherapy and some other cancer treatments are especially susceptible.[16] Soya lecithin also provides substances called choline and insitol, which help to improve liver function and are particularly important during chemotherapy. Soya also contains co-enzyme Q10.

Recent dietary studies into the effects of exchanging soya for animal products indicate a reduction in cholesterol levels of more than 20 per cent. Moreover, it is the levels of the 'bad' cholesterol – low-density lipo-proteins or LDLs – which are reduced. However, simply adding soya to a typical Western diet is unlikely to be sufficient to counteract high plasma cholesterol.[17] You must replace – not supplement – dairy with soya produce to achieve the benefits.

Replace milk with soya milk and cheese with tofu and use soya ice cream (or water ices or sorbets) instead of dairy ice cream. There are no half measures. As discussed previously, using skimmed milk or low-fat yoghurt is irrelevant and will not help to reduce your risk of cancer or your recovery from the disease, because some of the most likely cancer-causing agents are proteins or sugars, not fats.

Remember that soya contains plant oestrogens which protect the prostate and that one of the plant oestrogens – genistein – seems to prevent cancer through multiple mechanisms: not only is it phyto-oestrogenic, it is anti-angiogenic too, meaning that it actually prevents tumours from developing their own blood supply.[18] It is also a powerful antioxidant, increasing the activities of protective antioxidative enzymes in various organs with an important role in the removal of free radicals, which have been particularly implicated in cancer. Also, soya isoflavones have been shown in animal and other laboratory substances to inhibit the growth of cancer cells by inhibiting their DNA replication, interfering with their signalling pathways, reducing the activity of various enzymes that they need to grow and inhibiting the actions of a range of growth factors and chemicals called cytokines that cancer cells need in order to develop.[19] The vast majority of experimental studies into soya and cancer have shown that soya products prevent the growth of a range of cancer cells.[20]

There is only one problem with buying soya now: it has often been genetically modified. One of the reasons this has been done is so that it can withstand being treated with herbicides to destroy insects and weeds. So read labels carefully and buy only organically grown soya.

The soya bean is one of the most nutritious vegetables known. It is said that the soya bean was a gift to all generations of mankind from the sages and wise rulers of China. The first commercial use for the soya bean in the West, however, was as a source of oil for the manufacture of soap. This pattern of usage, so different from that in Asia, is at last beginning to change as more and more people appreciate the extraordinary health-giving properties of soya.

The soya bean is an environmentally friendly crop, too. One acre of land cultivated by conventional Western agricultural practices will feed an average adult for 77 days if it is used to raise beef. This may seem impressive, until you learn that the same acre can feed an adult for 527 days when it is devoted to growing wheat. However, if soya beans are grown on the same land, then it will yield enough protein to feed a person for over six years! The protein content of the bean when harvested is about 40 per cent, which rises to 50 per cent after it has been processed. Soya also contains a full range of proteins, whereas other plant foods contain only some. Hence many vegans depend on combining cereals and pulses to obtain the full range of the twenty amino acids necessary for good nutrition. The delicious traditional

Jamaican dish of rice and peas, which I ate a lot of when I worked there, is a good example.

Most of us are now familiar with soya milk, which can be purchased from all supermarkets. However, there are many other traditional soya products which you can enjoy.

Tofu, or bean curd, is made from soya beans. It has a higher percentage of protein than any other natural food, is very low in saturated fats, is entirely cholesterol free, and is inexpensive. It has been a staple food for millions of people in Asia for over four thousand years. Tofu is good for everyone, because it is so full of good nutrients, so low in bad nutrients and is easily digested. Puréed carrots and leeks with tofu can be used as a nutritious, easily digested food for babies and invalids.[21] Also, it can be cooked quickly in simple stir-fries or simmered in soup. It is made by precipitating soya milk, normally using calcium or magnesium sulphates so it is also high in some of the most bioavailable forms of calcium or magnesium. In their classical treatise on the subject, William Shurtleff and Akiko Aoyagi explain its revered status in the East. They point out that when Japanese connoisseurs speak of tofu they use many of the same terms we employ when evaluating wines. And when the new crop of soya beans arrives at tofu shops, ardent devotees sample the first tofu with similar relish to that of French vintners.[22]

Commercially, tofu is available in either 'silken' form (suitable for making low-fat, high-protein dressings and sauces) or firm, which can be used in an infinite number of ways: scrambled, marinated, smoked, barbecued, crumbled into salads, in burgers, sandwiches and soups, or even used in a dessert. Tofu may not taste good on its own but it is very good at absorbing almost any flavour or colour.[23] Tofu is ideal as a replacement for dairy cream or milk in many potato dishes. It can also be liquidised with a wide range of fresh juice and with honey to make delicious sweets and puddings.

Tempeh (pronounced 'tem-pay') is a fermented soya-bean product, made in the traditional manner for centuries throughout Indonesia. You can buy it in health-food shops and an increasing number of supermarkets. It is highly digestible, smells like fresh mushrooms and tastes remarkably similar to chicken or veal cutlets. Since the protein in tempeh is partially broken down by fermentation it is very digestible and particularly suitable for young children and the elderly. The easiest way to serve it is as wedge-shaped slices, pan fried until crisp and golden brown on both sides, with rice and a selection of vegetables.

Natto can generally be found in Chinese or Japanese grocery stores, though it is less readily available than tempeh. Like tempeh, it is made by fermenting soya beans, but in this case for less than 24 hours. The fermentation process makes the high-quality protein of the soya beans particularly easy to digest.

Miso, which is a fermented mixture of soya beans and other cereals, has a paste-like texture and is an important component of oriental macrobiotic diets. It has subtle, aromatic flavours and ranges in colour from brown to pale yellow. It is one of the staples of every Japanese and Chinese kitchen and is made by inoculating the basic ingredients with a mould before aging the mixture in cedarwood kegs for at least one year. It is commonly used as an ingredient in soups, sauces, dressings, spreads, casseroles and other vegetable dishes. In Japan, miso is used as a medicine in the same way that Jewish people use chicken soup; miso is much healthier, though. On no account should miso be boiled or cooked at high temperatures, because this will destroy its beneficial, health-giving substances. Unfortunately, synthetic misos, with various colourings and additives, have become widely available. Avoid such products and buy only traditional miso which contains many different beneficial enzymes and bacteria. Also buy only reputable brands because fermentation in un-hygienic conditions can lead to high concentrations of the micro-organisms thought to be responsible for stomach cancer. Also I buy miso only in waxed cartons, never in plastic (*see* p. 200).

Soy Sauce is an ancient and traditional Japanese seasoning which is now accepted the world over. It is a dark, rich sauce with a savoury, salty taste. Very little is required within a dish or serving. There are three types:

The first is the widely available commercial type, made by speeding up the fermentation process using chemical additives. It usually contains colourings and preservatives as well. I do not recommend this.

The second is called shoyu and is made by fermenting wheat and soya beans together for at least three years. It makes a delicious addition to most savoury meals.

The third is tamari, which is made by fermenting soya beans and salt for two to three years. It is less widely available than shoyu and has a very strong flavour.

Both shoyu and tamari contain enzymes similar to those found in our saliva, which help in digesting proteins and starches.

*   *   *

Many of these products are widely available, not only in specialist health-food and oriental shops but also, increasingly, in super-markets, so there is no difficulty in buying them. Since there are so many different types and flavours, it is worth experimenting until you find the flavours you enjoy most. Your brain will adapt to the change in taste and you will soon find you do not want to go back to dairy produce.

So what about yoghurt and all those healthy lactobacillus acidophilus bacteria it contains, which are so good for us? There is evidence that taking these bacteria increases immunity, prevents infections and increases vitamin production. Don't worry: it is easy to buy capsules of the bacteria, break them open, and sprinkle the contents on soya milk or other cold drinks. Hence you have the health benefits of the bacteria without the risk that consuming dairy products carries. Moreover, following the Plant Programme will favour the growth and survival of these helpful bacteria in the digestive tract.

If you do only one thing to cut your risk of prostate cancer, make the change from dairy to soya products. Remember that soya products reduce prostate-cancer risk, while milk and the growth factors and hormones it contains have been shown in experiment after experiment to promote the growth of prostate (and breast) cancer cells.

There is one concern about eating food full of phyto-oestrogen that some men have expressed to me: that is that eating the phyto-oestrogens in soya will feminise them. Despite exhaustive studies, there is no evidence of this.[24] Moreover a lack of male potency and reproductive capacity does not appear to have been a problem in China or other oriental countries over the many centuries they have used soya. Rather the reverse.

Since the publication of the first edition of *Your Life in Your Hands* in 2000, there have been many attacks on soya (frequently on untraceable and unattributable websites), many suggesting that soya causes cancer. There have also been recommendations from a few physicians, who really should know better, that people who have had prostate or breast cancer should not have soya. Many of the questions put to me express concern about this issue.

The anti-soya argument centres on the fact that soya contains phyto-oestrogens – but the fact is that most vegetables naturally contain phyto-oestrogens or substances that are converted to phyto-oestrogens in the gut. Such foods include berries such as strawberries, cranberries and bilberries, whole-grain cereals, seeds and spices, peanuts, cabbage, hops, tea and, of course, peas and beans (the legume family, to which soya belongs).[25] In general, phyto-oestrogens are found in the seeds, stems, roots or flowers of plants, serving as natural fungicides and acting as part of the plant's defence mechanism against micro-organisms.[26] Phyto-oestrogens are chemically and structurally similar to the mammalian oestrogen, oestradiol, and have oestrogenic properties. However, their oestrogenic activity is generally much less than that of human oestrogens (their oestrogenic activity ranges from 1/500 to 1/1000 of that of oestrodiol), and they have been found to be protective against prostate cancer.[27] All the experiments on soya-bean phyto-oestrogens (isoflavones such as genistein) continue to indicate that such chemicals help prevent the growth of prostate and other cancers by a variety of mechanisms.[28]

Of course, the dairy industry have tried to fight back, and as their propaganda about the need for dairy calcium to prevent osteoporosis increasingly founders,[29] they have latched on to the presence of substances called CLAs (*see* p. 136) in dairy products and the meat of ruminant animals such as cows and sheep, which they claim to be preventive against cancer. Interestingly, the amount of CLA in milk is boosted by adding extracted whole soya bean and linseed oils to a corn-alfalfa diet.[30] As queried in an article in the *Sunday Times*,[31] how much artery-clogging saturated fat would we have to consume to have enough CLAs to be protected against cancer?

CLAs are natural derivatives of the essential fatty acid, linoleic acid, which is found in vegetable seeds and oils produced from them, such as soya. Despite the extent to which CLA is promoted as a product of microbial metabolism in the digestive tract of ruminants, especially cows,[32] it is also found in other mammals and some birds.[33] It would be interesting to see research into CLA production in the intestine of people consuming diets high in foods such as soya, linseed, corn and alfalfa compared with that in people on a predominantly animal diet.

At this point I would like to re-emphasise that simply adding soya to a typical dairy-rich Western diet will *not* decrease prostate-cancer risk. It is absolutely essential to eliminate ALL animal dairy produce, including 'hidden dairy' such as casein whey and lactose. Other vegetable milks, creams and yoghurts, besides soya, are all OK, including coconut, rice, oat and pea milks, but I recommend only organically produced GM-free products.

I also emphasise that I am not advocating that people live on an entirely soya-based diet, and I continue to recommend the Japanese principle, on which *The Plant Programme* cookbook is based, of eating at least thirty different food substances every day. I also agree with the advice of the American Cancer Society that eating a balanced diet should include five or more servings a day of fruit and vegetables (though I think it should be much more – *see* Food Factor 2), along with foods from a variety of other plant sources, such as cereals, legumes, seeds and nuts; this is more effective than consuming one particular food in large amounts.[34]

MAKING THE BREAK FROM DAIRY	
If You Used To Do This . . .	*Now Do This!*
Take cows' milk in your tea or coffee	Use soya milk in tea, straight from the carton, or drink green tea with a slice of fresh lemon or lime. In coffee, heat the soya milk first to avoid curdling. Avoid dry 'creamers' or 'whiteners', which can contain synthetic chemicals or hidden dairy.
Put cows' milk on your breakfast cereal	Use soya, rice, oat or coconut milk, or pour fresh fruit juice over your cereal instead (I always do this at hotels).
Tuck into a bowl of ice cream	Enjoy high-quality sorbets or water ices. Or try one of the growing range of soya ice creams now available.
Douse your desserts in cream or custard	Most supermarkets sell small cartons of soya cream.

	One of the oldest brands of custard powder is dairy free! Simply prepare it using soya milk instead of dairy.
Drink glasses of milk or milkshakes	There is now a wide range of naturally sweetened fruit soya, rice, oat or coconut milks. Or make your own! See the recipes in *The Plant Programme*.
Use dollops of butter in cooking or served onto bread or vegetables	Use organic, first cold-pressed extra-virgin olive oil in cooking. Try herb-flavoured olive oil drizzled over toast or baked potatoes and lift your sandwiches with a spread such as tahini (sesame-seed paste) or houmous to replace butter and enhance your nutrient intake.
Eat masses of hard, soft or cottage cheeses	Several brands of dairy-free hard 'cheeses' are currently available in health-food shops, which can be used in cookery as well as simply grated or sliced. Double-check the labels to ensure the product is free from casein, lactose and other 'hidden' dairy ingredients. There are many soft soya 'cheeses' – available as tofu dips, spreads or patés. My favourite option is houmous! I know it's not soya, but it has similar benefits.

Dive into a daily dose of yoghurt	Soya yoghurt is widely available in plain and fruit flavours.
Eat dairy (made from cow) meat products such as burgers, sausages, luncheon meats, patés and pastes	A huge range of products are now available to replace meat. Look in the dry-mix, freezer, tinned or chilled-food sections of your health-food shop or supermarket. Although some of the products are based on nuts, most are based on soya.
Cook with dairy products	Soya milk or cream readily substitutes for dairy milk in recipes as varied as Béchamel sauce and creamed soups to rice pudding and quiche. Most recipes calling for butter succeed as well with olive oil or soya spread. The meat replacements mentioned above work well in traditional recipes, as do the cheese substitutes.

FOOD FACTOR 2: VITAL VEGETABLES AND FREQUENT FRUIT

The US National Cancer Institute is launching a publicity campaign to boost men's fruit and vegetable consumption from the the 'bare minimum' of five servings a day to nine servings a day. Only 4 per cent of men in the US consume nine servings. More than a third of the population eat only one or two servings, and 4 per cent eat less than that.[35] The official recommendation of five portions a day, especially when each portion can comprise a glass of (commercial) fruit juice and a tablespoon of dried fruit,[36] was always completely inadequate.

Based on this new information and many other findings described below, the second food factor is to increase the amount of vegetables and fruit you consume, noting that vegetables are even more important than fruit. The evidence that an abundant intake of vegetables and fruit can play an important role in reducing cancer incidence is becoming overwhelming.[37]

The list of anti-cancer chemicals identified in vegetables and fruit just keeps on growing (Table 5.1). The investigation of plant chemicals pioneered by Lee Wattenberg of the University of Minnesota in the USA has identified many agents that protect against cancer in laboratory studies.[38]

In addition to the phyto-oestrogens discussed above, plant-derived foods contain thousands of other phytochemicals, many of which have been investigated in laboratory and clinical studies to determine their effects on cancer risk and their mechanisms of action.[39] The Division of Cancer Prevention of the US National Cancer Institute is currently sponsoring more than 65 chemo-prevention trials, many of them concerned with food substances in relation to particular cancers. They include, for example, three trials of lycopene in preventing prostate cancer.[40]

In general, the outcomes of such studies highlight the difficulty of identifying single dietary components, such as beta-carotene, as preventative (*see* further discussion in Chapter 6, Lifestyle Factor 1).[41] This may be because substances such as beta-carotene are simply biomarkers for other protective components of vegetables and fruit, or because they may not react in the same way when separated from the chemicals with which they are associated in natural food substances.

I have always wondered why I have never seen or heard of a plant with cancer despite all the poisonous chemicals we pour on them, so perhaps in the same way that mankind discovered that some substances such as honey contain natural antibiotics because they do not readily 'go rotten', we should have realised long ago that plants contain anti-cancer agents.

Eat as many vegetables, including salad vegetables, as possible, and make sure they are fresh and ripe. Most vegetables and fruit include such vitamins as beta-carotene (which is the precursor of vitamin A and is especially rich in yellow and orange vegetables such as carrots, saffron, red and yellow peppers, pumpkins and sweet potatoes, and fruit such as peaches, cherries and apricots (including the dried variety). Beta-carotene has long been suggested to be protective against several forms of cancer, including by acting as an antioxidant. Other vegetables and fruit contain other carotenoids such as lycopene, vitamin C (most fresh or very lightly cooked vegetables and fruit) and vitamin E (most fresh fruit and vegetables), which stop our tissues being damaged by free radicals. Garlic and Brussels sprouts are also especially rich in antioxidants.

Lycopene is the much-talked-about antioxidant where prostate cancer is concerned. It actually binds to fats and lipids in the bloodstream, protecting against some of the worst aspects of Western diets. One study stated that seven to ten helpings of tomatoes per week reduced risks by 40 per cent; another suggested that 40 per cent of prostate-cancer sufferers eating these quantities showed relief of symptoms.[42]

Research suggests that lycopene is a more potent inhibitor of human cancer-cell proliferation than beta-carotene.[43] In addition to its powerful antioxidant properties, it suppressed IGF-I-stimulated growth of (breast) cancer cells. More recently, associations of lower bioactive IGFs with increased consumption of tomatoes and products containing tomatoes[44] have supported the results of earlier findings reported for Greek men.[45] The findings of the protective effect of tomato intake on prostate cancer have been reported in several investigations.[46] Interestingly, a small trial of lycopene-only supplementation found no difference in IGF-I levels between those taking the tablets and the controls – whereas in the case of the trials of beta-carotene pills rather than carrots, which had been shown to be protective, the pure chemical actually made matters worse.

Other good sources of natural lycopene include tomatoes (especially when cooked or sundried), strawberries, red grapes, peaches, pink grapefruit, red and yellow peppers and carrots. One large helping of freshly made tomato soup contains masses of lycopene (see the easy-to-follow recipe in The Plant Programme). I recommend against tinned or packaged tomato soups, since they frequently contain cream, whey or other dairy products and many tin cans are lined with a substance that can leach BPA, an endocrine-disrupting chemical (see p. 220). If you eat tinned baked beans, be very careful to read the label, because even some brands that claim to be in tomato sauce might be more accurately described as being in a milk or cream sauce.

Fresh red peppers, as well as being rich in lycopene, are a particularly good source of vitamin C, which strengthens the immune system and neutralises toxins. Other especially good sources of Vitamin C include papaya, berries, cherries and all citrus fruits. Salad vegetables, especially watercress, and raw or lightly cooked broccoli, are also good sources.

Plants, especially green leafy vegetables, avocados, beans, carrots, pumpkins, apricots, melons and newly sprouted shoots such as bean sprouts and alfalfa, are all good sources of folic acid, which is involved in making the copies of the chromosomes carrying the gene sequences when cells divide. This is the very point at which mistakes which could cause cancer are likely to happen. An adequate intake of folic acid is essential to protect your DNA during radiotherapy or chemotherapy. A great deal of evidence suggests that most Americans' diets are deficient in folic acid.[47] Deterioration in the elderly has also been attributed to folate deficiency.[48] Indeed, throughout the West, women wishing to become pregnant are advised to take folic-acid pills to avoid birth defects such as spina bifida in their babies.

Surely we should *all* be eating a diet that has adequate quantities of folic acid without having to resort to taking pills. As discussed previously, some of the chemotherapeutic drugs used to disrupt breast-cancer cells replace folic acid in cell division. I believe that it was drinking fresh juices high in folic acid as soon as I was able to after chemotherapy that helped me to recover so quickly and saved my hair from falling out. I drank about half a pint of green Bramley apple with fennel juice, about 50:50 apple-fennel, and about half a pint of carrot juice each and every day. I also ate lots of melon which is especially rich in folic acid. People who were treated with me who took folic-acid pills still lost their hair, but most of the people I persuaded to use juices kept theirs (though this does not work with some of the new chemotherapeutic agents with a different mode of action).

I have mentioned plant oestrogens in the context of soya several times in the book because of their protective effect against prostate cancer. Plant oestrogens are found in almost all fruit and vegetables and cereals. Vegetables such as soya, lentils, peas and beans, all legumes capable of fixing nitrogen from the air to make proteins, are rich sources of isoflavones. Typically oriental, Mediterranean and Latin American diets include large quantities of legumes and it has been calculated that a typical Western diet provides only about 3mg of isoflavones a day compared to the 30–100mg a day in oriental diets.

Red clover has particularly high levels of phyto-oestrogens called coumestans and, like chick peas (the basis of the Greek food houmous) and lentils, it contains all of the four important dietary isoflavones. Sunflower seeds and alfalfa sprouts also contain substantial quantities of phyto-oestrogen compounds.

Other rich sources of protective phytohormones include wild yam or sweet potato, and fennel, which contain both phyto-oestrogens and phytoprogesterones. Flaxseed has a high content of lignans, which are converted in the digestive tract into substances that help to regulate endocrine function. Much research on flax has been carried out by the FDA, the National Cancer Institute and the Canadian Food Protection Branch.[49] The recommendation is to take about one tablespoon a day of flaxseed in your diet for each 100 pounds of body weight (but be prepared to go to the loo more often!).

As well as being a good source of phyto-oestrogens, seeds can be good sources of minerals such as zinc, selenium and vitamin E. Sunflower and sesame seeds can be particularly good sources of zinc, which helps vitamin C work and accelerates healing.

After iron, zinc is the next most important trace nutrient needed by our bodies,[50] and it is an active participant in maximising the effect of several other antioxidants.[51] It is involved in more than 200 enzymes in the human body and is essential for healing, so it is important you have adequate zinc to help recover from surgery, radiotherapy and chemotherapy. Its value has long been understood by ancient civilisations. When American doctors thought that they had made a major breakthrough in identifying zinc as a crucial factor affecting recovery from injuries during the Vietnam war, it was pointed out that the remedy had been known to the Ancient Egyptians, as recorded in the Pyramids.

In men, its highest concentration in the body is in the prostate gland, suggesting zinc is particularly important for its proper functioning. Zinc is also involved in cell division, and in the way IGF-I is controlled. Researchers at the University of Illinois, USA have shown that a complex interactive set of factors are required to ensure IGF-I activity occurs only when conditions are right for cell growth, and they describe a discrete role for trace nutrients – especially zinc – in regulating IGF-I activity.[52] They have suggested that one of zinc's functions is to help to inactivate IGF-I. Good sources of zinc include crabs, snails and oysters (especially Atlantic oysters), as well as sesame seeds (best as tahini – a delicious spread made from sesame seed), pumpkin seeds, sunflower seeds or wheat germ. Brewer's yeast is a particularly good source of many trace elements including selenium, chromium and zinc and B vitamins which are essential for the skin and nervous tissue.

New research also indicates that selenium may play a crucial role in prostate health. In one trial, men consuming higher concentrations of selenium, 150mcg/day, had three times less risk of prostate problems than men taking 86mcg/day. One estimate suggests that the average intake of men in the UK is less than half that. Once again, it is best from natural sources. In addition to seeds and garlic, good sources include wholemeal bread, organic eggs, onions, broccoli and tomato, but I do not eat brazil nuts as a source of selenium for the reasons given on page 166.

I also eat sprouted seeds including soya, pumpkin and sesame (all rich in zinc), sunflower, alfalfa and lentil. They are all rich in vitamin C and other vitamins and minerals, as well as high-quality proteins. I generally buy mine already sprouted, but if you wish to sprout your own, here's how to do it:

- Buy organic seeds from health-food stores or supermarkets. Use only the clean, whole ones and discard the rest. NEVER buy seeds from agricultural merchants, because they may have been treated with chemicals which can be fatal if consumed.
- Use a jar large enough to hold at least half a litre of water, with a piece of cheesecloth or muslin held in place around the top with a rubber band.
- For every 100ml of water, use two to three tablespoons of seeds. First, soak them overnight in four times their own volume of (ideally filtered) water, until they have doubled in size. Then pour off the water.
- Keep the sprout container in darkness, and rinse the seeds two or three times a day. Make sure you drain them thoroughly by turning the container upside down, or they will rot.
- Throw away any seeds that have not sprouted after two days. The rest will be ready to eat after four or five days. On the last day they can be put into the light, but only for a few hours or they will become bitter.
- Most sprouts need a final rinse before being drained and stored in the fridge in a covered container. Some varieties have loose husks which need to be removed. Place such sprouts in a large bowl of water and agitate until the husks float to the top, then skim them off.

Vegetables and fruit also contain compounds, or their precursor chemicals, which have no known nutritional value but which have anti-cancer properties (*see* Table 5.1). They include indoles, isothiocyanates, dithiolthiones and organosulphur components (some of which are thought to be natural pesticides). About twenty years ago epidemiological studies showed that consumption of cruciferous vegetables, including bok choy, broccoli, Brussels sprouts, cauliflower, cabbage and kale, which contain dithiolthiones, was associated with a decreased risk of developing cancer. A synthetic dithiolthione called oltipraz has been shown to inhibit the development of tumours in laboratory animals. Like other beneficial plant chemicals, it interferes with cancer development in several ways, including by activating the liver enzymes that remove cancer-causing agents from the bloodstream.[53] Sulphoraphane, an isothiocyanate which is also found in cruciferous vegetables and is responsible for their sharp taste, is also thought to prevent cancer by activating detoxifying enzymes in the liver. In rats it blocks the formation of chemically induced cancers. Recently, research at Robert Gordon University in Aberdeen suggests that only raw broccoli offers any protective effect against colon cancer as measured by the amount of DNA damage in colon cells from laboratory pigs.[54] It is suggested that cooking destroys glucosinolates, which are the precursors of isothiocyanates produced in the colon, which are the substances protective against cancer. The degree of cooking of the broccoli is not described however. As indicated in the section on cooking it is best to eat vegetables which are as raw as possible (light steaming or stir-frying) although it is important to cook all meat and fish slowly and thoroughly (*see* Lifestyle Factor 3). All the cruciferous vegetables also contain good amounts of fibre, which helps to eliminate toxins and hormones such as testosterone.

Garlic and onions, chives and leeks (the allium family) are important in helping to protect against cancer. They contain chemicals similar to those used in anti-radiation pills (cysteine-like amino acids) and are particularly useful in reducing the effects of diagnostic X-rays and radiotherapy in the body. They contain powerful antioxidants (active against free radicals including those produced by anti-cancer treatments). Allicin, one of garlic's main biologically active components, created when garlic is crushed, has been shown to decrease proliferation of prostate-cancer cells in laboratory studies.[55] In addition to allicin, garlic also contains other powerful antioxidants such as selenium and germanium. Other research into cancer at universities in Pennsylvania and Texas in the USA has identified two other compounds active against cancer in crushed garlic: diallysulphide

and S-allyl cysteine. Current studies at the Memorial Sloan-
Kettering Cancer Center in New York indicate that it is effective
against prostate cancer, especially in the initial phases of the
disease, partly by improving the cell's ability to eliminate
carcinogens and partly by reducing the ability of carcinogenic
chemicals to bind to DNA. Preliminary studies at the same centre
have indicated that garlic also prevents prostate (and breast)
cancer cells from dividing, thereby limiting the growth of
tumours.[56] Garlic is also a natural anti-microbial agent, active
against a wide range of fungi, bacteria and viruses, and it was
used for these purposes in the First World War. You should have
at least two to three raw cloves of fresh garlic a day to prevent
and treat prostate and other types of cancer, and to ward off
infectious illnesses when your immune system is impaired from
cancer treatment. Many people worry about smelling of garlic but
if everyone eats it, no one notices – just as everyone who has
dairy products does not notice that they and others smell of sour
milk (a much more unpleasant smell to me)!

One of the problems if you have active cancer is in consuming
the amount of fresh fruit and vegetables needed to deliver
adequate quantities of anti-cancer chemicals to the sites of the
tumours. The best way to overcome this problem, is to extract
juices from the vegetables and fruits. This way, the active
compounds are separated from the large mass of fibre that you
would otherwise have to chew through and the anti-cancer agents
are made more biologically available to your body. Even if you
do not like certain vegetables, you can hold your nose and simply
drink the juice as if it is a medicine – it is! Naturopaths and some
doctors have been treating patients with fresh juices and raw food
to improve their health since the nineteenth century. The
therapy was pioneered in Germany and Switzerland before being
used by health clinics worldwide. Famous pioneers include
Father Kniepp, Dr Kellogg, Dr Max Bircher-Benner and Dr Max
Gerson. To make the quantities of juices needed you must invest
in a juicer (*not a liquidiser*). There are several available but when
I had cancer I found that the cheaper ones burned out quickly
and I therefore invested in a type normally used in commercial
juice bars – which I still use.

Carrot juice is good but do not drink more than a half-pint
glass a day or you may turn orange (I did – with orange palms
and an orange moustache, which was described grandly by one
of my doctors as carotenosis!). Do not have too much cabbage
juice either. Cabbage contains substances known as goitrogens

which can cause problems with the thyroid gland if taken in too large quantities, especially if it is eaten raw. It increases the requirement for iodine, which is essential for good nutrition (*see* p. 168) and for which the main source in the diet is seafood. The main green juice I drank every day when I was ill with cancer was made from green Bramley apple, celery and fennel, with small amounts of watercress.

If you're thinking of cheating by drinking bottled juices instead of freshly made ones, there is simply no point. If you cut an apple it immediately starts going brown (because it has oxidised) and you need the green unoxidised juice. The same is true for all juices. If you buy commercial juices they will be far more oxidised and chemically far less potent as anti-cancer agents. Also they may contain some type of preservative or have undergone some type of process to stop them going rotten (just think about it, how else could carrot juice be sold weeks after it is prepared?), so they will be chemically changed. The only exceptions are good frozen juices, not made from concentrates. I have discovered people with colon cancer changing the diet I recommend by eating vegetable pills instead of raw vegetables and their juices – a complete waste of time!

In addition to juices, you should have masses of fresh salads and vegetables. I cook vegetables by lightly steaming them (not by boiling) or just wilting them in a little extra-virgin olive oil (essentially cooked for a few minutes without water). This is an especially good method of cooking spinach, which is delicious if a few onions are softened in the extra-virgin olive oil first. I also eat lots of vegetable soups. One of the problems people complain of when they start to eat lots of fruit and vegetables is the number of times they have to go to the loo. Sorry, but that is what is supposed to happen – two to three times a day is normal, not two to three times a week! Also by not suffering from constipation you will reduce your chance of suffering from haemorrhoids (piles) and varicose veins. A good indication that your diet is correct is when your stools float rather than sink. You may also suffer from 'wind' but don't worry, after a few weeks of the diet recommended here the body will adjust and you will have no further problems with flatulence.

Whole foods are a complex package of essential nutrients with many benefits that cannot be found in bottles of pills. Whole foods really are greater than the sum of their parts. For example, natural foods contain enzymes that help break down the components of the food. Hence bananas are rich in carbohydrates and contain amylase, a carbohydrate-splitting enzyme. Natural carrot juice contains all sorts of substances that work with beta-carotene. Foods generally contain hundreds or thousands of substances (many of which have yet to be studied) that may be important for health. It has been suggested that the difference between natural vegetables and commercial juices or pills is similar to that between trees and paper. Be like Chinese people and eat everything when it is as fresh and ripe as possible.

With all this accumulated evidence on the beneficial effects of vegetables and fruit in protecting against cancer and other diseases, why did it take so long for us to be told? (*See* Chapter 7 for further discussion on this point.)

Organic food and pesticides
In the UK, organically grown food has its origins in the work of Sir Albert Howard who published *An Agricultural Testament* in 1940, advocating that Britain preserve the 'cycle of life' and adopt 'permanent agriculture' systems, using urban food waste and sewage to build soil fertility. The first person to apply the term 'organic' to food production was JI Rodale in his 1942 publication *Organic Gardening and Farming*. In 1946 the young Lady Eve Balfour was inspired by Howard to set up the Soil Association, a pioneering organic farming charity that is the major organic certification organisation in the UK today. In 1974 the Soil Association established the UK's first set of Organic Food Standards. These standards form the basis of EU regulation 2092/91, which lays down in detail how food must be produced, processed and packaged to qualify for the description 'organic'. The regulation also specifies detailed criteria for the inspection and certification of food producers and processors. In the USA, organic regulations have been developed on a state-by-state basis – currently there is no national organic legislation.

Sometimes, people who advocate organic food are dismissed as middle-class food fanatics, with no rational or scientific basis for their concerns. I'd like to tell you why this caricature is wrong and why it is so vitally important that you insist on as much high-quality organic food as possible, despite the efforts of organisations such as the Food Standards Agency to persuade us that there is no difference between organic and conventionally produced food.[57]

I believe it is particularly important to limit exposure to harmful chemicals. I also believe the food industry contributes significantly to modern health problems with their widespread use of pesticides, plant and animal hormones and other drugs, and genetically modified crops, some of which are designed to survive being dowsed with herbicides while other plants are killed off. Thus, even eating an apparently healthy diet can lead to an increasing burden of man-made toxins, many of which have not been properly assessed for their toxicity.

The establishment view is that a relatively small percentage of cancers are attributable to pesticides, following epidemiological studies that indicated that not more than 2 per cent of cancers are attributable to the use of pesticides.[58] If this is accurate, it is still a lot of cancers! However, this estimate preceded our knowledge of the endocrine-disrupting behaviour of certain pesticides (many of which are now banned or strictly controlled), so it is likely to be a serious underestimate of cases of, particularly, prostate and other hormone-dependent cancers.

According to Lang and Clutterbuck, animal studies have implicated about 50 pesticides as cancer-causing agents.[59] Many other pesticides are suspected of causing birth or genetic defects; and over 60 pesticides have been implicated in causing various reproductive effects.

A new study on women aged 55 or younger in one of Canada's largest fruit- and vegetable-growing regions, showed that women who have worked on farms are up to 9 times more likely to develop breast cancer than those who have never been employed in agriculture.[60] These findings raise further suspicions that the array of fungicides, herbicides and insecticides used on many farms is a factor in the 'huge increase in the rates of breast cancer' in Canada.

According to McMichael,[61] there has been a thirty-fold increase in global pesticide use and a nine-fold increase in chemical fertiliser use since the 1950s. This has increased food yield, but it has also caused widespread chemical pollution, destruction of wildlife and disturbance of ecosystems. As of the mid-1990s, US agriculture used about 365 million kg of pesticides per year, although even more than that, about 900 million kg of insecticides, were used in non-agricultural applications, including forestry, landscaping, gardening, food distribution and home pest control.

Fortunately, in the UK, more than seventy such products, including some that were in use for growing vegetables, have recently been cleared from garden-centre shelves because they have been banned by the EU – but why did it take so long? After banning DDT in the 1970s, followed by other organochlorines including the drins (aldrin and dieldrin) and many, many other pesticides, it might have been expected that there would have been a speedier reaction to limit our exposure. I am still left with the question: What are we still using today that in the future we shall find evidence to ban?

The alternative to the chemical nightmare of industrialised agriculture is to buy organically produced food, ideally grown to the standards of the UK Soil Association – their symbol is a circle with the words 'SOIL ASSOCIATION' around the top and 'ORGANIC STANDARD' round the bottom, and a sort of curly, triangular design inside the circle. Also, I object to buying so-called organically produced food, produced to no particular standard, which is then expensively flown in to supermarkets from across the world – long-distance air transport causes pollution too.[62] Choosing food that carries symbols such as that of the Soil Association also means you will avoid genetically modified food. If you are unable to obtain good organically produced food at your local supermarket, use a search engine on the Internet to identify local suppliers – who will often deliver to your door. If you cannot afford the additional expense of buying organically produced food for all your needs and cannot grow your own, make food that will not be cooked (such as salad, vegetables and fruit) your spending priority, since at least some of the damaging chemicals in pesticides break down during cooking and processing.[63] *See* further in Chapter 6, Lifestyle Factor 3.

Peel fruit if it is not organically grown, because unfortunately the skin, which is otherwise very nutritious, is often treated with chemicals and then waxed so the chemicals do not wash off. This is often the case with oranges, grapefruit and lemons and some heavily marketed commercial apples. Of course, it does not matter too much whether or not citrus fruit has been waxed if it is to be peeled, but it does if you are using it to cook marmalade or other food which uses the skin or the rind of the fruit. I avoid eating apples that have been treated in this way. I stick to English Cox's, and Bramleys which I have never found waxed. Just one important cautionary note: animal manure and waste are used as fertilisers in organic farming, so pathogens will remain on your foods unless you are particularly vigilant and wash all fruit and vegetables thoroughly before eating them.

Another problem with some organically grown food such as peanuts stored in hot, humid conditions, usually from developing countries, is that it may be contaminated with high levels of carcinogenic fungal substances called aflatoxins. If buying peanuts, simply buy them in their shells and discard the shells.

I have been eating organic for years and have never had a problem.

TEN KEY WAYS TO BOOST YOUR VITAL VEGETABLE INTAKE	
If You Used To Do This . . .	*Now Do This!*
Boil your potatoes and cabbages to death	Buy a stainless steel or bamboo steamer, add an inch of water in the pan, put on the steamer and fill it with veg. It takes about the same length of time to cook and you won't believe how much better it tastes!
Think crudités meant only celery sticks dipped in salt	Keep the celery sticks but add raw carrot sticks, raw broccoli and cauliflower florets, chunks of raw courgette and sweet pepper, cucumber, tomato, spring onions and on and on. Ditch the salt and add a dollop of houmous or soya yoghurt seasoned with chopped chives and herbs for dipping.
Turn up your nose at any vegetable except frozen peas	Lightly cook chopped veg in a little vegetable stock, blend and serve as a soup, flavoured with black pepper and herbs. It tastes delicious.
Think a salad was a careful arrangement of limp lettuce, shrivelled cucumber, a slice of tomato and half a boiled egg covered in salad cream	Aim to create a salad with at least five ingredients. Here is the 'add list' for one of my favourite salads: grated carrot and turnip, chopped spring onion, diced

	cucumber and courgette, red kidney beans or tiny cubes of marinated tofu, watercress and parsley, rocket, radicchio and Cos lettuce. Mix and serve with sunflower seeds and a little walnut or sesame oil with cider vinegar flavoured with herbs drizzled over each serving.
Throw the parsley garnish away	Make garnish from fresh, finely chopped herbs, such as parsley, coriander and watercress, and vegetables, such as tomato, onion and courgette. This will add valuable nutrients as well as colour to your meal.
Eat just one tablespoon of vegetables at each evening meal	I use the Rainbow Rule: fill one-quarter of your plate with white veg such as potato, parsnip, celeriac or turnip. These can be mashed, baked, roasted or steamed. Fill the next quarter with orange veg such as carrot, sweet potato or pumpkin; another quarter with yellow veg such as swedes, sweetcorn and sweet pepper; and the final quarter with greens. Alternatively use similar combinations to make vegetable kebabs, roast vegetables, salads or stir-fries. Also, add red tomatoes and peppers to your cooking whenever you can.

Think garlic was for rubbing inside the salad bowls	Whatever recipe you are reading, double the amount of garlic. Add crushed garlic to soups, stir-fries and casseroles, and to salad dressings, houmous and savoury sauces.
Reach for a dictionary whenever you heard the word 'brassica'	Add all the edible members of the cabbage family to your diet: broccoli, Brussels sprouts, cabbages of all sorts, cauliflower, collards, kale, kohlrabi. These are rich in calcium and phytochemicals known to be anti-carcinogenic. Eat some raw or lightly steamed every day.
Think vegetable juice meant gravy and that a pound of carrots would last a year	Push one half pound of organic carrots, well scrubbed, through your new juicer. Drink immediately. Tomorrow, do the same with celery and tomatoes.

FOOD FACTOR 3: PROTEINS

Undoubtedly one of the main differences between the Western and traditional oriental diets is the amount of animal protein in the former, while the latter is heavily based on foods of vegetable origin. Figure 3.3 shows how crucial this is to preventing and treating prostate cancer, so, if you wish to prevent prostate or other types of cancer, don't even think about going on a high-animal-protein diet to help weight loss. I advise people who have active cancer of the prostate (or breast or colon) to eliminate all animal produce from their diet until they are better, after seeking advice on how to eat a balanced vegan diet from experts at the Bristol Cancer Help Centre. For other people, unless they wish to follow a vegan diet, a small amount of animal protein in the diet is fine provided it is balanced by a similar amount of vegetable protein and lots of other vegetables and fruit as well.

Soya has a complete range of amino acids, and other pulses such as peas and beans, cereals (see below) and nuts are good sources of protein – without the unhealthy animal fat. All pulses are also very good sources of fibre, including a type that binds and inactivates free radicals in the gut and bloodstream. As discussed above, they are also valuable sources of phyto-oestrogens. Eat at least one good-sized portion a day.[64] Cereals are a good source of vegetable proteins that complement those in pulses and are discussed further under Food Factor 6 (see p. 183). Another good protein source is nuts. I eat lots (but never pre-shelled because they quickly become rancid; and groundnuts can be contaminated with carcinogens – see p. 162). I avoid brazil nuts which can contain elevated levels of the radioactive substance radium-226. When one of my colleagues told me this because he was concerned that I was eating so many, I did not believe him. After leaving some of the nuts in our detector overnight, I did!

Now my cancer is gone, I eat one small portion of animal protein a day. I eat fish but I am prepared to pay for wild or organically farmed fish, since this is less likely to contain antibiotic residues and other man-made pollutants (there has recently been concern in the press, for example, about high levels of cancer-causing chemicals in farmed salmon). Oily fish such as salmon, herring and mackerel are also rich in vitamin D, essential for healthy bones, and omega-3 fatty acids. Both vitamins A and D, found in oily fish and in fish oils, may work to reduce risk of prostate cancer and breast cancer by lowering blood levels of IGF-I.[65]

In the case of farmed fish, I particularly avoid farmed trout which may have been treated with steroid hormones to produce only female fish. If I eat salmon, I buy that produced to the standards of the Soil Association. This is much paler than most farmed salmon on the market, because it does not contain the artificial colouring agent which makes other farmed salmon so vividly pink; one such agent, canthaxanthin, has been implicated in damaging eyesight. The same additive is used to feed non-organically produced chickens to colour their skins and the yolks of their eggs.[66] Non-organically produced farmed fish can also contain antibiotic residues and toxic chemicals used to control sea lice and to prevent growth of other organisms on the cages in which the fish are kept. In the past, the latter have included tributyl tin, an appalling endocrine-disrupting chemical (*see* pp. 223–4).

Ensure that you buy the ultra-pure varieties which have had harmful chemicals such as PCBs (*see* p. 218) extracted. I take a teaspoon of Seven Seas cod-liver oil a day, the type which is labelled 'original and ultra-pure', which is slightly more expensive. By the way, do not expect your pharmacist to know the difference between standard fish oils and the ultra-pure varieties – you will have to search them out yourself.

I began to include small quantities of animal food in my diet because, after about eight months of eating only plant foods when I had active cancer, I began to feel low and I knew that meat was a good source of a range of bioavailable minerals. I eat only very small portions of young meat such as lamb, chicken or duck drumsticks and wild game such as rabbit or venison (organically produced meat from beef herds is also fine). Game generally has higher levels of nutrients and far lower levels of fat than concentrate-fed animals which have a sedentary life.

If I were an American, I would never eat beef or pork unless it was absolutely guaranteed to be organically produced. Growth-hormone implants based on male and/or female hormones have been used in beef production there for about thirty years. According to the Institute of Agriculture and Natural Resources at the University of Nebraska in the USA, implants are available for all cattle except calves less than 45 days old and breeding cattle. Some of the most potent hormone implants combine both male and female hormones. Such meat has higher levels of IGF-I than untreated meat.[67] A genetically engineered pig growth hormone – Porcine Somatotrophin, PST – is also available in the United States but I can find no evidence of the use of such products in the production of sheep meat.

One physician has been quoted as saying 'it is very likely that hormone residues in American beef is a factor in the early onset of puberty among girls in recent decades.'[68] It has been claimed that PST is safer than any of the steroid hormones banned by the European Union (but still used in America) because cooking destroys PST. However, this doesn't take IGF-I levels into account, nor does it address the problem of undercooked meat. Although the use of all such hormones is banned throughout Europe, on a BBC Radio 4 programme, British pig farmers complained that European farmers were allowed to feed their animals on sewage sludge – a practice forbidden in Britain! The message is clear. If you wish to eat pork, bacon or ham, eat organically produced British products, especially from traditional rare breeds such as Gloucester Old Spot and Tamworth pigs.

Other good sources of protein and essential trace nutrients include organically produced eggs. Eggs contain high levels of the amino acid cysteine used in anti-radiation pills so, in moderation, egg consumption will help combat the effects of radiotherapy and diagnostic X-rays. The sulphur in cysteine is in a form thought to de-activate free radicals and hence protect cells.[69] I ate one small organically produced egg a day while being treated with radiotherapy; I often eat organic eggs now, but never more than one a day.

Populations such as the Eskimos living on a predominantly fish diet have long been known to have less hormone-dependent cancer than those eating other animal fats. If properly cooked, seafood also contains lots of iodine, and iodine compounds (like those of zinc) are involved in ensuring that mistakes (which could cause cancer) do not occur during cell division in the body.[70]

The chemical element iodine has very unusual behaviour. It is called a conservative element, which means that it prefers to stay in water and hence, in the Earth's system, it ends up being concentrated in the oceans. This is why its main dietary source is seafood. The distinctive chemistry of iodine means that it is easily lost when processing and cooking food (Chinese people tend to cook fish in sealed containers and use the juices to make soup which keeps levels of iodine intake higher). Several components of our diet contain compounds called goitrogens which increase our need for iodine. The plant called rape, from which rapeseed or canola oil is obtained, contains goitrogens and I avoid this in my diet and anything that contains unspecified vegetable oils since this could include such oil.

To ensure I have enough iodine I take kelp tablets. All seaweed has high concentrations of iodine and other nutrients but it can also concentrate pollutants. I therefore try to buy kelp from countries such as Iceland, which has a low population, uses only natural geothermal energy, and is further away from most pollutant sources than any other supplier of seaweed I know of. A hundred years ago fish waste and seaweed were commonly used as fertiliser, but these have now been mostly replaced by inorganic fertilisers, including rock phosphate, which generally has low iodine content (but high levels of the potentially toxic element cadmium (now known to be an important endocrine disrupter)). Again, the Soil Association are careful to limit the amounts of cadmium and other toxic substances allowed in rock-phosphate fertiliser for food production and they totally ban the use of sewage sludge, which can have high cadmium levels.

Soils in most Western countries tend to contain much less organic matter because of industrialised agriculture, so they cannot hold iodine delivered to them in rain water, resulting in lower levels in crops. Taking kelp in my diet has improved my skin enormously. If I run out of tablets for any length of time my skin becomes rough, initially around my elbows, knees and buttocks, and the roughness gradually extends over progressively larger areas until I take kelp again, when the roughness retreats. Seaweed is also protective against radiation. Alginate, a mucous material extracted from seaweed, is a standard protective agent against radioactivity. Hence kelp and other seaweeds help reduce the side effects of X-rays and radiotherapy. Agar-agar, which is widely used to replace gelatine in vegan foods, can also be used in your diet as a source of iodine. Other seaweeds which I use include: arame, hiziki, dulse and wakame (which I add to some soups immediately before serving). Nori, which is commonly sold in sheets, can be used to wrap rice balls, sushi and many other foods. A lunch box containing this is available from at least one supplier of ready-to-eat meals – much better for you than grabbing a sandwich or baguette!

An extra bonus is that iodine is good for the brain. Iodine deficiency is a common cause of mental retardation and brain damage, the untreatable condition known as cretinism whereby children are born severely mentally retarded, because of their mother's iodine deficiency during pregnancy.[71]

PREVENTION FOR ORDINARY MORTALS For those without cancer but who wish to cut their risk or those who have recovered from cancer (like me). **Remember to keep total animal produce low.**	
If You Used To Do This . . .	*Now Do This!*
Breakfast Processed refined cereals with milk and white sugar	Organic muesli or porridge with a tablespoon of flaxseed, moistened with fruit juice previously

	sweetened with honey, raw cane sugar or molasses, or use rice, soya or coconut milk.
Fried sausage, bacon, scrambled eggs and fried bread	1. Grilled organic bacon (or vegetarian alternative), tomatoes and mushrooms brushed with, or softened in, olive oil. Toast or lightly fry bread in olive oil, or 2. Haddock poached in 50 per cent soya milk, 50 per cent water, or 3. Boiled or poached eggs on wholemeal, organic bread lightly fried in olive oil.
Toasted white bread and butter with marmalade	Toasted organic wholemeal bread with a good brand of soya spread and marmalade.
Commercial orange juice	Freshly made melon and raspberry juice or any other juice you enjoy.
Snacks and nibbles Commercial biscuits, especially those containing dairy (whey, casein, lactose, milk powder etc.)	Dried fruit, nuts, pumpkin seeds, bananas, dried coconut. Dairy-free sesame bars or other snacks from health-food stores. Dairy-free ginger nuts.
Main meals Meat cooked in butter or lard eaten rare or undercooked	Roast or grill meat slowly and thoroughly using olive oil, sea salt and black pepper, garlic and other herbs and spices to flavour.

Fast foods

Hamburgers, sausage, paté, prepared dishes from supermarkets	Eat veggie burgers or veggie sausages. Fish or eggs are the ultimate fast food. Steam or poach fish in water or white wine flavoured with ginger, onions, fennel or dill, or simply grill after brushing with olive oil and seasoning with sea salt, black pepper and herbs.
Eat mainly tinned peas	Lightly steam fresh peas, mange tout, asparagus, broccoli or any other vegetables and keep the juice to make soup or gravy. Don't add butter – use olive oil flavoured with herbs.
Chips, buttered or roast potatoes. Baked potatoes with butter or cheese	Scrub the potatoes before baking or steaming, then rub in olive oil and garnish with chopped parsley before serving. Eat with houmous or taramasalata instead of butter and cheese.
Milky sauces and cream soups	Replace the dairy with soya milk; or use potato as a thickener.
Thin soups	Miso-based soups (p. 146), or use simple vegetable broth.
Puddings	Choose from fresh fruit salads, water ices or sorbets, soya ice cream, tofu fruit puddings or other delicious

	puddings described in *The Plant Programme*. Use soya or coconut cream rather than dairy.
Cheese course	Substitute a salad course with pine nuts, sun-dried tomatoes and herb-flavoured olives, artichoke hearts and marinated tofu.
Commercial mayonnaise, salad dressing or salad cream	Make a base of 3–1 virgin olive oil to wine, cider, raspberry or balsamic vinegar, season with a pinch of sea salt and black pepper to taste and use herbs and garlic to ring the changes.
Cheesy or yoghurt-based dips	Replace with houmous, tahini or taramasalata.
After-dinner chocolates	Buy the organic, dairy-free, dark-chocolate version.
Milky tea or coffee	Substitute from lists in Food Factors 1 and 8.
Late-night milk-chocolate or malt drink	Check that it contains no dairy, then make it with soya milk instead of dairy, using raw sugar, vanilla or other flavourings you enjoy.

FOOD FACTOR 4: OILS AND FATS

One clue to the puzzle of why prostate cancers metastasise in those on a Western diet but not in oriental men eating their traditional diet was discovered when death rates from prostate cancer were compared with the annual fat consumption of men in a wide range of nations around the world. The nations included in the study ranged from Western industrialised nations to third-world countries in which most of the population lived a rural agrarian existence. The results showed that the death rate from prostate cancer was directly correlated with the fat content in the diet.[72]

There are good reasons to be cautious about studies like these, because of the types of fat consumed. There are two convincing prospective studies, however: the Physician's Health Study and the Health Professionals Follow-up (HPFU) Study. In both studies, dietary intake was recorded regularly and not based on patients' sometimes faulty memory. The findings suggested that the risk of prostate cancer was directly related to total fat intake, but the risk was associated with animal (including dairy products and meat), not vegetable, fat, so that the risk of metastatic prostate cancer is associated with dietary *animal* fat intake.[73]

It is important to note that prostate cancer is not the only human disease that appears to be associated with dietary animal fat intake. High-animal-fat diets have also been correlated with breast and colon cancer, heart disease and hypertension, and most cancer and heart charities recommend reduction in the amount consumed. Prostate-cancer patients and those people wishing to reduce their chances of developing the disease would be wise to reduce their intake of animal fat to an absolute minimum.[74]

Many people are confused about the type and quantity of oils and fat they should be eating.

At a meeting on Cancer Prevention at Bethesda, USA, it was noted that the move towards lower dietary fat had failed to distinguish between unhealthy, saturated fats and healthy fats – and this matters. Apparently, some tomato sauces available in health food stores have had olive oil removed so they could be labelled 'fat free'.[75] Also, we have been persuaded to buy spreads based on (usually altered and processed) polyunsaturated fats. Our bodies do need fats, but only in the quantities and forms which we would have consumed as hunters or gatherers. Let us try to sort out the unhealthy from the healthy forms of fat, because the right fat profile in your diet is crucial to good health.

Fats are solid at room temperature, oils are liquid. However, scientists often use the term 'fat' to include all oils and fats, whether they're solid or liquid. Chemically, fats are made up of three molecules of fatty acids and one of an alcohol called glycerol. The word 'triglycerides' is also used to describe fat – it means three ('tri') fatty acid molecules plus glycerol – triglyceride.

Fatty acids are, simply, acids found in fats. There are four major fatty acids: palmitic, stearic, oleic and linoleic. Remember, each molecule of fat contains three of these four fatty acids. It's the *combination* of these acids in the fat molecule that determines whether the fat is saturated, unsaturated, or polyunsaturated – words we've all heard a great deal in the past few years. Let me explain them.

Lipids (fats and oils) which are made from various combinations of fatty acids combined with glycerol, have long tails of carbon atoms (often fifteen to seventeen carbon atoms long) combined with hydrogen. Some fatty acids are chains of carbon atoms attached by single bonds and all their spare bonds are attached to hydrogen. They are therefore called saturated (with respect to hydrogen) because all their bonds are used up. Some have double bonds between carbon atoms and are called unsaturated. Unsaturated fatty acids can have one (monounsaturated) or many (polyunsaturated) double bonds between carbon atoms. Double bonds make fatty acids and lipids melt more easily, hence most oils are unsaturated while fats, especially animal fats, which are generally saturated, are solid at room temperature.

Saturated

Saturated fat is known to raise the level of cholesterol in your blood. The more you eat, the higher your cholesterol level, and the greater your chances of suffering a stroke or heart attack. Animal fat – butter and that in meat – contains lots of saturated fat. A few plant fats – principally coconut and palm oil – also contain significant amounts. Among all the controversies about foods, the message to minimise saturated fat in our diet has remained unchanged for more than thirty years, despite the marketing of dairy produce and red meat as sources of CLAs now. Similarly, the advice against consuming trans-fatty acids (TFAs), which can be formed during the manufacture of margarine, remains unchanged. I avoid all margarines including those claiming to be high in polyunsaturates because they have been hydrogenated (involving passing hydrogen gas through them under pressure, often in the presence of a nickel catalyst). This process can produce 'trans fats' which some nutrition experts believe are unhealthy and which have been implicated in breast cancer.[76] The Western diet typically contains large quantities of TFAs, which experimental evidence suggests impair essential fatty acid metabolism.[77] The TFAs are somewhat similar in structure and behaviour to saturated fatty acids, and the WHO recommends that manufacturers reduce the levels of TFA in spreads. Most spreads now state the amount of TFAs they contain: one organic soya spread my family uses contains only trace quantities.

Monounsaturated

Oleic fatty acid has eighteen carbon atoms and one unsaturated carbon bond. So it's called 'monounsaturated'. Ongoing research suggests that monounsaturated fat is much healthier than saturated fat. Experiments on humans show that switching from saturated to monounsaturated fat not only decreases the risk of heart disease, but may also lower your blood pressure. A major source is olive oil. This contains more than 80 per cent monounsaturated fats and is naturally resistant to oxidation, which means it is relatively safe for cooking and is also less prone to rancidity than other types of unsaturated fat.

I avoid rapeseed or canola oil. Canola has been bred from old varieties of rapeseed in Canada, and is reported to contain very low levels of erucic acid, which is suspected to have pathogenic potential in diets high in the original rapeseed oil in experimental animals.[78] Canola oil is now the most widely consumed food oil in Canada and is approved by the US FDA.

Polyunsaturated

Linoleic fatty acid has eighteen carbon atoms and two unsaturated carbon bonds. So it's called 'polyunsaturated'. Early research indicated that polyunsaturated fats lowered total and LDL cholesterol more than monounsaturated fats. The latest research, however, finds no difference in their cholesterol-lowering ability. However, the more polyunsaturated an oil is, the more it can be damaged by heat, air and light. Most polyunsaturated oils should only be used raw because, once damaged, they form free radicals. Good sources of polyunsaturated fats include sunflower and corn oil.

Essential fatty acids

The two classes of essential fatty acids, omega-6 fatty acids such as linoleic acid (which, when conjugated – or linked up – forms CLAs), and omega-3 fatty acids, continue to receive considerable attention. They are both necessary for good health, because they provide the catalysts for various metabolic functions (e.g. in the synthesis of prostaglandins, which are important as cell regulators and for the proper functioning of the immune system). They are called 'essential' because the body cannot make them, and they must be obtained from food sources. Most vegetable oils provide essential fatty acids to a greater or lesser extent.

Omega-6 fatty acids (e.g. linoleic acid) are found in vegetable seeds and the oils produced from them. Good sources include oils made from safflower, sunflower, corn, soya, evening primrose, pumpkin, walnut, and wheat germ.

Omega-3 fatty acids (e.g. alpha linolenic acid) are found in oily fish such as salmon, mackerel and sardines, and also in linseed (flaxseed), evening primrose, borage seed and soya bean oil. In addition to being protective against cancer, evidence is mounting that they are protective against a range of other conditions including coronary heart disease and high blood pressure, arthritis, eczema and psoriasis, BPH[79] and depression. The food supplement spirulina (a microscopic algae) contains both linoleic and linolenic acids – indeed the omega-3 fatty acids in oily fish are derived from such sources.

Gamma linoleic acid is a particularly good omega-3 fatty acid, enriched in organ meats such as liver (but eat only from organically reared animals) and in evening primrose oil – but do not have this in gelatine capsules (which are made from rendered dead animal carcasses).

Japanese researchers have shown that a deficiency of these essential fatty acids leads to an impaired ability to learn and recall information. Much new information suggests that the human brain, which contains much fatty material,[80] depends for optimal functioning on adequate supplies of omega-3 and omega-6 fatty acids and that their proportion in the diet is also important.

There has been a huge change in the proportion of omega-3 to omega-6 fatty acids, especially in the Western diet.[81] With settled agriculture, which began about 10,000 years ago, people started to rely on cultivated foods, and the consumption of omega-3-rich fish and wild game declined. With the industrialisation of the food industry in the twentieth century, there was an even more dramatic shift in the proportion of omega-6 fatty acids to omega-3 fatty acids in the diet, a situation made worse by the hydrogenation of oils to make them keep longer. A typical Western diet now contains sixteen times as much omega-6 fatty acids as omega-3, whereas a century ago our diet would have contained similar amounts of each type of fatty acid. The advice is to eat more of the foods that are high in omega-3 fatty acids such as fatty fish, walnuts, flaxseed and olive oil for health.

I will no longer eat dairy produce in any guise, ever, and I rely mainly on first pressed extra-virgin olive oil for everything from cooking to salad dressings. I never re-use the oil in cooking and I cook food slowly so that the oil is not damaged and the food absorbs the flavour. I avoid brands of margarine based on olive oil but which also contain dairy produce.

The only oils I use have been organically grown and extracted by cold pressing. There are three methods of extraction:

- Cold pressing. This is the traditional hydraulic pressing process where the temperature is kept low throughout and which therefore preserves temperature-sensitive vitamins. The end product is expensive, but the oil is nutritious and tastes and smells good. It may be more expensive but you consume less!
- Screw or expeller. This process involves the use of high pressure which generates high temperatures, thereby destroying vitamins. Such oil is dark, strong smelling and needs further refining and deodorising – and I do not use it.
- Solvent extraction, using solvents such as benzene, hexane or heptane and lots of other processing and chemical treatment. I avoid this at all costs.

All oils should be stored in dark opaque stoppered glass bottles in dark cupboards or pantries, to minimise oxidation, and ideally used cold in salad dressings. I prefer to eat whole flaxseed rather than the oil. According to Ingram and others[82] it is flaxseed – but not flax oil – that is rich in lignan precursors which are anti-carcinogenic, and it is also excellent for avoiding constipation – and hence piles and varicose veins.[83]

In many Mediterranean restaurants it is usual to have virgin olive oil flavoured with herbs to dip bread into. It is so much tastier and healthier than butter. I do this now if I have dinner parties. Usually my guests eat their bread dipped in flavoured olive oil with great relish, and I have noticed many of them have copied the idea. The Spanish, Italian and Greek people I know use olive oil with fish or tomato paste in their sandwiches (with salad), instead of butter or processed spreads on their bread. This is not only healthier but the sandwiches and snacks are much more delicious than those most people in the UK eat.

It is particularly important to obtain fats from fresh, unpolluted sources, since many of the most health-damaging pollutants, including some powerful endocrine disrupters, are highly fat-soluble. Large quantities can accumulate in the fatty tissue of farmed fish, fresh fish downstream of sewage works and dairy fat, for example.

I also try never to use oils from plastic bottles, since many of the potentially harmful chemical substances in plastics are fat soluble.

In summary, I never eat butter or margarine, but I use olive oil for cooking and a range of extra-virgin cold-pressed oils for salad dressings.

TEN WAYS TO MODIFY YOUR FAT INTAKE	
If You Used To Do This . . .	*Now Do This!*
Make your sandwiches with a thick layer of butter, then with a thick layer of peanut butter	Leave out the butter.
Spread your toast with a thick layer of butter or margarine	Drizzle a little organic, cold-pressed extra-virgin olive oil over your toast instead. It tastes delicious, especially with tomato paste or savoury food.
Buy oil labelled canola or unspecified 'vegetable' oil	Buy only cold-pressed extra-virgin organic olive, walnut, sesame or sunflower oils.
Prepare a fondue every weekend	Keep the little forks but switch ethnic loyalties and prepare a plate of raw and steamed vegetables with a selection of Thai, Japanese and Chinese dips.
Buy a cheese and pickle sandwich from your local supermarket every lunchtime	Buy a tub of their houmous instead, with a salad and a few baby pittas to dip into it.

Buy crackers and snack foods without reading the labels	Read all labels for fat and hidden-dairy content! Buy fresh and dried fruit and nuts instead of fatty, salty or sugary snacks.
Insist on eating popcorn while watching that film	Go ahead, but use an air-popper to make it. They make a good gift and require no fat. Add a little sea salt or your favourite spices.
Order the Four Cheeses pizza from your local	Try the Marguerita without the mozzarella, but request extra olives, capers, mushrooms, garlic etc.
Order the baked potato with butter, chilli con carne and cheese sauce	Order the baked potato with baked beans or houmous and a side salad.
Go crazy for any dessert topped with cream	Make some fruit sauce or drizzle a little organic maple syrup over your favourite non-dairy dessert.

FOOD FACTOR 5: SEASONING AND FLAVOURING

Healthy food doesn't have to be – indeed, *shouldn't* be – bland food. Until recently the main methods of preserving food were to add lots of salt, especially to meat and vegetables, sugar to fruit, and alcohol to a range of products. It has been said that the British, because they shipped so much food from their overseas territories, developed a particular liking for these tastes. Food naturally contains sodium so we do not need to add any to our food. Overuse of salt and sodium bicarbonate have been linked by Gerson to cancer and it continues to be implicated by some researchers in promoting certain types of cancer, including naso-pharyngeal (nose and throat) cancer.[84]

It is easy to learn to change your taste and you will find food tastes much better with far more subtle flavours when you reduce the salt. Oriental people, however, consume lots of salt in soya sauce, for example, so I do not think that cutting out salt is one of the most critical things to do in combating prostate cancer. It is, however, helpful to your health generally.

Many anti-cancer diet books recommend against the use of spices. Korean and Thai food, however, are very heavily spiced, but the rates of prostate and breast cancer in these countries are exceptionally low. In *The Plant Programme* many of the delicious recipes include spices since, by the time we wrote the book, we were aware of the use of many spices as anti-cancer treatments in traditional Indian Ayurvedic and Chinese medicine. Turmeric, for example, one of the main ingredients of curry powder, contains curcumin, which has been shown to have powerful antioxidant and anti-cancer properties, suppressing the proliferation of cancer cells. Curcumin has even been shown to help prevent cancer cells producing their own growth factors, which can happen in advanced cases of the disease. In particular, curcumin inhibits the growth of oestrogen-receptor-positive breast cancer.[85]

Real saffron made from crocus stamens and traditionally used to colour rice yellow contains carotenoids and has anti-free-radical properties – but never eat the horribly yellow (or pink) coloured food now sold as Eastern food in some shops, restaurants and supermarkets.

I grow fresh herbs such as parsley, thyme, chives, marjoram, rosemary and mint in a small patch in the garden and buy others from the supermarket. Herbs are good for you and help to make food taste delicious.

Substances useful for making delicious food, which stimulate the activity of an important detoxifying enzyme GST (glutathione-S-transferase), occur in celery seed, garlic, onions, ginger and turmeric.[86] Rosemary, sage, oregano and thyme are also strong antioxidants,[87] and rosemary and sage have documented anti-tumour activity.[88] Ginger contains more powerful antioxidants than even vitamin E,[89] and many other herbs and spices contain substances considered to be cancer-preventive agents.[90]

I use vinegar (wine or cider, preferably organically produced) with organic extra-virgin olive oil as the basis for delicious salad dressings. I never eat commercially produced mayonnaise, salad creams or other such 'glop'.

TEN HEALTHY WAYS TO SPICE UP YOUR FOOD	
If You Used To Do This . . .	*Now Do This!*
Shower everything with salt	Stop cooking with salt. Try seasoning your meal with tamari (wheat-free soy sauce) and extra herbs and spices.
Spread yeast extract on your toast	Spread miso on your toast for a similar-but-different flavour and added nutrient value.
Serve boiled carrots with a dollop of butter	Steam them and then toss in a light sauté of garlic and/or freshly grated ginger with organic extra-virgin olive oil.
Think black pepper is the only spice	Arrange a small collection of spices on the table including black pepper, chilli pepper flakes and Tabasco sauce. Visit your local ethnic grocer to explore a new world of spices, then experiment . . .
Use 'salad cream' and nothing else on every salad you are given	Mix finest olive oil with a herb-flavoured cider vinegar and freshly crushed garlic. Or drizzle a little freshly squeezed lemon juice and sesame or walnut oil over your salad. A splash of Tabasco will also lift the flavour.

Think boiled cabbage and potatoes were only there to soak up the gravy	Steam the vegetables very lightly then toss them gently in a light sauté of caraway seed and chopped garlic. Season with black pepper, to taste.
Think every soup needed a hefty dose of beef broth and monosodium glutamate (MSG) to be tasty	Make your soups with a strong vegetable broth including the seaweed, Kombu, which has flavouring and thickening properties similar to MSG but is healthier.
Think all vinegar was white or brown malt vinegar	Mix together organic cider vinegar and organically grown fresh herbs. Try tarragon, rosemary, basil or garlic. Some delicatessens sell raspberry and other delicious fruit vinegars.
Think that rice was a white and fluffy but rather bland way of bulking out the good stuff	First, change your brand of rice! Buy whole-grain, basmati or wild rice, and then zip up the flavour this way: heat 1 teaspoon olive oil in the saucepan and sauté one teaspoon of Chinese Five Spices. Stir in dry rice, then add the water and follow the usual cooking routine.
Roast onions tasted of cooked water	Leave small onions whole and slice larger ones in half. Then press two or three whole cloves into each onion and place in the

baking tray with potatoes,
parsnips and half the oil you
would normally use. Pour a
little warm water over the
veg before roasting.

FOOD FACTOR 6: CEREAL FOODS, SNACKS AND TREATS

Food is one of life's great pleasures, and the Plant Programme is not a hair-shirt regime! I eat sorbets and soya ice creams and organic dark dairy-free chocolate for occasional treats. Also, sometimes I eat the delicious soups sold in waxed paper cartons (but never in plastic pots) now on sale after checking that they contain no dairy products.

My favourite treat is fish and chips – 'the great British experience' – which I eat about once a week, although I remove all the batter unless I buy it from my local fish and chip shop, where they are kind enough to make it without milk and I know they change their cooking oil frequently. This is much better, on health grounds as well as taste, than cow burgers on white bread!

I eat masses of dried fruit of all descriptions. Prunes contain anti-cancer chemicals and figs are an excellent source of calcium. Pumpkin, sesame and sunflower seeds make delicious, nutritious snacks.

Most cancer-prevention diets include plenty of whole-grain cereal foods such as bread and pasta.[91] Clearly if you are intolerant of, or allergic to, gluten you may need to avoid food and drink based on one or more of wheat, rye and barley, although many people can tolerate some gluten-containing foods better than others (wheat contains the most gluten). Good substitutes include rice and corn, and some new scientific evidence suggests that oats may be safe.[92]

Whole grains contain a wide range of phytochemicals which reduce the risk of cancer.[93] The active phytochemicals are concentrated in the bran and the germ, so that refining wheat, for example, causes a 200- to 300-fold loss in valuable phytochemical content.[94] Tumour cells synthesise and accumulate cholesterol faster than normal cells, and one group of chemicals in whole-grain cereals (and fruit and vegetables) suppress tumour growth by limiting cholesterol synthesis.[95] Other anti-cancer substances in whole grains induce the production of the detoxifying enzyme GST.[96]

On the other hand, consuming highly processed bread and cereals that are too easily digested floods the body with sugar, stimulating it to produce high levels of IGF-I.[97] Acne is suggested to be an indicator of the over-production of IGF-I as a result of this process. (Several people following my diet have reported that their acne has disappeared, but I think giving up dairy produce helps this too.)

Undoubtedly, consuming lots of refined cereals can be harmful. Processing wheat to make white flour for white bread and many commercial pastries removes much of the proteins, vitamins and minerals, which are often used for animal fodder. In order to compensate, inorganic nutrients such as chalk (as a source of calcium), iron and vitamins are added back. Despite adding these vitamins, such processed flour has often lost much of its vitamin B6, vitamin B5 and molybdenum; nearly all of its vitamin E, cobalt and zinc; much of its chromium; and some selenium, too. The degradation of nutritional content is made worse by the addition of bleaches and 'improvers' such as potassium bromate, some of which have been shown to be toxic.[98] Always check the list of ingredients carefully when buying bread, and ensure that it is free of chemical additives. If I had the time, I would make my own bread with freshly purchased organic wheat or other cereals, using one of the bread-making machines which are now widely available, but my life is far too busy at the moment!

Do try to buy organic wherever possible because, unfortunately, much wheat is now produced mainly by monoculture methods under conditions as prairie-like as possible, with the liberal use of artificial fertilisers and pesticides.[99]

Try to eat only organic wholemeal brown bread made with stone-ground flour. I eat many other types of organically grown cereals including porridge and oatcakes, organic whole brown rice and wholemeal brown organic pasta in my diet, all widely available in health-food stores and supermarkets. Despite some recently published versions of anti-breast-cancer diets there is nothing wrong with muesli providing it is based on organic produce and provided it is not the commercial 'muesli' made with sugar or milk-derived components. Also use rice, oat or soya milk or fruit juice rather than dairy milk to moisten it. If you are staying in a hotel use the juice from fresh fruit salad or if there is none use the juice from the prunes which are almost always on the buffet. Just one thing – it is important to eat zinc-containing protein (such as meat or eggs) at least eight hours after eating food such as cereal which contains high levels of substances called phytates, which can bind zinc, making it unavailable for absorption. Interestingly the fibre in flaxseed has been shown in experiments not to bind zinc.[100]

TEN HEALTHY TREATS	
If You Used To Do This . . .	*Now Do This!*
Tuck into a giant bag of crisps	Pour a small handful each of sesame, sunflower and pumpkin seeds into a bowl and munch them instead.
Leave a trail of sweet wrappers around the place	Mix your own blend of organic dried fruits such as figs, dates, apricots, mango and raisins, and place little bowls or cartons of them in handy places: the car, your desk, near the phone . . .
Eat sweet and sticky desserts	Take an organically grown orange, slice it in half and use a grapefruit knife to slice around the segment edges. Sprinkle the sliced surface with a tiny pinch of nutmeg or cloves and a hint of maple syrup. Bake for about fifteen minutes.
Reward yourself with sweet and sticky desserts layered with cream	Take an organic Bramley apple, remove the core and fill it with raisins, chopped banana, cinnamon and a little maple syrup. Place it in a dish and bake it for about fifteen minutes. Serve with soya cream or soya ice cream.

Eat whole variety packs of snack crackers	Buy rice cakes and oatcakes and arrange them on a plate with a little houmous, tofu dip, tahini or home-made salsa.
Get a sweet craving at least twice a day	Soak a mixture of chopped organic dried fruit in filtered water overnight. Eat a small bowlful dressed with a little rose water and chopped pumpkin seeds.
Get a serious snack attack once a day	Fight back with a piping-hot baked potato filled with houmous or dairy-free baked beans. Sometimes a bean salad will do the trick.
Blow out on ice cream and chocolate	Go ahead, but with soya ice cream and dairy-free dark chocolate instead.
Eat a packet of biscuits every day	Pack your own stack of oatcakes spread with home-made jam. Sweet, crunchy and very nutritious.
Eat toast made with white bread and whatever until the whole loaf is gone	Buy only wholemeal organic loaves made with organic flour and be fussy about what you spread on them. Try tahini, barley miso, mashed banana or olive paté.

FOOD FACTOR 7: SWEETENERS
Use raw cane-sugar molasses, unrefined honey (preferably wild) or maple syrup as sweeteners. Refined white sugar (called 'pure, white and deadly' by Professor Yudkin) is just empty calories

stripped of nutrients; I never eat it. A natural herbal substance called Stevia, which has been used as a sweetener and flavour enhancer in Paraguay for centuries and is also suitable for diabetics, is now available from good health stores.

I avoid any products containing man-made sweeteners such as aspartame,[101] cyclamates, or saccharin, or refined sugar. I do so because some of these artificial sweeteners have been linked in laboratory studies to a range of diseases.[102] Artificial sweeteners are frequently found in soft drinks, over-the-counter drugs and prescription drugs, vitamin and herbal supplements, yoghurt, confectionery, some processed cereals, sugar-free chewing-gum, some desserts, some ready-made meals, some milk-shake mixers, sweeteners, and some instant teas and coffees. So read all labels carefully!

Traditionally, Chinese children have eaten very few sweets. Their treats were pumpkin seeds or dried fruit.

FOOD FACTOR 8: WHAT TO DRINK

As I mentioned earlier, I drink freshly made vegetable and fruit juices from organic produce. Clean, pure water is also fundamental for good health. Unfortunately the only way of providing adequate water now, in areas of high population density, is to recycle it by treating or reprocessing water at sewage works. Indeed, we joke that when people drink a glass of water in the East End of London, ten people have previously drunk the same water! During treatment, the water is filtered through progressively finer material to remove particles, microbes and chemicals and it is often mixed with other water to dilute harmful chemicals so that their concentration falls below legal requirements. Finally, chlorine is added to kill microbes.

The problems of recycled treated sewage water commonly used as the principal drinking-water supply in urban areas (*see* further under Lifestyle Factor 6 in Chapter 6) continue to be a revelation to many medical professionals – or so it seems to me. For example, I remember a TV interview in which a senior cancer specialist from a famous London hospital accused me of putting cancer patients to unnecessary trouble in advising them to filter and boil their water before drinking it. It emerged that he had no idea that levels of natural and synthetic oestrogens (the latter from the female contraceptive pill) and other endocrine-disrupting chemicals in water from sewage-discharge systems could be so high in the UK that 100 per cent of the male fish downstream of such discharges are feminised.

Reprocessed drinking water can contain many other harmful chemicals, including benzene and cancer-causing organic chemicals, pesticides and disinfection by-products such as trihalomethanes (THMs) and haloacetic acids (HAAs). More rigorous limits for disinfection by-products are being legislated for in America.[103] For these and other reasons I do not drink water straight from the tap. Nevertheless, I continue to advise against bottled water since some bottled waters can contain such high levels of radioactivity or nitrates that they would be illegal if they came out of the tap. This is important advice when travelling. For example, the Indian government has ordered a revision of national safety standards for drinking water after the Centre for Science and Environment in New Delhi found pesticide residues in bottled drinking water that were 36 times higher than the maximum limits set by the European Commission.[104]

I use tap water but I filter it through charcoal into a glass jug. I have found it impossible to buy a filtration unit made completely of glass but the plastic is hard and when thoroughly washed is unlikely to release into the water the high concentrations of phthalates associated with soft plastic. After filtering I always boil the water before drinking it to remove or further reduce harmful chemicals and to take out germs not removed by water treatment. These can occur in tap water and bottled water from shallow sources, and I always add tea or herbal teas to try to further remove pollutants (lots of organic plant matter absorbs harmful chemicals onto the surface, removing it from the liquid that you drink). This takes out or reduces many harmful chemical residues, which, if they are given the opportunity, will sorb on to something such as charcoal or organic matter instead.

It is particularly important to boil water before drinking when undergoing chemotherapy because technically such patients are regarded as immunocompromised. Over the past fifteen years or so it has become apparent that a protozoan parasite (related to the malaria parasite) called Cryptosporidium, can cause severe sickness, vomiting, dehydration and diarrhoea in immunocompromised people, with symptoms which can persist indefinitely (although the gastroenteritis it causes usually clears up on its own in healthy individuals). In 1993 more than 400,000 people were affected and several people died after Cryptosporidium breached a water filtration plant in Milwaukee, Wisconsin. Prevention involves boiling (including of bottled water if it is from shallow sources), and frequent and thorough hand washing and bedding changes. Infection has been reported via pets, livestock and wildlife.[105]

I never drink coffee but I drink lots of Chinese, Japanese or Korean green tea with no milk (if you use lemon or lime, remove the peel first unless you are using unwaxed organic fruits). Extracts of green tea have been shown to prevent cancer in experimental animals. The chemicals thought to have anti-cancer properties in green tea are polyphenols known as cathechins including epigallo-cathechin-3 gallate, an antioxidant that accounts for much of the solid materials in brewed green tea.[106] It is thought that the well-known anti-cancer activity of green tea is because it inhibits one of the most frequently over-expressed enzymes in human cancers, called urokinase.[107]

Evidence of the cancer-protecting properties of green tea continue to emerge. Recent studies have confirmed that epigallo-catechin-3-gallate has a protective role against several types of epithelial cancers, including prostate cancer.[108] Experimental studies on mice with a type of prostate cancer that mimics a progressive form of human prostate cancer showed that an infusion equivalent to six cups of green tea a day for humans significantly inhibited the development and spread of the cancer and increased overall survival. It has also been suggested that green tea is a stronger antioxidant than vitamin C.[109] Green tea also helps to neutralise free radicals.

Drinking fluid this way is exactly what the Chinese do. When I first worked in China, I used to wonder what the jam jars with strange looking bits in the bottom were in the front of taxis. Eventually, I realised they were jars of green tea! Chinese, Japanese and Korean green teas used to contain fewer pesticides than commonly produced black tea, although this may no longer be true, as they become increasingly Westernised. In China, green tea is valued for its digestive properties and for assisting circulation and regulating body temperature. Preparation of black teas, unlike green teas, involves fermentation.[110] Black tea can contain twice the amount of caffeine (as theine) when compared to coffee; the tannin content of black tea can also inhibit iron uptake, and brewing black tea oxidises the cathechins, according to some authors, destroying any beneficial effects.[111] I recommend drinking at least six cups a day of organic green tea certified by the Soil Association (and buy Fair Trade, which guarantees a better deal for Third World producers, whenever you can).

I also use herbal teas, mostly peppermint or camomile with honey (many people do not like the taste of pure camomile at first). I also use fruit teas – but sparingly because some are so acid that if I drink too much they give me cystitis. Also some contain artificial chemicals of the kind used to flavour jellies and sweets (the give-away is that they are called 'fruit flavoured') and I avoid these.

Alcohol has been incriminated in prostate cancer, although, observing the quantities of rice wine and moutai (the Chinese equivalent of strong spirits) drunk by Chinese men, it is difficult to believe that it can be an important factor.

Oliver and others[112] found that those with prostate cancer were more likely to be heavy alcohol consumers (22 units a week or more) than those without the disease (19 per cent v 26 per cent), but the studies were carried out on Western men likely to be eating a typical Western diet.

Studies are also being carried out in Sweden to assess the effects of alcohol on IGF-I and the proteins which can inactivate IGF-binding proteins.[113]

Alcoholic beverages such as red wine can contain hidden animal-produce ingredients which it would be difficult to take account of in such studies. Also, if wine is stored in plastic-lined vats it can contain an endocrine-disrupting chemical bisphenol A (BPA).[114] According to the website of the Vegan Society,[115] many wines on sale have been fined – that is any sediment in them has been cleared (I can remember when wines had to be decanted to remove any sediment) – using one of the following: animal blood, bone marrow, chitosan (from the hard parts of insects and crustacea such as shrimps and crabs), albumen (egg white), fish oil, gelatin (obtained by boiling animal tissues such as skin, tendons, ligaments or bones), isinglass (a fish's swim bladder), milk or milk casein (precipitated from milk). Non-animal alternatives used in wines labelled as vegan include limestone, clays and silica gel. But remember that wines labelled as vegetarian may have been fined using casein (milk protein). In the case of beer, isinglass is used especially for real ales. Keg, canned and some bottled beers are usually cleared without the use of animal substances. The production of spirits generally does not appear to involve the use of animal substances (vodka is filtered using birchwood charcoal). The Vegan Society website[116] gives a list of good sources of vegan alcoholic beverages. I continue to drink organically produced cider, perry, beer and occasionally organic vegan wine. I avoid all diet drinks since these are likely to contain man-made sweeteners. Some ciders also contain man-made sweeteners.

I drank very little alcohol before I had cancer and I had none during treatment. I drink some alcohol now.

When I had active cancer I drank no black tea or alcohol and I never drink coffee. One of the benefits of removing these substances from my diet when I was ill was that I felt less anxious (without caffeine) and less depressed (without alcohol). Some of my fellow patients who felt the need to drown their sorrows noticeably fared badly and many were clearly depressed. You should certainly avoid alcohol during chemotherapy.

THIRST QUENCHERS: TEN DRINKS TO DELIGHT YOU	
If You Used To Do This . . .	*Now Do This!*
Start the day with a hot black one	Make it a hot yannoh instead. This is the finest cereal 'coffee' on the market. Try brewing it with 2–3 pods of cardamom and a few whole cloves.
Drink strong milky tea all day long (as I used to do)	Try switching to rooibos tea, available at health-food stores. It is strong, caffeine-free and tastes good with soya milk.
Drink black tea with sliced lemon	That's better, but better still try green tea or a strongly flavoured herbal tea such as nettle or dandelion.
Treat yourself to a Starbuck's hot chocolate	Order it made with soya milk. When you make it yourself, try making it with carob instead. This is a chocolate-flavoured bean that is tasty and nutritious but caffeine-free.
Guzzle cola all day long	Buy sarsaparilla concentrate from a health-food shop or herbalist and dilute to taste with sparkling mineral water.

Swig soft drinks by the gallon	Dilute natural fruit or flower cordials, such as elderflower, with sparkling mineral water. If you have active cancer, prepare freshly made vegetable and fruit juices and down as many as you can.
Enjoy a jug of iced coffee now and then	Brew the yannoh and cardamom, above, and leave to cool. Pour a little into an ice-cube tray and freeze. Blend the cooled yannoh with cold soya milk, whisk and serve with an ice cube.
Lead a single-handed campaign to double the government recommendations for intake of alcohol	Switch to the types of alcohol from the vegan website, and drink in moderation.
Spend huge amounts on fresh juices from the chill cabinets in your supermarket	Make fresh juices with your own juicer and organic fruit and veg. Try melon, apple and celery, pear, apple and fennel, carrot and parsley, and so on.
Think carrot juice was a cure for sunburn	Make your own with organic carrots. Add a quarter pint of carrot juice to a half pint of cold soya milk, stir well and serve with a straw.

THE PLANT PROGRAMME

A recent report from the Royal College of Physicians asks doctors to pay more attention to nutrition status, something they have neglected in the past and which can cause many health problems and delay recovery. It can also increase health-care costs. Their report calls for nutrition to be tackled seriously and included in undergraduate and post-graduate training of doctors and other health-care staff.[117] Hear! Hear! – and about time too!

In the meantime, *The Plant Programme* gives full details of what to eat and what not to eat for those with prostate (or breast) cancer, and provides dietary regimens for those suffering from active cancer and for those wanting to avoid getting these cancers or having recurrences. There is space here for only a brief summary.

The basis of the dietary recommendations in the Plant Programme is:

1. To reduce the intake of natural hormones and growth factors from food

How?

- Eliminate **all** dairy produce, including hidden dairy, from cows, sheep or goats.
- Cut down on the amount of animal food eaten – the total amount of animal food such as meat, fish and eggs should comprise less than 10 per cent of daily intake for the prevention of cancer, and should be eliminated as much as possible by those with active cancer.
- Eat only organically produced meat or game that is thoroughly cooked, in order to break down hormones, growth factors and pollutants (but do not burn it because this will form other damaging carcinogenic chemicals).
- Replace animal protein, especially dairy, with soya-based food, and meals combining cereals, pulses and nuts.

2. To reduce the intake of man-made chemicals for which there is evidence for, or a suspicion of, carcinogenicity, especially endocrine-disrupting chemicals

These are suspected of promoting cancers of the reproductive organs, including the prostate and breast, and also testicular cancer and cancer of the womb and ovaries. Endocrine-disrupting chemicals are persistent and accumulate in the food chain, becoming particularly concentrated in certain foods.

How?

- Avoid all dairy produce, untreated fish-liver oils and farmed fish such as salmon, unless it is organically farmed.

- Eat only organically produced meat, especially in the case of fat meats such as pork and duck, and even then remove the fat and the skin.
- Do not use plastic, especially soft plastic wrappings, or eat food from cans with plastic linings.
- Filter tap water through charcoal, then boil it and store in glass bottles.
- Drink liquids stored in glass with cork or aluminium seals, but not in plastic bottles.
- Never have 'diet' drinks, or other food or drink that contains man-made sweeteners such as saccharine or aspartame.

3. To increase the proportion of food that is protective against cancer

How?
- Eat as much fresh organic vegetables and fruit as possible, especially red vegetables such as tomatoes, red peppers and chillies; cruciferous vegetables such as bok choy, cauliflower and broccoli; and orange vegetables, including peppers, carrots and pumpkin.
- Eat lots of fresh herbs.
- Eat vegetables as fresh and raw as possible and have at least five large portions of fruit and vegetables as salads or juices every day. The UK Government recommendation of five portions a day, which includes prepared fruit and vegetables is completely inadequate for healthy living – one portion should be at least one piece of fruit or half a cup of raw vegetables.
- Eat a diet rich in phyto-oestrogens including soya and other beans and peas, whole-grain cereals (especially flax), nuts and berries (the best are cranberries), and sprouting seeds (such as alfalfa).
- Eat spices, many of which have antioxidant properties. Turmeric, in particular, causes cancer cells to commit suicide.
- Eat lots of garlic, which has anti-cancer properties and other health benefits, and onions and chives.
- Drink lots of green tea.

4. To ensure that you consume adequate quantities of the key nutrients in a bio-available form, so that a significant proportion can be absorbed by the body

This is especially true of nutrients such as zinc, iodine and folic acid, which play a crucial role in cell division in the body (which is when the errors that cause cancer are most likely to arise).

How?
- Eat more fresh or lightly cooked vegetables and fruit, nuts and seeds, seaweed, wild or organically produced fish and shellfish.
- Have some brewer's yeast and kelp every day (follow the instructions on the packet or bottle and ensure you take the correct dose).
- Have some ultra-pure cod liver oil every day.

5. To reduce the amount of free radicals in the body which are capable of damaging DNA

How?
- Yet more fruit and vegetables and whole grains.
- Take a good-quality selenium supplement.
- Eat garlic, fresh herbs and spices.
- Drink lots of green tea.

6. To eliminate or reduce to a minimum food that has been refined, preserved or overcooked
In such foods, the content of fibre, vitamins, minerals, natural colours or other natural constituents have been removed or reduced. Be especially vigilant in avoiding man-made chemical substances, including artificial vitamins or minerals.

How?
- Cut out or cut down on manufactured convenience food, especially anything with 'E' numbers in it. Frozen foods are usually OK and there is an increasing range of organically produced food available in bottles, jars and cans, which are fine occasionally.
- Cut down or cut out refined sugar – use molasses, rice or maple syrup or honey.
- Use brown unrefined flour, pasta and rice.
- Ensure everything is as fresh, natural and unaltered as possible.
- Cut down on or, ideally, cut out salt – use a little sea salt if absolutely necessary.
- Substitute green tea and herbal teas such as camomile, fennel, peppermint and clover for black tea and coffee.

- Do not binge on alcohol, but enjoy an occasional good-quality organic wine recommended on the Vegan Society's website, or have a small good-quality malt whisky.
- Eat good freshly made food to avoid the need for vitamin or mineral supplements.

7. To provide the nutrients to help your body withstand and recover from surgery, radiotherapy and chemotherapy

Many drugs, including those used in chemotherapy, destroy vitamins. Stress means you need more vitamins, while antibiotics can prevent them being absorbed.

How?
- Eat unrefined food, including whole-grain cereals.
- Drink as much freshly made fruit and vegetable juice as possible.
- Garlic, seaweed and organic eggs contain substances that help repair DNA.
- Take brewer's yeast, which is a good source of B vitamins, folic acid and minerals.

8. To provide maximum choice and variety, so that healthy eating can be maintained without too much reliance on any one food substance

How?
- Have at least thirty different ingredients a day.
- Use herbs and spices to add flavour.

All this might sound a bit daunting, but when you have adjusted and are preparing and eating the great meals described in *The Plant Programme*, I believe you will be a convert for life – especially when your health and appearance begin to improve. Anyway, in that book we have done all the hard work for you. All you need to do is make the delicious meals described and follow the simple point-scoring system to help prevent or treat prostate cancer.

6 The Lifestyle Factors

There are important things, apart from diet, that you can change to help cut your risk of prostate cancer. In this chapter I discuss eight lifestyle factors, from strategies for coping with stress to ways of avoiding harmful substances in your environment.

LIFESTYLE FACTOR 1: VITAMINS, MINERAL SUPPLEMENTS AND FOOD FORTIFICATION

Most vitamins (A, B complex and folic acid, C, D, E and K) and several minerals, including selenium, zinc and iodine, are considered to protect against cancer, partly because of their antioxidant properties. Zinc, for example, helps to maintain epithelial and tissue integrity and acts as an antioxidant.[1] A new study published in the *Journal of the American Medical Association* asserts that nearly all adult Americans have dietary deficiencies in one or more vitamins and should be taking multivitamin supplements.[2] The American diet is such that this is unsurprising. See, for example, the comparison of the American and Chinese diets reported by researchers from Cornell University, USA, Oxford University, UK and Beijing University, China.[3]

One of the first experimental and observational studies to show that taking vegetable or other pills does not help involved beta-carotene. In a study beginning in 1985, beta-carotene was included in two large long-term trials sponsored by the National Cancer Institute in the USA. Previous epidemiological studies had suggested that diets high in beta-carotene (for instance, from carrots) reduced lung-cancer incidence. In the trial studies, daily doses of beta-carotene in combination with either vitamin E or vitamin A were administered for several years to tens of thousands of people thought to be at high risk of developing lung cancer. What happened? The rate of lung cancer in those taking the pills increased in both trials![4]

A recent Canadian study also showed that women who took large doses of vitamins and minerals during conventional treatment for breast cancer were more likely to relapse and die than women who did not.[5] The five-year survival rate for patients prescribed vitamin C, beta-carotene, niacin (vitamin B3), zinc, selenium and coenzyme Q10 was 72 per cent, compared with 81 per cent for the control group. Over a ten-year period, those who took large doses of vitamins and minerals were 10 per cent more likely to die. The investigators were surprised with the results, because they were expecting that the patients prescribed vitamin and mineral supplements would have a 25–30 per cent increase in survival rates.

In an editorial article in the *BMJ* in July 2002,[6] consideration of the value of daily doses of multivitamin tablets concluded that regular consumption would probably do no good unless your intake was inadequate as a result of poor diet. The article recommends only folic acid for women before and after conception (but if you eat enough green leafy vegetables – or fruits such as melon – this is unnecessary), and perhaps vitamin D in elderly people. In the case of cancer, the article refers to unexpected results that more people receiving supposedly protective supplements died than people receiving placebos.

The vice chair of the panel of US Preventive Services Task Force has also stated that there is insufficient scientific evidence to support the notion that taking certain vitamins will prevent cancer. She pointed out that people should strive to eat the healthiest diet possible and that nutrients from supplements may not offer the same benefits that they do when consumed as part of a healthy diet.[7]

In the UK, the Food Standards Agency has suggested that many people could be damaging their health by taking vitamin and mineral supplements in doses that are too high. The agency's expert group on vitamins and minerals has spent four years looking at the evidence on the potential harmful effects of taking high doses of 34 vitamins and minerals that can be bought over the counter. It found enough evidence to suggest safe upper levels for 8 of them and suggested guidance on 23. It also issued statements on three minerals. Two supplements – beta-carotene and chromium – were found to have the potential to cause cancer in some people and should be avoided by smokers and those who have been exposed to asbestos. Chromium picolinate supplements may also cause cancer and should be avoided.[8]

Other evidence against taking pills involves zinc, which, as discussed earlier, is crucial for prostate health. Men who took more than 100mg a day of zinc supplements were found to have more than twice the risk of advanced prostate cancer. These levels are far above the recommended doses. However, in the USA, a significant number of men take higher than the recommended levels of zinc supplements, partly because of their supposed benefit in preventing colds. Again the message is clear: DO NOT take man-made vitamin or mineral supplements. Have them as nature intended – as part of a good diet.[9]

Selenium status can often be marginal to deficient in UK diets and it is important for immune function generally and as an antioxidant. It works best in conjunction with vitamin E, since both are antioxidants and can increase the production of antibodies by up to thirty times,[10] greatly enhancing your immune response. Selenium is essential to health, though required only in minute quantities. Although it is not certain at precisely what level selenium begins to cause adverse effects, it has been found that doses of 900 micrograms (0.9 milligrams) per day can make hair and nails fall out and affect the nervous system.[11]

Vitamin D, which is stored in fat, is also considered to be protective against prostate cancer (*see* p. 118), but consuming large quantities in tablets can produce toxic effects.[12] Vitamin D forms in the skin under the influence of solar ultraviolet light, so that outdoor exercise wearing light clothing in sunny weather is usually adequate. Good food sources include oily fish and eggs, and only vegans living in cold climates or the housebound elderly need consider taking supplements. In the latter case I would recommend the ultra-pure versions of fish-liver oils.

According to Oakley, as many as 350,000 deaths from coronary heart disease could have been prevented over the last decade in the UK if the government had fortified flour with folic acid when the evidence was first published.[13] This suggestion, however, neglects the fact that many people suffer from coeliac disease and therefore would not benefit. Moreover, according to Reynolds fortifying flour with folic acid understates the potential risks to the nervous system. Experimental studies confirm that folates cause convulsions if the blood-brain barrier is circumvented.[14] I am totally opposed to fortification of our food or water, whether by folic acid or fluoride. It is likely to be driven by a vested-interest group, and someone will be cashing in.

In general, I prefer to eat whole foods because, as I have indicated, problems often arise when we try to separate food into constituent parts. Moreover, vitamin/mineral pills are often synthesised from coal or petroleum derivatives. Also, taking too much of one or other man-made supplement can cause a deficiency elsewhere in the diet. For example, taking the trace element molybdenum blocks copper intake. The body knows how to deal with nutrients from natural foods, but may absorb too much or too little from man-made chemical supplements.

Food such as fruit, vegetables and whole grains contain hundreds of antioxidants (and other phytochemicals) and at least some of them work together (i.e. synergistically).[15] The protective effect of a mineral-vitamin-phytochemical-rich diet is best obtained from the consumption of adequate amounts of fruit, vegetables, legumes and whole-grain produce[16] based on a good, well-balanced diet such as the Plant Programme.

The food supplements I use

I do use supplements, but these are not man-made synthetic substances of the type discussed above: they are foods that are naturally enriched in trace nutrients. I continue to take kelp* to avoid iodine deficiency and also brewer's yeast,* which is a good source of many trace elements such as iron, and of B vitamins which are important if the body is to synthesise important compounds such as co-enzyme Q10, which is essential to the optimal functioning of all cell types and is also an antioxidant. These are all natural and not synthetic substances. I now take balanced omega-3, omega-6 vegetable oils* daily and Seven Seas ultra-pure cod-liver oil*, which I store in a cool, dark place. Also I took tablets containing selenium and vitamins A, C and E when I had active cancer. I always follow manufacturers' instructions.

If you must take man-made minerals, vitamins, supplements or any pharmaceutical products, do ensure that they are not in a lactose matrix.

LIFESTYLE FACTOR 2: FOOD PACKAGING

Food packaging is very important. A recent report, on the abundance of chemicals that mimic the female hormone oestrogen, from the authoritative British Institute of Environment and Health (IEH) has suggested that a group of chemicals called phthalates seriously disrupt reproduction in animals (including damaging the testes in males). Scientific experiments suggest that certain phthalates may also cause cancer.[17] One of the main sources of phthalates identified in the report is soft plastics such as those used to wrap and cover food. The chemicals leak from the plastic into the food, and then accumulate in our body fat. Try whenever possible to buy food in good old-fashioned brown paper bags – be prepared to make a fuss if necessary. One of my friends

---

* Follow the manufacturer's instructions for all of these and do not exceed the recommended amount – the quantity of tablets or oil depends on the brand.

dumps all plastic wrappings at supermarket tills although I have never dared go as far as that. If you find it impossible to buy food not pre-packed in plastic, and this is increasingly difficult, try to wash food as thoroughly as possible or in the case of vegetables peel or scrape off the surface which has been most in contact with the plastic. Unfortunately the chemicals concerned are fat soluble, so it is best to avoid them if possible since they are difficult to remove by washing. This is of particular concern if you are buying oily fish. My fishmonger now wraps my fish in paper or foil.

My advice is to minimise consumption of water or juices sold in plastic bottles, food purchased in cans, and wines stored in vats[18] lined with plastics, which can contain the endocrine-disrupting substance bisphenol A (BPA). Try to eat fresh or frozen food, and drink wines stored in oak.

LIFESTYLE FACTOR 3: COOKING

Love it or hate it, cooking is an essential part of our diet and lifestyle. In amongst all the aromas and sizzles, it has an effect on the food that can be enhancing or potentially destructive. For instance, it changes starches, proteins and some vitamins into forms that the body can absorb readily as well as releasing nutrients in some foods, which are otherwise unavailable – like the amino acid tryptophan in cornmeal. Cooking of some foods is necessary to destroy toxic substances such as those found in red beans, and cooking also makes some foods more palatable. However, it can destroy and leach fragile nutrients in food, although there are ways in which you can reduce this nutrient loss.

The style of cooking recommended in the Plant Programme ensures that fresh, wholesome ingredients are cooked in the healthiest way possible and served as soon as possible. Two very important rules are:

- Never use a microwave cooker, because free radicals are formed in the food.
- Never use a pressure cooker, because it destroys vitamins and other important nutrients.

The way meat is cooked is important. My mother and all her generation of British women were taught to cook meat thoroughly, and that meant slowly. For all sorts of reasons, including preventing cancer, I will not now eat undercooked meat under any circumstances. Meat is a poor conductor of heat and if it is not cooked properly hormones in it (whether natural or introduced by man) will not be destroyed. Even if it is well-cooked, steroid hormones such as those used in the USA may survive.

Cancer-promoting chemicals (heterocyclic amines (HCA), the most abundant of which is known as PhiP) are likely to be formed in burned meat, while cancer-promoting chemicals including hormones will remain intact in the relatively raw meat inside. I never eat meat that could contain ground-up dairy animal, such as hamburger or sausages. (Remember, official figures show that dairy-cow meat contains even more IGF-I than milk.) Amounts of HCA range from very low in poached, steamed or stewed meat and fish to very high levels in grilled or barbecued meat. PhiP has been linked to prostate, breast and colon cancer.[19] High levels of HCA also occur in pan-fried meat.[20] Other toxic by-products of interaction between sugars, fats, and proteins also form when food is cooked at too high a temperature.[21]

In the last few years there has been concern about the presence of a potentially cancer-causing chemical called acrylamide in certain foods, especially fried food, including chips and potato crisps. The levels of acrylamide in some foods are compared with the US Environmental Protection Agency (EPA) limit for this chemical in water in Table 6.1.

Research first announced by Swedish scientists in April 2002 and subsequently confirmed by studies in Norway, Switzerland, the UK and the USA shows levels in certain foods well above the

Table 6.1: Levels of acrylamide in foods, in micrograms per serving	
Water, 8oz, EPA limit	0.12
Boiled potatoes, 4oz	<3
Taco shells, 3, 1.1oz	1
French fries, uncooked, 3oz	5
French fries, baked, 3oz	28
Breakfast cereals, 1oz	6–7
Tortilla chips, 1oz	5
Corn chips, 1oz	11
Potato crisps, 1oz	25
French fries, 5.6–6.2oz, and potato wedges, 6.2, purchased from fast-food outlets	39–82

Data from http://www.cspinet.org/new/200206251.html

WHO guideline values for drinking-water quality.[22] Swiss researchers have also reported relatively high levels of the substance in ground roast coffee.[23]

Studies to date suggest that a minimum temperature of 120°C is needed to form acrylamide in food, although the levels increase at temperatures between 140° and 180°C. Scientists have found a ten-fold difference between normal and overcooked chips.[24] Some scientists in North America have suggested that the substance forms at high temperature by interaction of a natural amino acid called asparagine with certain sugars such as glucose.[25] Experts recommend a diet with plenty of fresh fruit and vegetables to help to counteract the problem.

Increased incidences of tumours have been observed in rats orally exposed to acrylamide. In the USA, levels of acrylamide are highly regulated.[26] The EPA has classified acrylamide as a probable human carcinogen,[27] and it is classified as a substance which may reasonably be anticipated to be a carcinogen by the US Department of Health.

Previously, concern about acrylamide had centred on occupational exposure (through the skin, or inhalation of dust or vapour) during its manufacture and use by industry, and environmental exposure.[28] Acrylamide is used in the manufacture of adhesives, dyes, soil-conditioning agents, products for sewage and waste treatment, chemical grouting, the manufacture of non-iron fabrics, crude-oil production, and the processing of paper and pulp, and some ores and concrete.[29] Some home appliances and parts of cars and other vehicles are coated with acrylamide resin and other acrylics. Acrylamides are also contained in some cosmetics and soaps (in which they act as thickeners), and in dental fixtures, hair-grooming preparations and pre-shave lotions.[30] In a report published in 1997, it was stated that no information about the natural occurrence of acrylamide was found in the readily available literature.[31]

All this information tends to suggest that acrylamide might be expected to occur at low levels in the environment in industrialised countries, from man-made sources.[32] It is a water-soluble, rather than fat-soluble, substance,[33] with a high water solubility which increases with temperature.[34]

Despite the statement by the UK Food Standards Agency[35] that frying and baking create high levels of acrylamide in a wide range of food, the high levels could reflect environmental pollution. Initially, some foods may contain the chemical as a contaminant, especially if it is used as a soil conditioner, and more may be added during processing if the food comes into contact with acrylamide-containing substances. When food is fried, the acrylamide will not be dissolved out into the fat and it is likely to become more concentrated in the food as water is lost in cooking. On the other hand, where food is boiled, the highly soluble acrylamide is likely to be lost to the cooking water. My advice remains the same as for avoiding other harmful man-made chemicals in food and drink. In other words, ignore the advice of the Food Standards Agency[36] and eat as organically as possible, following the methods of preparation and cooking set out here. Also, my advice for avoiding harmful substances generally (*see* pp. 224–8) would seem to apply to acrylamide.

In summary I lightly steam vegetables in a stainless-steel or bamboo steamer, or stir-fry lightly after first dipping vegetables in boiling water like the Chinese do. Fruit and vegetables should be eaten as raw as possible in order to preserve the vitamins and enzymes they contain. I use only organic extra-virgin olive oil to soften or gently fry vegetables. Any meat I eat is cooked slowly in the oven or under a grill and the fish I eat is just lightly grilled. I add no additional fat or salt to meat or fish, which I cook slowly with herbs or garlic and occasionally black pepper or other spices, for flavouring. I do not own a microwave and try to avoid food cooked or heated in one. Unlike normal heating, microwaving food works by vibrating water molecules in food. This generates free radicals and I suspect would not destroy as many 'bad' chemicals as ordinary cooking (although I have been unable to find any data on this). There is no comparison between the taste of a jacket potato cooked in the traditional way and the soggy unpleasant-tasting equivalent prepared by microwaving.

Here are some general guidelines:

- If you cook with fat don't let it become so hot that it starts to smoke. At this temperature the essential fatty acid linoleic acid is destroyed.
- Fats which have been used for cooking once should be discarded, since the linoleic acid and vitamins A and C will have been lost; they may have been chemically altered and become potentially carcinogenic.
- If you boil food, steam it instead and do so for the minimum amount of time; then use the water for stock. The fragile water-soluble vitamins as well as some minerals leach into cooking water, which is why soups are so nutritious.

- Don't add bicarbonate of soda to cooking water, even if it is recommended in cookery books for cooking pulses. It destroys B vitamins.
- Prepare food immediately before cooking – remember that vitamin C is destroyed once cells are damaged in vegetables – and for the same reason try not to chop them too finely. Scrubbing vegetables is better than peeling them.
- Once prepared, immerse the vegetables in boiling water straight away before stir-frying.
- Use pans with close-fitting lids and avoid using copper pans which encourage oxidation and vitamin C loss. I use stainless-steel pans and bamboo baskets for steaming.
- Once food is cooked, eat it straight away. Keeping it warm will result in further nutrient loss, which is why eating out too frequently may be less healthy for you.

LIFESTYLE FACTOR 4: DEALING WITH STRESS

The word 'cancer' is terrifying to most people, and in *Your Life in Your Hands* I described the horror I felt at discovering I had breast cancer. But remember that new medicines have been developed that effectively relieve most of the worst symptoms of cancer, including pain and nausea – including that caused by treatment. Modern prostate-cancer treatments are effective and are given with an increasingly significant chance for a positive response.[37]

In an article entitled 'ABC of psychological medicine: Cancer',[38] White and Macleod point out that cancer is the most feared of diseases and causes considerable psychological distress, including depression and anxiety, in patients and their families, and even in health professionals who care for them. A diagnosis of cancer can precipitate feelings similar to bereavement (it is worth noting that a recent study showed that people who profess stronger spiritual beliefs seem to resolve grief more rapidly than people with no spiritual beliefs[39]). Severe and persistent depressive disorder is up to 4 times more common in cancer patients than in the general population, and occurs in 10–20 per cent of people affected by the disease. Feelings of loss may be reaction to perceived loss, for example of sexual potency in the case of prostate cancer, the role in family or society, or impending loss of life. Anxiety can manifest itself as apprehension, uncontrollable worry, restlessness, panic attacks, and avoidance of people and of reminders of cancer. Patients may overestimate the risks associated with treatment and the likelihood of a poor outcome.

Anxiety can also exacerbate or heighten perceptions of physical symptoms that patients can interpret as cancer symptoms, and post-traumatic-stress symptoms occasionally follow diagnosis or treatment that the patient has found particularly frightening. Certain cancers and treatments are associated with specific fears. For example, patients may develop phobias and conditioned vomiting in relation to treatments such as chemotherapy.[40]

Distress is more likely to occur at specific points in a patient's experience of cancer. These include:[41]

- *Diagnosis*, when doctors should explain that feelings such as shock, anger, disbelief and distress are normal.
- *During treatment*, especially at times when treatment appears to be failing.
- *At the end of treatment*, because of the fear that the cancer might recur.
- *After treatment*, because of fear of recurrence and misinterpretation of symptoms (such as believing that pain associated with a muscle strain represents a recurrence of cancer).
- *Recurrence*. Most patients report recurrence of cancer as more distressing than receiving the initial diagnosis.

The principles of treatment[42] to help such patients involve:

- A clearly identified principal therapist to coordinate care.
- Sympathetic interest and concern.
- Effective symptomatic relief.
- Understanding the patient's concerns and needs.
- Collaborative planning of continuing care.
- Good information and advice.
- Involvement of the patient in treatment decisions.
- Involvement of family and friends.
- Early recognition and treatment of psychological complications.
- Clear arrangements to deal with urgent problems.

Let me turn now to some of the things that I found helpful and some that I did not.

The idea that cancer could be cured by thinking positively had always seemed ill-founded to me. One of the particular problems with the 'think positive' approach is that people who do not get better often feel guilty that they are not trying hard enough, and this is sometimes reinforced by well-meaning friends. In the book

You Can Heal Your Life by Louise Hay, there is a list of diseases and their probable causes. In the case of cancer, the probable cause is given as 'deep hurt, long-standing resentment, deep secret or grief eating away at the self; carrying hatreds; what's the use.' The advice is to develop a new thought pattern as follows: 'I lovingly forgive and release all of the past. I choose to fill my world with joy. I love and approve of myself.' This may be admirable as a general attitude to life, but when it comes to preventing cancer I prefer a more rational approach, based on science.

It has also been claimed that there is a particular personality type that is likely to be affected by breast cancer. Much has been written about the 'cancer personality' especially by Lawrence LeShan, an American psychotherapist. According to LeShan, the typical personality had an emotionally deprived youth, followed by a period of fulfilment in an intense relationship or all-involving work, followed by the loss of that relationship or work at which time the cancer occurs. The other main characteristic is the person's inability to express anger, particularly in their own defence; such a person is often described by others as being like a saint. LeShan believed that this pattern fitted 76 per cent of his patients. This is certainly not a description of me or my life and I cannot think of anyone else I know who has had breast cancer who fits this description!

All carefully controlled research indicates that this theory is wrong. The concept is unhelpful, and again tends to lead to feelings of guilt. As indicated earlier, the problem is one of chemistry and is rooted in the Western diet. The book *Wild Swans* by Jung Chang provides a vivid example of the high levels of stress that Chinese women have suffered in the past, yet they retained low breast-cancer rates except when they have changed to a Western diet.

A recent systematic review of the influence of psychological coping on survival and recurrence in people with cancer[43] supports the view that positive thinking is not key to fighting cancer. It found that most of the studies that investigated fighting spirit or feelings of helplessness or hopelessness found no significant associations with survival or recurrence. The authors conclude that people with cancer should not feel pressured into adopting particular coping styles.

Also some people feel guilt that their cancer is some form of punishment. I certainly felt that but, as I now say in all the many lectures I give, cancer is not brought about by a wrathful God.

Almost all cancers, and certainly prostate cancer, have far more rational explanations, as discussed in this book.

Because stress has been implicated as an important factor in cancer generally, people can become worried and hence more stressed by problems so that a vicious circle is set up. Over the last ten and a half years I have faced up to some extremely stressful situations in my family life and at work, and yet my cancer has not returned – because fundamentally it was a problem caused by harmful chemicals from my food and the environment causing problems in my body. Now my diet and lifestyle are sound, I cope much better with stress.

However, for your health and general well-being it is helpful to reduce the stress and distress in your life as much as possible, and there is scientific evidence that stress has physiological effects suggesting it is worthwhile working on methods of reducing sources of stress. The chemical changes in the body caused by stress would need a book in themselves. Hormones from the adrenal gland as part of the body's 'fight or flight' mechanism increase the amount of blood sugar available, boost heart rate and slow down digestive function to enable us to run or fight. Too much for too long, however, can affect the immune system. As mentioned earlier, prolactin levels also increase as a result of stress.

When humans are confronted by an important loss or change in their lifestyle – such as a diagnosis of breast cancer – their emotions are likely to follow a pattern which is well known to counsellors and others trained to help with our emotional well-being. Initially, denial, shock, numbness and grief may be experienced, followed by resistance, gradual acceptance and depression before beginning to let go of the old reality and adjust to the new one. People differ in the intensity of their emotions and the time taken for each part of the cycle. Indeed, in the case of cancer some people simply give up hope and never leave the 'trough of despair'. This can be a particularly serious problem with prostate cancer, I suspect, because of the fear of impotence and incontinence. Some people remain in denial, and I receive much correspondence from people intending to refuse conventional medical treatment and simply follow my programme. I always advise against such a course of action in the strongest possible terms.

In my case, when confronted with problems I tend to move to the 'what can be done about it' stage very quickly, and of course one of the frustrations with being confronted with a diagnosis of prostate (or breast) cancer is that according to orthodox medicine the answer is, 'nothing'. If you have heart disease you can follow a diet and exercise plan, if you have an infectious illness you can take tablets and rest, but with prostate cancer you are told there is nothing you can do.

I totally disagree with this and with doctors who advise that you simply accept your fate because it will bring peace. On the contrary, you must be empowered to help yourself and, as I have explained, there is a lot you can do to help yourself with crucially important changes in diet and lifestyle. The diet itself, in addition to helping you fight cancer directly, will help your state of mental and emotional well-being by providing greatly improved nutrition.

Several complementary and alternative medicine treatments have been suggested to improve the well-being of patients with cancer. These include: mind-body programmes for stress; acupuncture or acupressure for nausea; tai chi and other gentle exercise techniques to improve strength; therapeutic massage and relaxation techniques to reduce stress; and herbal medicines for depression and anxiety.[44]

Let us look at some of the particular problems associated with coping with prostate cancer, such as incontinence and impotence.

Concerns about sexual potency are often of very great concern to men with prostate cancer (*see* Chapter 1) and it is important to discuss worries with partners because they are affected as well. Partners are usually concerned about how to express their love during and after treatment. Suggestions that may help a man cope better include involving his partner as soon as possible after treatment, openly communicating feelings, needs, and wants, and seeking the support of others.[45] Some marriages and family relationships break down following the wife and mother suffering from breast cancer, and I have heard of many such cases. However, I cannot think of a single case where this has happened with any of the prostate-cancer sufferers who correspond with me.

Some other coping strategies include psychotherapy which, according to MIND, the mental health charity, is particularly helpful in understanding, and coming to terms with, past events.

Cognitive therapy teaches you to trace the building of frightening scenarios backwards and stop at the facts. This can help to develop a more sensible, rational, less frightening vision, which is especially useful for cancer patients. Again according to MIND, cognitive therapy is about learning to think and behave in positive ways. It is a type of behavioural therapy which is helpful in overcoming negative thinking. If you think this would be helpful, ensure that you consult an expert in cognitive therapy, since most GPs have had little training in this field.[46] My psychotherapist also taught me how to be more assertive without being aggressive, which helps avoid situations where one is affected by negative emotions. For example if you calmly but clearly state your concerns or dislikes, many situations that lead to negative emotions can be avoided. There are many excellent books on cognitive therapy and assertive behaviour which are well worth reading.

I have to say that I found counselling of the type based on trying to release pent-up emotions far less helpful than psycho-therapy or cognitive therapy. The analogy I would use about my counselling sessions is that of a pond in which emotions had settled to the bottom and the water had cleared, and every week I was encouraged to put in a large stick and stir it around until I became upset. Counsellors are trained never to give reassurances and by repeating answers to 'how do you feel about that' or 'what is your worst fear' you may be giving your brain only negative feedback and reinforcing fears. Many people find counselling helpful – it just did not work for me. Also self-help and support groups made me feel that I was 'wallowing in cancer', although others have found attending such groups useful.

The person I found most helpful was a lady who has become one of my dearest friends – Peggy Heason who is a trained hypnotherapist. I found sessions with her extremely beneficial. Also, having brought up her family through difficult situations she has so much common sense and she was prepared to reassure me where she could. But above all she was always there for me. She was not as emotionally involved as my own family so she was better able to help me. If you have cancer or any other serious problems in your life, my advice is to find yourself a Peggy Heason. I went to relaxation sessions with her and I also used her relaxation tapes a great deal.[47]

The basis of many techniques to reduce stress and tension start with relaxation. First, turn off the telephone, doorbell etc. so you will not be interrupted. Then turn off the light or draw the curtains and lie flat (I do this without a pillow – at most use only one) and make sure you are warm and comfortable. Then systematically relax each part of your body, beginning with your toes, then your feet, your lower legs, gradually progressing up through the body. Repeat until you feel totally relaxed. This way you relax each bit of you from toe to top. There are several good relaxation tapes based on these methods, but Peggy Heason's was the one that I found the best. At the same time I used diaphragm breathing, which is very relaxing. When we are anxious we tend to take lots of shallow breaths by breathing using only the ribcage. Diaphragm breathing is a technique to ensure you are using your full lung capacity by using the large muscle called the diaphragm at the base of the lung cavity to suck in and expel air. You simply place your hands on your abdomen and make sure that they go up and down as you breathe in and out.

Used with imagery you can accompany your relaxation by imagining yourself walking through a beautiful calm garden listening to the birdsong or walking along a beautiful beach with waves gently crashing on the sand. It is possible to buy tapes to guide you through imagery and relaxation but do listen to them first. I found some voices on tapes that I bought incredibly irritating. It is important to find ones that you enjoy and find helpful because you will probably use them many times. Many such tapes are readily available from health and new-age shops. Some include affirmations (quiet verbal instructions) and subliminal messages to your body. I also learned meditation, which I still use. Despite being such a simple method, it clears worries out of the mind and allows deep relaxation. I chose the word crystal, and I repeat it continuously in my mind and visualise the crystal sparkling. After a time one feels truly relaxed. I found meditation difficult at first because I am normally a busy-busy sort of person but the technique really does clear my mind and helps me in my work especially in solving problems.

I now find yoga helpful as well. There is a great deal of evidence of the effectiveness of such techniques in reducing stress and the physical symptoms that this creates in the body. Several of the methods lower blood pressure, for example.

Another technique sometimes used for cancer patients is visualisation, a technique made famous by the Simontons in the USA. This involves imagining your body killing the cancer, removing the debris and finally visualising situations where you are well and whole again. I found visualisation techniques unhelpful but others feel better for using them.

What I learned was how important it is that you understand how distressed your family is, if your relationships are to survive cancer. They will all react differently. They are having to come to terms with their own distress, fears and anxieties about your illness as well as helping and supporting you. They have different personalities with different capabilities and methods of coping. Try not to dump your fears, feelings and anxieties onto them – they may be too close and too frightened and upset already and families can quickly enter damaging downward-spiralling emotional situations.

Try instead to rely on others who care but are not so close that their fears become amplified and spiral out of control. A group of my friends, all professionals with busy lives, each gave some of their time to take me to hospital and stay with me during radiotherapy and chemotherapy treatments. Somehow they worked together as an efficient team, each giving the help and the time they could spare to provide me with a wonderful cocoon of total care. When they asked me how they could help I managed to shed my typically British reserve and independence and tell them.

Working with your friends is a two-way process and can be so helpful. If you want to do something for a friend with cancer, ask them sincerely how you can help and show that you mean it. All sorts of practical things – doing some shopping, going with them for treatment – means so much at such times.

Some friends simply cannot cope. This is a common experience for cancer patients. Try to understand that these people do care about you, but they just do not know how to cope themselves. Do not allow yourself to become bitter. Let them back into your life when they feel able to cope.

The level of fatigue after cancer treatment is the largest factor in predicting a return to work. Nearly two thirds (64 per cent) of cancer survivors in a study of 235 patients were back at work within 18 months. The duration of sick leave depended on diagnosis, treatment, age, physical complaints and workload.[48]

During my illness, I found it helpful to keep working and I took the minimum of sick leave. This gave me a sense of purpose and took my mind off my problems. Many other friends and colleagues with cancer or with partners with cancer have also found the routine of going to work helpful in coping with the disease. Of course, this depends on the type of work you do, the working environment and your personality, and it requires a supportive boss and colleagues. Friends and colleagues showered me with flowers, messages and cards, and they telephoned me a lot – this type of support can be very important in maintaining morale, although other cancer sufferers prefer just to be left alone.

I think that the best way of coping emotionally can be summed up by quoting a friend and former colleague, Dr Chris Evans, whose wife, Norma, sadly died of cancer in 1995, 'I learnt during the four years that Norma was ill that we all react differently. There is no right or wrong way. There are people out there who can help and people who are going through the same thing. These people can suggest a range of coping strategies, but friendship, openness and love are at the heart of most.'

The big dos and don'ts[49]

- Do not believe the old adage 'cancer equals death'. Today, many cancers are curable; others can be controlled for long periods, during which new treatments may become available.
- Do not believe that you caused your cancer. There is no evidence linking specific personalities, emotional states or painful life events to the development of cancer.
- Do rely on strategies that helped you solve problems in the past, such as gathering information, talking to others and finding ways to feel in control. Seek help if they don't work.
- Do not feel guilty if you can't keep a 'positive' attitude all the time. Low periods will occur, no matter how good you are at coping. There is no evidence that these periods have a negative effect on your health. If they become too frequent or severe, though, seek help.
- Do use support and self-help groups if they make you feel better. Leave any that make you feel worse.
- Do not be embarrassed to seek counsel from a mental-health professional. It is a sign of strength, not weakness, and it may help you to tolerate your symptoms and treatments better. I recommend against pills for anxiety wherever possible. I am still suffering the after-effects of such treatment ten years on (see Lifestyle Factor 5).
- Do use any methods that aid you in gaining control over your emotions, such as meditation and relaxation.
- Do find a doctor of whom you can ask questions and with whom you feel mutual respect and trust. Insist on being a partner with him or her in your treatment. Ask what side effects to expect and be prepared for them. Anticipating problems often makes them easier to handle if they occur.
- Do not keep your worries to yourself. If the person closest to you can cope, involve them. If they find it difficult you may need to involve a group of friends so each can give you some support. If all else fails, phone the Samaritans and talk to them of your fears. Ask a close friend to accompany you to visits to the doctor when treatments are to be discussed.

- Do explore spiritual and religious beliefs and practices that may have helped you in the past. They may comfort you and even help you find meaning in the experience of illness.
- Do not abandon your treatment in favour of an alternative method, especially those which make no sense and are irrational. But do change your diet and lifestyle in the ways described here to help to overcome your disease and withstand treatment.

LIFESTYLE FACTOR 5: SLEEPLESSNESS AND FATIGUE

One of the common problems of cancer sufferers is that of sleeplessness. Ten years on, I am still affected by this problem. In my case, it was probably made worse by the strong tranquillisers I was prescribed to make me sleep when it was thought that I was terminally ill.

Alternative techniques for helping people to sleep include herbal substances, but I have found these to be ineffective.

Methods I have found to be helpful include the use of acupressure cones, which can be bought from high-street chemists and applied to the acupuncture sleep points on the wrists as shown in the accompanying leaflets. One tip is to buy travel bands instead, since, unlike the cones, they can be re-used many times. They work on the same principle as the cones, but are intended for use on different acupuncture points on the wrists, to prevent nausea. I use them with the studs placed on the sleep pressure points, which saves money and avoids using yet more plastic.

I listen to self-hypnosis tapes, available widely in bookstores and health food shops (mine come from Peggy Heason, *see* p. 210). I also find it calming to have a bowl of organic porridge with a little soya milk before going to bed (though this may not be suitable for those with a gluten allergy); oats were the traditional treatment for hyperactivity in children and are still used by herbalists to help overcome benzodiazepin, valium, alcoholism and some other types of drug addiction.[50]

LIFESTYLE FACTOR 6: AVOIDING HARMFUL SUBSTANCES IN YOUR ENVIRONMENT

Cancer cells are relatively big and when they spread they usually get trapped in the first network of capillaries – the very fine blood vessels that take blood to and from all the tissues in our bodies – that they encounter downstream of their origin. The first highly vascularised organ encountered by blood leaving most organs in the body is the lung, except in the case of the intestine from which the blood supply goes to the liver first. Hence, in the case of all types of cancer, the organs to protect from secondary tumours as much as possible are the lungs and liver. Protecting the pelvic bones and other bones is particularly important in the case of prostate cancer.

The effects of exposure to harmful chemicals depend on the dose, the duration, how and when you are exposed and the presence of other chemicals. The main task of the lungs is to exchange 'old blood' containing carbon dioxide created by body processes for 'new blood' invigorated with fresh oxygen. They can cope with some dust particles and bad chemicals but if you overwhelm them with harmful chemicals (for example from tobacco smoke; or if you live in a city environment where the air usually contains high levels of car, aeroplane and other exhausts containing benzene, a potent cancer-causing agent, as well as many other cancer-causing agents) they are far more likely to become diseased with primary lung cancer. Also, they are far less likely to be able to fight against invading cancer cells trying to establish secondary tumours.

The liver is an amazing organ, responsible for eliminating poisonous chemicals, including those produced by our own metabolism, from the body as well as manufacturing all sorts of important enzymes and other chemicals essential for our bodies to function. The liver detoxifies our system and produces anti-cancer chemicals. My strategy was, and continues to be, to have as many good nutritious substances as possible to help my liver to help me and to keep it as unburdened as possible with pollutants in my food, applied to my skin or inhaled.

One of the main sources of pollutants to try to eliminate is tobacco smoke. It is estimated that smoking tobacco causes approximately 30 per cent of all cancers in the USA alone. Smoking tobacco not only causes cancer in the lungs but it is also implicated in many other types of cancer too.

One study, which focused on men younger than age 65, calculated that, even after taking account of ethnicity and prostate cancer in close relatives, the risk of prostate cancer increases by 40 per cent when men smoke. The effects are worse in heavy smokers who have smoked for a long time. For example, smoking two packs a day for 20 years was found to double a man's risk of aggressive prostate cancer – but if he had given up smoking for ten years before 40 years of age, he was no more likely to develop prostate cancer than if he had never smoked.[51]

Oliver and others[52] found, however, that men with prostate cancer were more likely to report a lifetime history of non-smoking, while other studies have also found no association between smoking and prostate cancer.[53] Oliver and others conclude that the effects of smoking on prostate cancer are unclear when studied in isolation from other factors.[54] I find it hard to believe that smoking is such a key factor in prostate-cancer risk, since many Chinese men smoke so heavily and prostate cancer rates there are so low. On the other hand, cigarettes contain a lot of cadmium, which is a carcinogen and seems to make testosterone more dangerous in its effects on the prostate gland.[55] It is also an endocrine-disrupter and is particularly damaging to bones,[56] which need to be specially protected in prostate cancer. Other authors have also indicated that there is a positive association between smoking history and IGF-I levels.[57]

I think it sensible to try not to smoke, and try to avoid passive smoking. If people ask you if you mind if they smoke in your presence, just say 'yes'. If you smoke and are addicted to nicotine and find it difficult to give up, you can reduce your risks by having nicotine as patches or by chewing nicotine-impregnated gum – it is the tar in tobacco which contains the powerful cancer-causing agents, not the nicotine.

I am now going to tell you about some other damaging chemicals in the environment, before advising you on how to cut your exposure to them. The concentration of many of them, especially the endocrine-disrupting chemicals, can actually be measured by their effects on cancer-cell cultures. Many are persistent and fat soluble and bioaccumulate up the food chain, becoming especially concentrated in milk and oily fish.

CANCER HAZARD: POLYCYCLIC AROMATIC HYDROCARBONS (PAHs)

Because so many combustion processes favour production of PAHs, they can be abundant in the environment from sources such as engine exhausts, cigarette smoke, grilled food, and coal and wood smoke. Coal tars and petroleum residues such as road and roofing asphalt and many contaminated land sites such as old gas works also have high levels of PAHs.

They deserve special attention because, as well as acting as endocrine disrupting chemicals (EDCs – discussed on p. 220), some of them cause cancer in other ways. They have particularly sinister chemical properties in the body because, as the liver tries to eliminate them, their oxidised metabolites can react chemically and become permanently inserted into the structure of DNA, introducing mistakes into it. It is this property that makes some of the PAHs so carcinogenic.

The complicated name of this group of chemicals refers to the fact that they comprise more than one ring of carbon atoms. Benzene, which is the basic single ring structure of carbon atoms with hydrogen atoms attached from which PAHs are built up, is itself a very powerful carcinogen. Some PAHs, including benzo(a)pyrene, the molecules of which comprise an arrangement of five benzene rings and which is concentrated in tobacco smoke, are well known to be the precursors of cancer-causing breakdown products.

Benzene has special regulations for its use in laboratories in order to meet Health and Safety regulations. So it always strikes me as strange that we are allowed to be exposed to this dangerous chemical every time we fill our cars with petrol or walk down the street and breathe in car exhaust fumes.[58] Typical tests on exhaust fumes from cars show that they emit about 10mg of benzene for every kilometre travelled.[59]

CANCER HAZARD: DIOXINS

The major source of dioxin in the environment (95 per cent) used to come from incinerators burning chlorinated wastes. Dioxin is formed as an unintentional by-product of many other industrial processes involving chlorine, such as chemical and pesticide manufacturing, pulp and paper bleaching, and the production of polyvinyl chloride (PVC) plastics. Dioxin is the primary toxic component of Agent Orange. It was one of the main contaminants at Love Canal, New York State and was the basis for the evacuation at Seveso, Italy, and the Bhopal disaster in India.

Dioxin is a general term that describes a group of hundreds of chemicals that are highly persistent in the environment. The most toxic compound is 2,3,7,8-tetra-chlorodibenzo-*p*-dioxin or TCDD. The name dioxin is also used for the family of structurally and chemically related polychlorinated dibenzo-para-dioxins (PCDDs), polychlorinated dibenzofurans (PCDFs) and certain polychlorinated biphenyls (PCBs). Some 419 types of dioxin-related compounds have been identified but only about 30 are considered to have significant toxicity, with TCDD being the most toxic.[60]

TCDD dioxin is, in fact, one of the most toxic chemicals known. According to the September 1994 report of the US

Environmental Protection Agency (EPA), not only does there appear to be no 'safe' level of exposure to dioxin, but levels of dioxin and dioxin-like chemicals have been found in the general US population that are 'at or near levels associated with adverse health effects'. The EPA report confirmed that dioxin is a cancer hazard to people; that exposure to dioxin can also cause severe reproductive and developmental problems (at levels 100 times lower than those associated with its cancer-causing effects); and that it can cause immune system damage and interfere with regulatory hormones so that it is an EDC endocrine disrupter.

Chronic exposure of animals to dioxins has resulted in several types of cancer. The IARC (International Agency for Research on Cancer) announced in February 1997, that the most potent dioxin, 2,3,7,8-TCDD, is now considered a Class 1 carcinogen.

Dioxin is fat-soluble and bioaccumulates up the food chain; it is found mainly (97.5 per cent) in meat and dairy products.[61] The North American intake based on a total exposure of 119pg (picograms)/day is as follows: dairy products and milk, 34 per cent; beef 32 per cent; chicken 11 per cent; pork 11 per cent; fish 7 per cent and eggs 3 per cent. Milk in the UK also contains dioxins and PCBs.[62]

Extensive stores of waste industrial oils with high levels of dioxins exist throughout the world. Long-term storage of this material may result in releases into the environment and the contamination of human and animal food supplies. Dioxins are not easily disposed of, and incineration at temperatures above 850°C remains the best available method (temperatures above 1,000°C are required for large amounts). Further information on dioxin is available on several websites, including those of the WWF (World Wide Fund for Nature), the WHO and the US EPA.

CANCER HAZARD: POLYCHLORINATED BIPHENYLS (PCBs)
PCBs are a family of man-made chemicals that contains 209 individual compounds of varying toxicity. Commercial formulations of PCBs enter the environment as mixtures consisting of a variety of PCBs and impurities. They have very high chemical, thermal, and biological stability and low vapour pressure, and are good electrical insulators and fire retardants. Between the 1930s and 1970s these properties led to their widespread use as coolant-insulation fluids in transformers and capacitors; for the impregnation of cotton and asbestos; as

plasticisers; and as additives to some epoxy paints. The same properties that made the extraordinarily stable PCBs so useful also contributed to their widespread dispersion and accumulation in the environment. The manufacture of PCBs was discontinued in the US and their uses and disposal were strictly controlled after 1976.

It has been estimated that since 1929, a total of 1.2 million tons of PCBs have been manufactured,[63] of which 31 per cent (370,000 tons) has so far escaped into the environment. However, 780,000 tons of PCBs are still in use in transformers and capacitors, or have been sent to landfills. Thus the amount that could potentially be released into the environment is approximately twice that already released.

PCBs enter the body through contaminated food and air and through skin contact. They are particularly enriched in fatty food, including milk.[64] Fish have been implicated, but a survey of fish products reported in 1997 indicated that fish-liver oils contained higher concentrations of PCBs and dioxins than fish-body oils, so fish is safer than fish oils – though it is now possible to buy purified oils with greatly reduced levels.[65] Exposure from drinking water is minimal.

It is known that nearly everyone has PCBs in their bodies, including infants who drink breast milk containing PCBs.[66] Animal experiments have shown that some PCB mixtures produce adverse health effects, including liver damage, skin irritations, reproductive and development effects and cancer. Some PCBs cause mutations in cells and they are endocrine disrupters.

While the risk of PCBs in producing cancer in humans cannot be clearly defined, the available evidence provides a basis for concern.

The FDA specifies PCB concentration limits of 0.2 to 3 parts per million (milligrams PCB per kilogram of food) in infant foods, eggs, milk (in milk fat), and poultry (fat). The American EPA guideline for drinking water ranges from 0.005 to 0.5 micrograms of PCBs per litre of water, which is associated with the risk of a person developing cancer of between 1 in 10,000,000 and 1 in 100,000.

In Britain, levels of PCBs in soils peaked in the late 1960s but have now fallen to 1940s levels and between 1982 and 1992 the estimated UK dietary intake of PCBs declined significantly.[67] Disposal of PCBs from discarded electrical equipment and other sources remains a problem.

CANCER HAZARD: ENDOCRINE-DISRUPTING CHEMICALS
(EDCs)

One of the ways in which many pollutants are now implicated in causing cancer is in the way they have been shown to mimic hormones or otherwise disrupt our endocrine system, so they are called endocrine-disrupting chemicals (EDCs). Because prostate cancer is considered to be a hormone-dependent cancer, EDCs are of particular significance to its prevention and treatment.

EDCs are defined by the UK Environment Agency as 'naturally occurring or synthetic substances that interfere with the functioning of hormone systems resulting in unnatural responses'.[68] They cause problems, including by 1) mimicking the natural hormone and producing a similar response by the cell, 2) binding to cell receptors and preventing a normal response and 3) interfering with the way natural hormones and receptors behave. Perhaps of most concern is the evidence that EDCs or their breakdown products can directly damage DNA to alter the cell cycle, affect repair processes, or interfere with cell-to-cell signalling – all processes implicated in the initiation of cancer.

Concern about this group of chemicals has mushroomed since 2000. The concern reflects 1) the discovery that a range of widely used man-made chemicals, including substances used in detergents, herbicides, pesticides, plastics, the female contraceptive pill and by-products of other industrial and waste-disposal processes, to which we are exposed daily, can act as EDCs,[69] 2) hypothetical links to an increase in disorders of reproductive development and function in the human male and in some species of wildlife,[70] and 3) the striking coincidence between human exposure to these chemicals and the increase in prevalence of a range of hormone-dependent human reproductive cancers (prostate, breast, endometrial, testicular and ovarian). Some of the substances have been used in household and personal-care products and even in the manufacture of children's toys and teething rings. Countries around the world are phasing out the use of many of these substances of concern.[71] In addition to oestrogen-mimicking substances, EDCs are thought to include substances that block oestrogen, mimic or block androgens (male hormones) and possibly also mimic or block thyroid hormones.

There are now many sources of information on EDCs. For example, a new database (REDIPED), launched in 2002 by the

Department for Environment, Food and Rural Affairs in the UK, provides information on 79 confirmed or suspected EDCs.

Because EDCs are related to hormones an infinitesimal quantity can have a negative effect.[72] Some persistent EDCs can accumulate in the body and be passed from one generation to the next.

Some researchers have suggested that xeno-oestrogens are unlikely to cause harm because we are already exposed to phyto-oestrogens. Humans and their pre-human ancestors have been eating phyto-oestrogens for millions of years, however, whereas most xeno-oestrogens have been around for, at the most, a few decades. Moreover, bioaccumulative persistent xeno-oestrogens and other endocrine disrupters accumulate in body tissues to much higher levels than phyto-oestrogens.[73] All of the epidemiological and other research I have read suggests that phyto-oestrogens are protective while xeno-oestrogens are potentially very harmful.

SOME OTHER HAZARDOUS ENVIRONMENTAL CHEMICALS

The occurrence of pharmaceuticals in the environment and the extent to which they pose a risk to the environment and humankind has also received considerable attention since the early 1990s. An initial risk assessment for the UK,[74] of more than sixty compounds thought to account for more than half of the known tonnage of pharmaceutical consumption, suggested that the substances of most concern were paracetamol/acetaminophen, aspirin and dextropropoxyphene (pain killers), fluoxetine (antidepressant), oxytetracycline (antibiotic), propranolol (for heart disease and migraine), aminotriptyline (for neuralgia) and thioridazine (for adult schizophrenia).

Recently the United States Geological Survey carried out the first nation-wide reconnaissance of the occurrence of pharmaceuticals, hormones and other organic contaminants in water.[75] The most frequently detected compounds were coprostanol (faecal steroid), cholesterol (plant and animal steroid), N,N-diethyltoluamide (insect repellent), caffeine (stimulant), triclosan (disinfectant), tri(2-chloroethyl)phosphate (fire retardant) and 4-nonylphenol (detergent breakdown product). More than one of the contaminants was commonly detected in samples, and there were as many as 38 in some samples. Little is known about the potential interactive effects that occur from such complex mixtures and their breakdown products and their overall effect on human health and the environment.

Other monitoring programmes in Europe and the Americas have detected painkillers, cholesterol regulators, antiseptics, chemotherapy agents, antibiotics and hormones in water.[76] One of the problems is that conventional sewage-treatment technologies vary greatly in their ability to remove drug residues and, in some instances, have even been shown to increase the bioactivity of the pharmaceutical residues.[77] Activated carbon filtration, which is used by some states in the USA, continues to be one of the most effective known methods of removing drug and other contaminant residues from drinking water. Please see the section on Food Factor 8 'What to Drink' in Chapter 5, to reduce your risk of taking in harmful substances through your drinking water.

HARMFUL GASEOUS SUBSTANCES
Brominated flame retardants (BFRs), widely used for fire-proofing everything from televisions and computers to carpets and curtains, are now known to be persistent, bioaccumulating and toxic – and have been detected in human breast-milk samples![78] Harmful gaseous substances are increasingly of concern in buildings and vehicles. The Hamburg Environment Institute has analysed gaseous emissions from household and office appliances such as computer mice and mobile phones.[79] They have also tested carpets and wallpaper. Their study identified a hundred compounds emitted from the products tested, including carcinogens and EDCs. Also, volatile organic compounds can reach particularly high levels in new cars.[80] A useful leaflet entitled 'Volatile Organic Compounds (Including Formaldehyde) in the Home' has been posted on the website of the UK Institute for Environment and Health.[81]

The problem of synthetic chemicals in our food, air and water has not been helped by the fact that many doctors take little or no interest in the environment and they often do not know much about the chemicals used in industry, agriculture or even in the home environment, or their effects. For example, an article in the October 1999 issue of the *BMJ* implied that crop yields would go on increasing, but there was no mention of the input of chemicals that this would require.[82] Nor was there any mention of the pesticides and other chemicals that have been used to achieve the increase in yield in the past. I have served on committees and attended many meetings concerned with the environment and health. Usually all the environmentalists sit through the presentations given by medical specialists. However, the doctors used to leave before any of the papers on the environment were presented (we now mix up the papers in sessions to prevent this happening). Thank goodness for doctors such as Professor AJ McMichael at the London School of Health and Tropical Hygiene, author of the book *Planetary Overload*[83], who has developed a broader vision of the causes of ill health related to the environment – including as a result of industrialisation of agriculture – and pollution.

According to a report entitled 'Chemicals in the European Environment: Low Doses, High Stakes', published by the European Environment Agency (EEA) and the United Nations Environment Programme (UNEP) in 1999, there are now many thousands of (man-made) chemicals on the market, and little is known about their fate or impact on people or the environment. Monitoring of a few of these substances is required by law in the US and Europe. Moreover, since much of the monitoring involves analysis of water samples and the compounds of concern are generally not water-soluble, the monitoring schemes are likely to underestimate their true impact and presence in the environment. The Royal Commission on Environmental Pollution's Report 24 'Chemicals in products: safeguarding the environment and human health' takes this further and states that 'ignorance outweighs knowledge at every stage in our understanding of synthetic chemicals.'

In some cases, for example that of pesticides, release to the environment has been deliberate. In other cases releases have been an unfortunate side effect of the use of substances by the manufacturing industry. In addition, harmful organic chemicals have accumulated in the environment because of energy generation, especially the combustion of fossil fuels. In some cases chemical releases have caused major incidents, for example the release of dioxins at Love Canal in Niagara Falls, New York State and Seveso, Italy – but contamination is usually a more insidious process.

Dairy milk does contain oestrogen and testosterone, although it has been suggested that the levels are so low that cows' milk oestrogen is biologically insignificant.[84] Yet for some of these chemicals, even very low levels can cause severe biological damage. One illustration of this was the problem caused by the effects of a chemical called tributyl tin (TBT) on dog whelks on Britain's south coast. The chemical was developed for use in paint to coat the underside of ships to prevent 'fouling' or the growth of creatures such as barnacles that increase friction and thus slow down ships and boats. The levels of TBT in water were only of the order of five parts in a millionth of a millionth of seawater and were barely detectable. Nevertheless, in the 1980s, over a wide area of Britain's south coast where minute traces of the chemical occurred, female dog whelks died when their egg tubes became blocked by their own eggs because they had developed male organs which had overgrown their female organs. It is difficult to comprehend that such an infinitesimal amount of a substance could, in the open sea, have such a profound effect: but it did. Unfortunately, the chemical is still licensed for use on larger ships including those used by the British Navy. Interestingly, TBT's mode of action is thought to be by blocking the conversion of testosterone to oestrogen in organisms because it inhibits aromatase. Aromatase inhibitors are now being widely prescribed for breast cancer, and I have yet to meet an oncologist who has heard of the damage caused by TBT.

Let me quickly summarise how I and many other earth and environmental scientists see the situation.

Life on Earth has evolved in a complex interrelationship with the environment for at least 3,500 million years. Modern man, whose body chemistry has developed over that period of biological evolution, has appeared in the last ten-thousandth of the planet's history (equivalent to the last ten seconds on the 24-hour clock). In the past fifty years or so (much less than a fraction of a second on the 24-hour clock) we have set about dramatically changing the types and proportions of chemical molecules in the environment.

In particular, we have reconfigured organic chemicals, which were the basis of all life, into new 'organic' substances to use in industry and industrialised agriculture. In some cases the new 'organic' substances, which range from plastics to pesticides, their by-products or their metabolites are the antithesis of life. Some of the new chemicals and their by-products are implicated in causing cancer. Chemicals which disrupt the endocrine system whereby chemical messengers or hormones control our physiological function are of particular concern in hormone-dependent cancers such as those of the prostate.

Making sense of it all – the practicalities
Here is some practical advice to cut down your individual exposure to such chemicals and that of society more generally,

although it is impossible to do this completely. Indeed, many of the chemicals of concern are distributed across the globe and are even found in the blubber of seals and other creatures at the polar regions.

My advice is to have as few man-made chemicals in your life as possible. Never use perfumed soap, aftershave, deodorant or similar products. Most women I know find highly perfumed men a joke. I recently read the label on some expensive shower gel marketed by a prestigious company, to find that it actually listed phthalates – one of the main groups of endocrine disrupters implicated in the feminisation of fish – among the chemicals it contained. Moreover, research by Professor John Sumpter of Brunel University, London, now suggests that parabens could be an EDC (*see* p. 220).[85] With cosmetics, as with all other products, read the label, and remember: the simpler and more old-fashioned the better. As a 1960s teenager, I cannot be without my make-up, but I buy hypoallergenic products which are unperfumed and generally contain fewer damaging chemicals.

I do not add chemicals other than simple salts such as Epsom salts to my bath water. Even familiar man-made chemicals are often eventually shown to cause problems. A report in the magazine *Nature* suggests that a commonly used antibacterial agent, Triclosan, may work by causing mutations in bacteria.[86] Triclosan is used in many antibacterial soaps, lotions, mouthwash, toothpaste, plastic toys, socks and cutting boards. I prefer to use good, old-fashioned simple soap that will bind with dirt, fat-soluble chemicals and 'germs' and wash them away.

I do not use chemicals to stay young artificially. Some doctors in America and at some London clinics are reportedly providing their patients with human growth hormone to prevent ageing. A study published in the *BMJ* in 1998 reported that high natural levels of the hormone could lead to premature death from cancer. Also, growth hormones available to athletes and body builders must be of concern.

Many other cancer-causing agents have been identified, mainly as a result of occupational exposure – of, for example, factory workers, painters and decorators and hairdressers – to high levels of particular chemical substances. Some of the most dangerous chemicals implicated include benzene (used in the manufacture of some furniture and rubber and emitted from some types of fresh paint and car exhausts), formaldehyde (often used as a preservative, for example on fabrics in new cars, clothes and furnishings and in some cosmetics and shampoos) and hair dyes.[87]

Avoid dark-coloured hair dyes, some of which contain chemicals suggested to cause cancer, when applied directly to the scalp. Anyway, men with grey hair usually look much more distinguished than those with dyed hair. Discuss with your hairdresser any chemicals they use on your hair and ensure they have checked the information on their carcinogenicity.

One of the alternative therapies I question as a treatment for cancer is aromatherapy, especially if you are undergoing chemotherapy. Your liver already has a massive job to do to clear out all the unwanted chemicals and dead cells and other debris from the treatment without having to deal with other powerful chemicals. The skin is the body's largest organ and a proportion of many of the things we put on it are absorbed into the bloodstream.

In aromatherapy a carrier oil such as almond oil (thought not to be absorbed by the skin) is used as a base and an essential oil which normally evaporates (and has molecules that can pass through the skin), is added to achieve particular effects. Some of the oils absorbed through the skin are concentrated extracts of powerful chemicals. Many people wrongly believe that because the essential oils used in aromatherapy are extracted from plants and flowers they cannot be harmful, despite being delivered in high concentrations through the skin. In nature they are at low concentrations as part of a total fruit, flower or leaf. Many of the 'essential' oils have never been tested scientifically for their side effects, but medical research has shown that camphor, hyssop and sage oils can have such serious side effects as causing fits. Limonene – the lemon-smelling aromatherapy oil – is known to be capable of causing kidney damage. Basil oil which is said to lift mood, and tarragon oil also contain a chemical called estrogole which causes cancer in rodents. Dr Sharon Hopkiss of the Department of Pharmacology and Toxicology at St Mary's Hospital Medical School in London has been quoted as saying that many oils used in aromatherapy are extremely potent natural agents.

Remember that the characteristic smell of a new car reflects the fact that it is emitting nasty chemicals such as plasticisers and brominated flame retardents. If you have a new car, make sure it is well ventilated when you use it. The only car I drive is an old Land Rover of 1973 vintage with an engine converted to use lead-free petrol. If anything goes wrong, we simply buy a new part and put it in. Any volatile organic chemicals used in manufacture or sprayed on its interior will long since have evaporated. Even so, I try to use it as little as possible and to travel by public transport. The chemicals emitted by cars, even when well tuned and running optimally, include many hazardous substances such as benzene (*see* John Pearson's book *The Air Quality Challenge*).

If you paint your house or have it painted, ensure it is well ventilated (some of the oil-based paints used in Britain are now banned in Scandinavia). New furniture, curtains and upholstery can be important sources of toxic chemical fumes, including BFRs. Vinyl chlorides (PVCs) should also be avoided as much as possible. In an article in *The Times* of 11 November 1999 by Martin Fletcher, it was reported that the European Commission had called for an emergency ban on soft PVC toys, including rattles and dummies which babies suck, because they contained dangerous chemicals – phthalates again.

Also be careful of gardening chemicals. If a plant in my garden is going to die, so be it. I feed it with composted household waste to help it survive but I minimise any use of chemicals around the house or in the garden. My garden has lots of different wild bird species, butterflies, ladybirds, toads and hedgehogs. The degree of biodiversity in my garden compared to those of many friends who use chemicals says a great deal about the damage our use of chemicals does to the animals, so why do we think that we will be unaffected? I have already discussed problems associated with pesticides implicated in reproductive cancers generally. To avoid irresponsible use of chemicals in the environment, I never buy or give cut flowers. It is much better to give a garden plant. In my garden, Susan's rose, Eileen's buddleia and Georgina's astilbe remind me of them every year. Many organophosphates, well known to be damaging to the central nervous system, are now known to be EDCs. Aside from sheep dip and shampoos to kill headlice, many familiar products are based on these substances, including many insecticides, sprays and treatments for lice or fleas on pets including flea collars. Avoid all such products, and never use aerosol sprays for hair, deodorants, cleaning, gardening or any other purpose because of the increased risk of inhaling man-made chemicals.

Use wood, glass, ceramics and natural mineral materials in the home, stainless steel, enamel or toughened glass for cooking, and aluminium foil to wrap food. Whenever possible, use natural materials for clothing and furnishing with as few plastics or man-made fibres or other chemicals in your life as possible. Also, always wash and thoroughly rinse new clothes before wearing them to remove preservatives. Minimise the use of detergents and ensure they are thoroughly rinsed from crockery and clothes before use. Ideally, use the ecofriendly varieties. You might find it strange that someone who has spent her professional career working as a geochemist should try so hard to avoid chemicals in everyday life. Like many of my colleagues, I have a healthy respect for what chemicals can do to biological processes and so try to minimise my exposure.

If you have good, nutritious food and reduce exposure to pollutants, you will find your skin and general appearance improves without the need to add polluting man-made chemicals to your body or the environment. We can all reduce our personal risk from hazardous chemicals and by doing so we help the environment generally, with cleaner air, water and soils and hence more wholesome food. To most natural scientists this is all just common sense.

So, whenever you read or hear a new advertisement for a new 'personal care' product, man-made fabric or garden spray for example, think very carefully whether you really need it. Almost certainly you do not. People who avoid such products are frequently portrayed as odd especially by those wishing to sell us products that we do not need, in order to make money. No one looking at me, spending time with me or visiting my home would think I was a crank. Unless pointed out to them they probably would not notice anything is missing or different. Indeed, people comment on how normal I am (presumably despite being a scientist)!

All of the factors described in Chapters 5 and 6 are easy to control in your own surroundings. I travel a lot internationally and here are a few tips to help you maintain the Plant Programme while on your travels.

AWAY FROM HOME

1. When travelling, allow plenty of time for every aspect of the journey. Do not allow yourself to become stressed or upset by delays. If flying, try to fly at night to cut your exposure to cosmic radiation.
2. Count out the number of kelp, brewer's-yeast and red-clover tablets to cover your entire time away, prepare small bottles of your oils and take a small pot of dried soya milk (normally sold in cans for babies and infants). Take herbal tea bags and enough fruit to see you through until you can find a local supply.

3. When flying, ensure you order a vegan meal and check that the travel agent uses the code VGML, as other codes can include dairy. Drink lots of boiled water flavoured with your own herbal tea bags to avoid dehydration. Drink beer to make you sleepy.

4. Travel only on 'No Smoking' flights or in 'No Smoking' train compartments.

5. When you arrive at your destination, locate the nearest fruit and vegetable stall or shop and buy fresh supplies daily. In many countries these must be washed in boiling water before eating. This is really a brief immersion (use the hotel sink) similar to the blanching process used in cooking.

6. Before you travel, look up key words in a dictionary and jot them down in the language of the country you will be visiting. For example, in France 'soya' is 'soja': having a small number of ready-translated words to hand is very helpful. Ask your hotel where to buy the items you need using the written version if necessary. There will usually be a supermarket near your hotel where you can buy supplies, including beer.

7. Research the local cuisine and check which dishes you will be able to eat without problem or fuss.

8. Tell everyone you are terribly allergic to dairy produce and insist that you have none at all. (I have found this is most difficult in France.) If all else fails you can remove the cheese, or scrape off the yoghurt or cream etc. – I do so ostentatiously!

9. Be inventive in avoiding dairy produce. For example, at the breakfast buffet use prune or other fruit juice to moisten your cereal.

10. If you have trouble sleeping in a different time zone, camomile is soothing and beer usually makes me sleepy.

LIFESTYLE FACTOR 7: EXERCISE

Outdoor exercise in daylight, which increases levels of a particularly beneficial form of vitamin D, may be helpful against prostate cancer, and other forms of gentle exercise, especially some types of yoga or tai chi, may be helpful in coping with stress and building strength.

LIFESTYLE FACTOR 8: SEXUAL ACTIVITY

Prostate cancer affects a gland that is under the control of male hormones, suggesting the possibility of a relationship between the disease and the levels of male hormones in the blood and sexual activity. Evidence for this includes findings that patients with prostate cancer have an increased likelihood of having had a sexually transmitted disease, to have had more sexual partners and possibly to have a greater libido than men without prostate cancer. This study, twenty years ago, involved only a small number of people, but more evidence emerged in 2001 confirming the possible link between sex and prostate cancer, linking numbers of partners and lack of condom use with an increased risk of prostate cancer. Circulating levels of the male hormone testosterone have been measured in patients with prostate cancer and compared with levels in patients with normal prostates and those with BPH. Recent evidence suggests slightly higher levels of testosterone in prostate cancer patients than in healthy men.[88]

Personally, from the many men I know affected by prostate cancer I think it most unlikely that promiscuity is a factor, unless a viral infection is involved and they have just been unlucky, as in the case of cervical cancer in women – though documenting the sexual behaviour of others is notoriously difficult! Also, there is other evidence that risk of prostate cancer results from a lack of sexual activity: one study reported that men who ejaculated most in their twenties, thirties and forties had about a third less prostate cancer risk than men in the lowest category of ejaculation. In the absence of a sexual partner, masturbation was recommended.[89]

I suspect that if sexual activity influences prostate health at all it is a relatively minor factor compared with diet and other lifestyle factors such as exposure to harmful chemicals.

7 Information, Misinformation and Money

I am convinced that our lives really are in our own hands. Much of the advice given to us, even from some government sources, cannot be regarded as reliable, because of the overwhelming influence of vested-interest groups such as the food and pharmaceutical industries. We must, therefore, rely very much on ourselves and our own efforts in safeguarding our health, and try to distinguish objective, unbiased information based on good science from data biased by commercial or political interests. This chapter gives some advice on how to do this.

As I wrote in the first edition of *Your Life in Your Hands*, much of the scientific evidence presented here is widely known by groups of researchers, so why have we, the public, not been told? Let us look first at dietary factors.

Many elements of the Western diet, such as the high levels of saturated fats in some dairy products and meats, have been known to cause ill health for decades. Yet even this has never been clearly communicated to the public. For example, I have never seen butter or fatty meat products carrying any form of health warning. In presenting the results of the China study that I discussed in Chapter 3, Campbell and Junshi showed that even small intakes of food of animal origin are associated with significant increases in chronic degenerative diseases, including several types of cancer.[1] These are findings very clearly confirmed by all the research results into prostate cancer, breast cancer and osteoporosis that I have studied over the last ten or eleven years and published in a series of books.[2] Campbell and Junshi noted that in the West, reduction in fat consumption was being achieved by using lower-fat foods e.g. low-fat dairy foods: while their central fruit-vegetable-cereal recommendation appeared to have received little attention. Concerned by this highly selective distortion of their important message, the scientists speculate that pressure from food-industry lobbying groups influenced both the media (and hence the public) and also policymakers.

According to an article entitled 'Food industry obfuscates healthy eating message'[3] this continues to this day. Apparently, food giants are still going to enormous lengths to obfuscate US government health messages on healthy eating. To counteract this type of problem, one US-based organisation is now sponsoring 'Clean Science in Regulation' to explore establishing a proper relation between an independent scientific community and the business community. The centre wants to prevent regulated industries from attacking and discrediting valid scientific information and to examine issues, such as bias in advisory committee membership, and conflicts of interest in the sponsorship of scientific studies in product regulation. One quote from Dr Marion Nestle of the Department of Food and Nutrition Studies, New York University, sums up the situation clearly: 'Food is big business, $1.3 trillion . . . and the food industry will do everything to make sure that no regulatory agency and no nutritionist ever suggests eating less . . . and what [we] should eat less of'. In the diseases I have looked at, one of my main concerns is the consumption of dairy produce. I should like to examine the politics of this in a little more detail.

DAIRY IN THE DOCK
As discussed in Chapter 4, in addition to the mounting evidence that dairy products are clearly implicated in prostate and breast cancer and are an important factor leading to osteoporosis, the industry is implicated in a very wide range of diseases including serious infectious illness.

To quote from an article in the *Sunday Times*, 'In reality, the modern high-yield dairy cow is a pitiful ramshackle embodiment of market-driven exploitation. The new UK model, so help us, is the American Holstein battery cow. A shed-housed fermentation vat on legs, teats dragging on the ground, it's a sight to frighten children'.[4] The article includes a photograph of 'a large-uddered milker, one of the grotesque products of the modern dairy industry'. The article goes on to point out that farmers have not been able to resist the genetic promise (of developing such creatures) – a 2 per cent compound increase in milk yield annually.

In the UK, the dairy industry has been immensely damaging to our economy, especially tourism, as a result of BSE and the foot-and-mouth crisis of 2001, and yet it continues to be heavily subsidised under the European Common Agricultural Policy. In fact, the EU's support for dairy farmers amounts to around £11 billion per year, which works out as about £1.40 per day for each cow. Put another way, the average EU cow now receives more than the income of half the world's population.[5]

Concerns about marketing cow's milk to replace breast feeding have been around for many years. The late Dr Benjamin Spock, in *Baby and Child Care* (the United States' bestselling book, other than the Bible, over the past fifty years), after recommending that no one consume cow's milk and cataloguing a host of ills associated with milk consumption (heart disease, cancer, obesity, antibiotic residue, iron deficiency, asthma, ear infections, skin conditions, stomach aches, bloating and diarrhoea), concludes: 'In nature, animals do not drink milk after infancy, and that is the normal pattern for humans, too ... Children stay in better calcium balance when their protein comes from plant sources.' Dr Spock recommends human mother's milk for baby humans.

Dr Spock's book has been hugely influential. A great deal of his advice has been followed conscientiously by parents in America and all round the world. Why has his simple advice on milk not been followed equally conscientiously? And why has it taken about fifty years since Dr Spock's book was published for the UK Department of Health to endorse the resolution passed at the World Health Assembly in May 2001 that babies should be exclusively breast fed for the first six months of life?[6]

One of the reasons action has taken so long is perhaps illustrated by the example of the recent prosecution of SMA Nutrition, part of Wyeth, one of the world's biggest manufacturers of infant formula milk. This company was fined and ordered to pay legal costs after being convicted of six separate breaches of illegal advertising direct to consumers. In what is thought to be the first case of its kind, Judge Rod Ross described the company's breaches as 'cynical and deliberate' and said the company had 'deliberately crossed the line to advertise to a vulnerable section of the public.'[7]

I have certainly come under strong personal attack for my anti-dairy statements. For example, 'Jane Plant's statements are truly unfortunate. A study describing a single case history, particularly when it is the author's own, is scientifically unacceptable and lacks any objectivity', says Gregory D Miller, PhD, FACN, vice president of nutrition research for (guess who?) the US National Dairy Council. He continues 'There is no scientific evidence ...'[8] Those of us in the UK know how little statements beginning 'There is no scientific evidence ...' mean after the BSE–new variant CJD problem that we have experienced.[9] What the US National Dairy Council website attacking my book *Your Life in Your Hands* totally fails to mention is that the book contains more than 600 references, mostly from the peer-reviewed literature, medical textbooks and websites such as those of the WHO. I have become accustomed to such attacks that are deliberately misleading. As an experienced scientist, I am quite prepared to listen to proof if specific facts are wrong and to change my book accordingly. In the three years since it was first published, however, I have received no such comments.

The study most frequently quoted against my books and in favour of the health benefits of dairy products is the Harvard Nurses' Health Study (HNHS), which purported to show the benefits of dairy products.

Dr RM Kradjian, in his book *Save Yourself from Breast Cancer*,[10] has much to say about the Harvard study in relation to breast cancer. In Appendix 1 of his book, he strongly criticises the methodology of the study, documenting several serious technical flaws in the scientific methodology. He concludes:

> When one carefully dissects this report, it is revealed as a very peculiar piece of work. The problem is that very few physicians, American women, or members of the press seem to have read the article in close detail; nor did more than a handful apparently read the twelve pages of remark-able supplementary material. They were apparently com-forted by the names – Harvard, National Institutes of Health, and the American Cancer Society – and looked no further.

He himself discourages all use of cows' milk and all other dairy products. He notes that human beings are the only mammals on Earth that continue to drink milk after weaning. 'Despite the fact that milk drinking is widespread among Westernised people, it is a truly bizarre habit.' Appendix 2 of his book is entitled 'Research Funding: an incentive for bias'. The first question is 'Who sponsored the Harvard Nurses' breast-cancer study?'

> At issue is the funding of university studies and university researchers by interested food-industry groups. Such fund-ing could clearly result in pressure on those investigators to deliver conclusions that are acceptable to the sponsors, should the investigators hope to continue receiving funds from those sponsors.

Much of the following section of the Appendix describes how he repeatedly contacted the Freedom of Information Office at the (US) National Institute of Health, but was unable to obtain an answer to the simple question 'Is the food industry involved in the funding of the Harvard Nurses' Health Study?' After a year of persistent probing, he had received 'only a verbal acknowledgement from one of the authors that the dairy industry is involved in "some part of the study" '.

In the UK, even one of our main cancer-treatment centres defends consuming dairy produce. The leaflet 'After Treatment' produced by the Royal Marsden Hospital and issued to a breast-cancer sufferer in 2002 dismisses dietary therapy and claims that there is no scientific evidence to support exclusion of dairy products from the diet. Clearly the authors of the leaflet have not read the extensive scientific reviews such as those by Outwater and others[11] and the European Commission[12] or the more recent review by Yu and Rohan[13] or the many, many other scientific references cited in my books.

Many people find it difficult to reconcile the advice given by me and others such as Kradjian with the very conflicting advice given by their own doctors, nurses and dieticians. I think this is mainly just the conservatism of the profession, but according to one source:[14]

> The dairy industry has a powerful hold on the nutrition industry in this country [the USA]; it pays huge numbers of dieticians, doctors, and researchers to push dairy, spending more than $300 million annually, just at the national level, to retain a market for its products. **The dairy industry has infiltrated schools, bought off sports stars, celebrities, and politicians, pushing all the while an agenda based on profit, rather than public health [my bold]**.

Let me finish this section with some extracts from reviews of *Your Life in Your Hands* posted on the Amazon.com website. One reviewer, a physician, writes: 'This book is a must read for any breast cancer activist and any health care professional who treats breast cancer in women. It is surprising that the book has not gotten more publicity and attention. I suspect the American dairy industry may have had something to do with that.'

A second writes: 'No wonder the dairy industry hates this book. Others have said this book is as important as Rachel Carson's *Silent Spring*. I agree.'

In *Your Life in Your Hands* I warned about the consequences of the privatisation of science. Interestingly, the *Sunday Times* article I quoted above in relation to the dairy industry makes the same point:[15]

> Of course, commercial science will look to where it's paid. 'CLA research was actually got going by the American meat and dairy industry', says Dr Campbell [Dr T Colin Campbell, one of the most eminent dietary epidemiologists in the world], 'and it's very depressing when people start looking into little components of this and that. Let's face it, if dairy products contained all the good things that fruit and vegetables do, we'd be tired of hearing about them by now.'

FRUITFUL ORGANIC ARGUMENTS

It is unfortunate in the UK that the Food Standards Agency and the Advertising Standards Agency do not pursue the claims of the Dairy Council with the same vigour that they have applied against organic food producers. Let me once again quote from the *Sunday Times* article:[16]

> 'Taken all together – the welfare and environmental issues, and the adverse health evidence – it points to a fundamental change in British agriculture', says Rayner [Dr Mike Rayner, a nutrition and heart specialist at Oxford University]. 'But there's huge reluctance on the part of the farming community, and the Food Standards Agency doesn't even have it on its agenda to move us away from an animal-dependent system to a more plant-based agriculture. It makes no sense.'

So why is the UK Dairy Council being allowed to make claims that 'A natural fat [CLAs] found in milk, cheese, yoghurts and butter may soon prove to contain anti-cancer properties', when, as the *Sunday Times* article (*see* p. 232) points out, 'the proportion of CLAs is only 1 in 120 parts of saturated fat; ergo, to come by a significant amount of CLAs, you'd have to eat artery-choking amounts of the fat stuff'?[17]

In Chapter 5 I have argued that one of the best ways of limiting the ingestion of toxic man-made substances is by eating organically grown food, ideally produced locally to the standards of the Soil Association.

FALSE CLAIMS[18]

Last year [2001], in an attempt to clamp down on false and misleading claims, the Advertising Standards Authority (ASA) issued guidelines for advertisers on claims about organic food. This was prompted by several complaints received by the ASA about organic claims made by well-known names, including Tesco and the Soil Association. The new guidelines state that:

- Advertisers can't claim that organic food is 'safer' or 'healthier' than conventional food, unless they have convincing evidence that this is the case.
- Organic food can't be described as 'environmentally friendly' or 'sustainable', as all managed food production systems cause some environmental damage.
- Claims that organic food uses no chemicals, pesticides or artificial additives can only be made if this is the case.

The following is an edited extract of an article in *Which?* magazine,[19] discussing the advantages of organically produced food:

One of the most common reasons our shoppers gave for choosing organic food was to avoid pesticides. Organic standards allow the use of some approved pesticides but these are mostly from natural sources. There's little data on pesticide residue levels in organic food, but the government's pesticide residue monitoring programme (see *Which?*, September 2001, p24) includes a limited number of organic samples, and residues are rarely found in those tested ... Processing can significantly reduce the levels of residues. Washing and peeling alone has been shown to reduce levels by 50 to 90 per cent in apples, carrots and potatoes. Cooking and other types of processing involving heat can reduce levels further ...

Also, by restricting the use of artificial fertilisers and pesticides, organic farmers and agricultural workers reduce the risk of harmful health effects to themselves as well as the risk of environmental damage associated with more intensive pesticide use.

Organic food can contain food additives (E numbers) and processing aids, but the list is more restricted – around 35 additives are approved, compared with hundreds in conventional food. Artificial sweeteners are banned and only natural flavourings and colourings are allowed ...

In spite of all the evidence to the contrary, the UK government has taken action, mainly through the Food Standards Agency, to argue that there are no health benefits to eating organically produced foods. The following is an edited extract from another article in *Which?*[20]

> The health benefits of eating fruit and vegetables are clear. The government wants us to eat at least five portions a day. To encourage this the Department of Health has introduced the National School Fruit Scheme, with the aim that, by 2004, all schoolchildren aged four to six will be receiving a piece of free fruit daily.
>
> But fruit and vegetables tested still contain pesticide residues. Although most residues fall within legal safety levels, figures show 72 per cent of apples and 81 per cent of pears have residues. And, in December [2001] it was reported that 61 per cent of grapes and 63 per cent of kiwi fruit contained toxic chemicals. Exposure to pesticides may be linked to increasing cancer rates and other health problems – young children, in particular, may be more vulnerable.
>
> The Food Standards Agency (FSA) has even established a working group to look at the 'cocktail effect' of multiple residues.
>
> With these concerns, you'd expect the current and long-standing advice to wash and peel fruit as 'a sensible additional precaution when preparing fruit for small children' to be emphasised or improved. Instead, the FSA wants to ditch the advice because its 'misinterpretation' could imply that 'only organic fruit should be supplied to the National School Fruit Scheme' – according to a leaked memo.
>
> However, the FSA told *Which?* that it was 'coincidental' that the advice was being reviewed prior to the launch of the school scheme and that it 'wasn't a trigger' for the review.
>
> *Which?* thinks that the FSA approach isn't good enough and asks the government to be more transparent about its motives.

Based on known levels of pesticide residues in some fruit and vegetables, *Which?* magazine urges the continued adoption of precautionary washing and peeling – which also reinforces good hygiene – to remain in place.

Let us now look at some of the reasons for the failure of modern medicine to prevent more cancer.

Prevention, screening and evidence-based medicine

One of the other problems in dealing with cancer is the industrialisation of medicine, which increasingly depends on costly drugs and other invasive and often unpleasant treatments. The term 'evidence-based medicine' seems to be one of the main pillars of this type of approach.

Writing in the *BMJ*,[21] Richard Smith pointed out that thirty years ago patients who had heart attacks were kept in bed for days, which killed them. He continued:

> Women giving birth used to be given an enema and had their pubic hair shaved – both procedures being unnecessary. The history of medicine is mostly a history of ineffective and often dangerous treatments. This is why the term 'evidence-based medicine' has become so popular.
>
> Unfortunately there is still no evidence to support most diagnostic methods and treatments. Either the research hasn't been done or it is of too poor a quality to be useful. Patients might want to read medical research in order to understand if evidence exists to support the treatments they are undergoing.
>
> ... one of medicine's most important – and simplest – questions [is]: 'Does a treatment work?' [This is certainly a problem for prostate-cancer sufferers.]
>
> ... The best way to be sure that you are comparing the same sorts of patients at the same time is to 'randomise' the patients to one treatment or another. To exclude 'bias' (which might, for example, lead a doctor to put all the sicker patients into one arm of the trial) neither the doctor nor the patient should know who has got the active treatment, making the trial 'double blind'.
>
> **Because the benefit from most medical treatments is so small and so hard to detect**, you need very many patients in the trial. Although 'double blind randomised trials' are considered the best way of determining whether a treatment works, **many of them have been poorly conducted and have given misleading results [my bold]**.[22]

The problems of recruitment of appropriate patients to randomised trials has been raised by Corrie, Shaw and Harris.[23] They found that even when a trial was available, eligibility criteria excluded over half of patients. It is a common criticism that the outcomes of trials for new treatments are superior to those subsequently encountered in standard clinical practice. Trials with broad entry criteria that better reflect everyday life will help with recruitment of patients[24] and probably yield more meaningful results.

More recently, Wald and Morris[25] have emphasised the need for synthesising different categories of evidence to obtain a quantitative summary between the cause of a disease and its risk, and the extent to which the disease can be prevented. These authors point out that, in addition to randomised trials, the results of which can be limited by factors such as dose, treatment duration and the limited age range of subjects, data from observational epidemiological studies are required. Their method, they suggest, is like putting together the pieces of a jigsaw puzzle.

According to Professor Waxman, from whose book *The Prostate Cancer Book*[26] I have quoted extensively, there are three forms of cancer research:

- Laboratory research to establish the molecular basis for disease from the study and analysis of cells and tumour samples.
- Pharmaceutical research, carried out by the pharmaceutical industry to develop new treatments for cancer.
- Clinical research.

But what about epidemiology, diet, nutrition, lifestyle, environmental pollutants and other hazards? In other words, what about a genuine attempt by the medical profession to *prevent* prostate and other cancers – and not by the introduction of yet more screening methods?

A report from the Health Development Agency (the NHS body responsible for promoting more healthy lifestyles) entitled 'Where's the Research on Preventing and Reducing Ill Health', states that only 0.4 per cent of studies into such issues as smoking, heart disease and cancer looked at prevention rather than cure.[27] Chaturvedi points out that medical students aim for a lucrative private practice; those opting for studies in prevention are considered academically unsound.[28]

The UK National Cancer Research Institute has produced what is thought to be the world's first detailed breakdown of cancer research in any country. It estimates that funding of more than £250 million ($390 million) from 15 leading charities and government organisations goes towards cancer research in the UK every year.[29] The analysis showed that most of the funding is spent on the country's most lethal cancers, including those of the prostate and breast. The study also showed that the biggest proportion of spending (41 per cent) goes on basic biological research, the results of which supposedly can be applied to any cancer. The next largest share (22 per cent) goes on research into treatment, while only 16 per cent is spent on research into causes. Research into prevention, care of patients, and survival attracts the least funding.

Health professionals really do need to think more clearly about empowering their patients to help themselves by providing them with good scientifically based information. They should try always to bear in mind the comment of Malcolm Alexander, director of the Association of Community Health Councils: 'The health service is an organisation made up of very powerful clusters of professions and other groups. The patient is actually in a very weak position.'

A doctor friend of mine describes the UK's National Health Service as the 'National Illness Service'. He is right to do so. In my own subject of environmental chemistry the whole approach would be regarded as an outdated 'end-of-pipe' solution. This approach is now discredited in favour of using a full-life-cycle analysis to avoid pollution at all stages, from raw-material extraction, refining and manufacturing to end-of-life disposal of products and beneficial after-use of land.[30] In medicine, such an approach would involve placing far more emphasis on prevention, where prevention means giving people clear, truthful, readily understandable information about healthy diet and lifestyle, whereas in conventional medicine, 'prevention' frequently seems to mean no more than 'early detection – a battery of screening tests, a considerable proportion of which involve using ionising radiation or the injection of potentially harmful chemicals.[31] This merely serves to generate yet more jobs and money in the pharmaceutical, medical-equipment and medical industry. Screening is potentially extremely lucrative and problematical.

In an editorial in the *BMJ*,[32] Richard Smith wrote:

Have you thought of buying your significant other a whole body scan? It's the most fashionable of gifts and perhaps particularly suitable for a 50th, 60th, or even 40th birthday.

You might be giving your loved one the supreme gift of extra years of life. Unfortunately, you may be more likely to give him or her a lorry load of anxiety and a series of invasive, painful, and unnecessary investigation.

Whole body scanning is currently being intensively marketed in the United States and the enthusiasm will surely spread. The 'sell' is simple. You might have something horrible lurking in your body. The scan will show it and allow early treatment. Or the scan will give you the all clear, providing the perfect excuse for an expensive dinner.

The problems lie in medicine's difficulties in defining normality, the devil of 'false positives', and our limited understanding of the natural history of disease. The commonest way of defining normal is that the measure lies within two standard deviations of the mean. So in a set of measurements from a normal population 5 per cent will be classed as 'abnormal'. The whole body scan will produce hundreds of measurements. So you have almost no chance of emerging as normal, but which abnormalities signify serious disease?

Moreover, this screening practice could potentially put enormous costs on the NHS, as the results of screening carried out privately are brought to the NHS for investigation.[33]

Let us look in more detail at some of the other fundamental sources of the problem.

PHARMACEUTICALS – SOME PROBLEMS

The pharmaceutical industry is very profitable (US drug sales grew 12 per cent to $220 billion in 2002[34]), and hence very powerful. An article released in May 2002 and entitled 'Drug companies maintain "astounding" profits'[35] states that pharmaceuticals ranked as the most profitable sector in the US annual 'Fortune 500' ranking of America's top industries. The pharmaceutical industry topped all three of *Fortune* magazine's measures of profitability. This is the third decade that the industry has been at or near the top in all these measures. Of course, there is nothing at all wrong with profitability itself – only with the abuse of the power that profits can bestow.

The *BMJ*, from which I have quoted extensively in this book, now asks all contributors, including editorial writers, to sign a declaration of competing interests. In the case of original publications, declarations of funding sources and competing interests are required. This has allowed the association between competing interests and author's conclusions to be investigated using a study of randomised clinical trials published in the *BMJ* between January 1997 and June 2001.[36] Financial competing interests were defined as funding by for-profit organisations and other competing interests as personal, academic or political. The results showed that authors' conclusions were significantly more positive towards the experimental intervention in trials funded by for-profit organisations alone than in trials without competing interests or in trials funded by both profit and non-profit organisations. The association between financial competing interests and authors' conclusions was not explained by the quality of the methods used, the statistical power, the type of experimental intervention, involving pharmaceuticals or non-pharmaceutical approaches, or medical speciality. The authors concluded that randomised clinical trials significantly favour experimental interventions when financial competing interests were declared. The authors could not see why their findings applied only to the *BMJ*, and pointed out that the other major journals publish a far higher propor-tion of trials funded by the pharmaceutical industry than the *BMJ*.

In a poll conducted by the *BMJ* on its website (bmj.com), 96 per cent of the 1,479 people who voted would like to see all financial relationships between doctors and drug companies conducted with transparent contracts that are disclosed to patients.[37] The poll was conducted after the *BMJ* published its theme issue 'Time to Untangle Doctors from Drug Companies'.[38]

In the US, also, researchers have claimed that most randomised trials of new treatments published in leading medical journals are reported in a potentially misleading way, with statistics designed to make the results more positive than if other statistical tests were used.[39]

The problem seems to have become much worse, at least in the US. Industry supported 62 per cent of biomedical research in the US in 2000, almost double the proportion in 1980, while government support declined. About a quarter of academic investigators have affiliations to industry that could influence research and publication, according to a review in the *Journal of the American Medical Association*.[40]

Concern about links between the pharmaceutical industry and experts were also raised in a recent study carried out by researchers in Toronto, Canada. They claim that most guidelines on clinical practice are written by experts with undisclosed links to the pharmaceutical industry. For example, in a survey of nearly 200 authors of 44 clinical guidelines, 87 per cent of respondents admitted to financial links with one or more pharmaceutical companies,[41] and one new American company called Time-Concepts LLC is offering doctors $50 (£34) each time they listen to a short sales pitch from a drug company representative.[42]

One of the problems of pharmaceuticals can be unforeseen adverse side effects. Doctors are warned generally to be wary of starting their patients on newly approved drugs, because of the high rate of adverse side effects that go undetected until late in the post-marketing surveillance period. More than 10 per cent of new drugs approved by the US Food and Drug Administration (FDA) have serious side effects that are not discovered on initial testing and marketing.[43] In the UK, a yellow-card system is used by doctors to report such problems in order to monitor drug safety.

Jeffrey Aronson, a consultant clinical pharmacologist, has drawn attention to the need for guidelines for reporting anecdotes of suspected adverse drug reactions.[44] There are many such anecdotes. Of the 3,252 citations in the 24th volume of the *Side Effects of Drugs Annual*,[45] in which the world literature on adverse drug reactions and interactions for 2000 was critically reviewed, about a third (1,075 citations) were anecdotes; in contrast, there were only 45 systematic reviews. The hierarchy of clinical evidence, however, emphasises large randomised controlled trials and systematic reviews; in this scheme anecdotal reports are ill favoured. Nevertheless, anecdotal reports of adverse reactions should be published, for they have different functions to randomised controlled trials, a fact that is not emphasised by the evidence hierarchy.

Aronson goes on to say that anecdotal reports of suspected adverse drug reactions and interactions often do not contain all the information that they should – such as formal assessment of the likelihood that the event was an adverse drug reaction, possible mechanisms, and reviews of previous cases. Of course, it can be difficult to obtain high-quality data when an event occurs, but often a more assiduous approach would help. We need formal guidance on what is required. Standardised guidelines on reporting randomised controlled trials have been developed,[46] but no similar guidelines exist for anecdotal reports. Uniform presentation would also facilitate systematic review of suspected reactions.

It has been suggested that adverse effects of drugs get trans-
lated from patient language into doctor language and then into a
coding language – like Chinese whispers: a large proportion of the
cards sent in by drug companies 'tend to classify the same things
under different names so it won't look so alarming'.[47]

Another increasing concern is the direct marketing of pharmaceuticals to patients, including via the Internet. According to a
recent article in the BMJ, a fifth of Americans contact their doctor
as a result of direct-to-consumer drug advertising.[48]

The drug companies have expressed the wish to inform
patients,[49] and the chief executive of the Association of British
Pharmaceutical Industries states: 'My feeling, from the pharmaceutical industry, is because we are the providers of medicines
that people get from the health service, we should not be
excluded from [giving information to patients], provided we do it
in an objective way.' He denied suggestions that this might stoke
demand for certain drugs.

All this sounds very worthy, but will they also give the
downsides of treatment such as short-term and long-term side
effects?

New Zealand is one of only two countries that allow drug
companies to advertise directly to the public; the other is the
United States. GPs in New Zealand are petitioning the health
minister to ban the advertising of prescription drugs to patients.[50]
They claim that such advertising causes many problems that are
bad for doctors, the economy, and patients. They have estimated
that it cost the country $1.56m in less than one year to switch
people to a new asthma inhaler after it was widely advertised on
television, and the switch was not necessarily good for all
patients. But because patients had seen it advertised they were
determined to have it, spending some of New Zealand's health
budget along the way. Professor Les Toop, who heads the
campaign for a ban, stated: 'GPs are particularly upset by the
misleading content of many of the advertisements and the
commercial pressure this puts them under to prescribe advertised drugs, even when they're no better than existing alternatives or are not suitable for the patient.'

Fortunately (in my view) moves to allow drug manufacturers
to advertise directly to particular groups of patients have been
rejected by European Union health ministers.[51]

In the UK, the General Medical Council has issued new
guidance on the standards expected for research carried out in
the National Health Service, universities and the private sector,[52]

while the US government[53] has joined the American Medical Association and the drug industry in efforts to control drug-company handouts to the medical profession – but the recommendations are voluntary.

There is also concern about links between pharmaceutical companies, charities and patient organisations.

CHARITIES, PATIENT ASSOCIATIONS AND RESEARCH

Writing in the *BMJ* on the subject of industry funding of patients' support groups, Paola Mosconi wrote that declaration of competing interests is rare in Italian breast-cancer associations. The following is an edited version:[54]

> Herxheimer reported and commented on relationships between pharmaceutical companies and consumers' and patients' associations.[55] This is a 'hot' topic: the debate on transparency of fundraising for voluntary health associations is far from being resolved, and consumers' umbrella associations have an increasingly important role in discussing health at a European level.
>
> In Italy, at least among the 100 breast cancer associations belonging to the Italian forum of Europa Donna, transparency of fund raising is rarely discussed and few data are available. Using a standardised self-administered questionnaire on the characteristics of breast cancer associations, information on the sponsorship of 67 of them indicated that although most of the funds come from individual donations, one third received funds from pharmaceutical companies.
>
> In the same survey it was found that only five breast-cancer associations had been open and transparent about sponsorship by pharmaceutical companies.
>
> These data confirm the concern expressed by Herxheimer and by Hirst[56] on the independence of consumers' and patients' associations, and support the need for more public funding for organisations participating in the debate on public health.

Another article in the *BMJ*, entitled 'A hot flush for Big Pharma'[57] tells 'How HRT studies have got drug firms rallying the troops':

> In 2002 the powerful New York-based Society for Women's Health Research, whose 'sole mission is to improve the

health of women through research,' held a celebrity gala ostensibly celebrating women's 'coming of age'. It was entirely underwritten by [pharmaceutical company] Wyeth. In a *Washington Monthly* article entitled 'Hot Flash, Cold Cash,' journalist Alicia Mundy reported that only a few days after the Wyeth themed gala the company donated a quarter of a million dollars to the society.

Several weeks later, in July 2002, [negative findings about HRT were made public after the huge US Women's Health Initiative (WHI) study was prematurely halted by its safety monitoring board[58]] Wyeth was in a tailspin. They found support from the society, whose high profile chief executive and her staff went on national radio and television talk shows attacking the findings of the WHI study and its authors. 'Instead of taking the side of its constituents,' Mundy observed, 'the society seemingly took the side of its donors – and of Wyeth in particular.' As they fervently downplayed the negative findings of the WHI study and urged women not to abandon their HRT, the society's staff failed to disclose their substantial links to Wyeth and other drug companies. Similar activities and non disclosures are under investigation in Australia, after a complaint about the involvement of a well known doctor, Susan Davis, in HRT promotion.

Another investigation in the US has discovered that three key organisations, the United Seniors Association, the Seniors Coalition, and the 60s Plus Association, have all received substantial contributions in recent years from the drug industry: 'When the pharmaceutical industry speaks these days, many Americans may not be able to recognise its voice. That's because the industry often uses 'front groups' that work to advance its agenda under the veil of other interests'.[59]

I have been asked countless times since *Your Life in Your Hands* was first published about donations to cancer charities. I recommend that any charitable donations should be given to highly reputable charities. The research charity I would choose is Cancer Research UK, which is headed by a distinguished doctor and has an impeccable track record of research. I also commend the charities concerned with caring, such as Macmillan Cancer Relief, Marie Curie Cancer Care, the Bristol Cancer Help Centre, Positive Action on Cancer and the various hospices. Before giving any donations to cancer charities, do consider what proportion of their funds are devoted to administration, or the acquisition of capital assets such as buildings, the merchandising of consumer goods, and what proportion is actually spent on cancer prevention and/or care.

MEDIA AND ADVERTISING

The *BMJ* in an attack on media spin distorting the outcomes of medical studies, entitled 'The operation was a success (but the patient died)'[60] pointed out that the previous week one simple health message had dominated the US media: radical prostate surgery for prostate cancer saves lives. The media were reporting the results of a Swedish trial,[61] yet the trial showed no such thing. The trial concluded that although radical surgery did reduce death from *prostate cancer*, there was no significant difference between surgery and watchful waiting in terms of overall survival (because of death from other causes). A companion study found that the surgery also failed to improve the men's quality of life.

The interaction between the pharmaceutical companies and the media is well shown in the case of HRT. According to Griffiths,[62] we have a medical profession that is mostly pro-HRT although expressing some concern about the long-term side effects of the treatment.

According to the article quoted above ('A hot flush for Big Pharma'),[63] the pharmaceutical public-relations machine will be doing all it can to limit the fallout from studies published in 2003 in the *New England Journal of Medicine*[64] and the *Lancet*[65], just as it has been since the first damning results from long-term HRT studies were released last year. After all, billions of dollars in global sales are at stake.

According to the article, the tireless promotion of HRT by manufacturers is often held up as the ultimate case study in pharmaceutical marketing. In 2001 global sales amounted to $3.8bn (£2.4bn). But after the first wave of publications from the WHI study, Wyeth, which accounts for more than 70 per cent of the global market, saw its share price plummet. The stock, which traded as high as $58.48 (£36.48) in May 2002, fell by almost half to a low of $28.25 in July.

HRT promotion has depended heavily, although covertly, on industry involvement with scientists. In the 1960s American physician Robert Wilson wrote the influential *Forever Feminine*, extolling the virtues of HRT as a virtual fountain of youth for the 'dull and unattractive' ageing woman. In an article in the *New York Times* last year (10 July 2002), Wilson's son conceded that Wyeth paid for his father's book and promotion of HRT.

According to a *BMJ* article, positive reporting bias about new treatments may occur for several reasons. Beyond the seemingly universal desire to believe in cures, which may underlie some of the bias in such media reports, are corporate interests, the author suggests. Journalists seeking experts for comments often turn to seemingly credible and disinterested groups, such as professional associations, non-profit health groups, and patient organisations. The article goes on to say that many journalists do not realise, or fail to report, that many groups receive substantial funding from vested interests. Hospitals in North America, facing brutal competition, have, the article suggests, started buying contracts with television stations to feature them 'in news reports'. A poll of 300 news directors found that 43 per cent felt that such payments create pressures to exert improper influence. Dr Ivan Oransky, who teaches medical journalism at New York University, believes that the sort of investigative reporting that is standard, for example, in political coverage is lacking in medical and science reporting, with too many journalists reporting researchers' assertions uncritically.[66]

A recent development in America is the sponsored news programme, and it may be queried whether these are a new form of paid front for the pharmaceutical industry.[67] What many viewers of these news-magazine-style programmes may not realise is that health-care companies, including pharmaceutical and biotechnology companies, are paying directly for videos and suggesting the topics to be covered, according to a report in the *New York Times*. That article named a number of senior American broadcasters as having worked for a company funded by pharmaceutical giants to make video material. The celebrity journalists were reportedly paid up to $100,000 for one day's work, broadcast as news on public television stations across the country.

That pharmaceutical companies devise clever ways to market their products is hardly surprising. But let us hope that any counter attack that they make on the findings of research or the adverse health effects of HRT, for example, is subjected to the same kind of scrutiny that HRT itself is now under. We should all be very sceptical of some recent articles with headlines such as 'HRT "scare" will waste GP's time, doctors claim' and 'Don't panic: it's a medical treatment not a lifestyle drug'.[68]

In general, it has been said, newspapers, under-report randomised trials, emphasise bad news from observational studies, and ignore research from developing countries.[69]

WHERE DOES THE FAULT LIE?

Instead of trying to prevent disease (based on good dietary advice), we continue to treat disease with pills and potions, surgery or other expensive invasive methods to suppress symptoms. Communicating problems in our diet and lifestyle that affect our health is typically done poorly – or not at all – and usually without proper, clear advice on how to change our behaviour.

In the first edition of *Your Life in Your Hands* I asked why. I raised concerns about wealth creation being more highly regarded than quality of life, the lack of an adequate knowledge of science in Parliament and the civil service, especially after the privatisation of much science in the late 1970s and 1980s, but I had no idea how serious the problems were. In the case of prostate cancer, which is such an unpleasant disease for men, the situation is, I believe, particularly serious. The whole approach to chronic illness, it appears to me, avoids antagonising special interest groups, and it maintains the material wealth of (and jobs in) sectors such as farming, agrochemicals, the food industry, pharmaceutical research and the manufacture of medicines and medical equipment. But would it not be better to communicate facts as they are known, clearly and simply so that people can make their own choices and prevent disease? Would it not be better to create jobs in sectors working for the well-being of society and the environment, for example, in growing wholesome, nutritious organically produced food, with medical professionals being concerned more with health education, disease prevention and monitoring than dishing out pills? The fact that many of the doctors I know do not eat healthy diets suggests they do not know the importance of good nutrition.

Very few of my friends who are medical professionals seem to know much about food chemistry and I have often seen consultants and junior doctors at busy hospitals eating junk food. It is my impression that they are all so busy that they do not have time to eat a proper lunch, probably because they work such long hours under intense pressure. All my observations tell me that most doctors are unaware of the likely connections between the food we consume, chemicals in our environment and prostate (and breast) cancer. Instead, much of their knowledge is based on the literature they are bombarded with about new drugs and procedures. I think it is unrealistic to expect clinical doctors, who are incredibly busy trying to meet targets imposed on them by politicians to assuage public concern, to root out all of the scientific literature on prostate cancer, but surely doctors' training could be improved. My son is training to become a doctor, and so I am aware how full the curriculum is, but far more proper science and far less sociology would be my prescription for producing better doctors.

My answer to the question of 'whose fault is the prostate- and breast-cancer epidemic?' is that it is all our faults – especially the relatively well-educated people in society. It remains my view that we are the ones who must make the changes that will reduce both our personal and societal risk of suffering from these diseases.

The research for this book impressed upon me strongly what an unpleasant disease prostate cancer is. Not only that, but the decisions about whether to opt for watchful waiting or for one of the other treatment options – all of which may have unpleasant physical and emotional side effects – are far from easy. How much wiser it would be to concentrate on prevention rather than risk the need of a 'cure' or the anxiety and risks of watchful waiting. And yet society continues to emphasise the search for cures. The point is well made by a story attributed to Joseph Malins (1895) about a dangerous cliff and the debate whether to erect a fence at the top of the cliff, to prevent people falling off, or keep an ambulance down in the valley:

A collection was made to accumulate aid
and the dwellers in highway and alley,
gave dollars and cents, to provide . . . not a fence,
but an ambulance down in the valley.

'For the cliff is all right if you're careful', they said,
'and if folks ever slip and are dropping,
it isn't the slipping and dropping that hurts,
it's the shock down below when they're stopping.'

So for many a year, as these mishaps occur,
quick forth do the rescuers sally,
to pick up the victims who fall from the cliff
with the ambulance down in the valley.

Then one made a plea: 'It's a marvel to me
that you'd give so much greater attention
to repairing results than to curing the cause;
why, you'd much better aim at prevention.

'For the mischief of course should be stopped at its source.
Come, neighbours and friends, let us rally:
it makes far better sense to rely on a fence
than an ambulance down in the valley.'

'He's wrong in his head', the majority said.
'He would end all our earnest endeavour.
He's the kind who would shirk this responsible work,
but we will support it for ever.'[70]

OUR LIVES IN OUR HANDS

In this book I have given information to reduce individual risk of
prostate cancer, but the only long-term, final and lasting answer
to these scourges of our Western lifestyle is to *change* that
lifestyle. We have to develop greater awareness of, and sensitivity
to, the impact of our lifestyle choices on our own health, that of
our fellow beings, and that of our planetary home. Let me quote
from Professor McMichael from the London School of Tropical
Hygiene and Health and Dr Powles of Cambridge University;
their paper in the *BMJ* states:[71]

> Population size and the material intensity of our economies
> are now so great that, at the global level, we are disrupting
> some of the biosphere's life support systems . . .
>
> Recent attempts at 'full cost accounting' estimate that the
> demands of the current world population already exceed
> global carrying capacity by approximately a third . . .
>
> Accordingly, a shift of emphasis from income to other
> types of wealth . . . is particularly important if we are to
> maximise human well-being while minimising consump-
> tion which leads to degradation and pollution of the planet.

What they are saying is this: if we are to survive as a healthy
species, we must change our values and emphasis from material-
ism to other measures of well-being. We need increasingly to put
more value on good food, education, the arts, beautiful unspoilt
environments populated by diverse species other than man,
friendships, social interaction and health than on 'things'.

Looking back, I realise that I have changed my diet and
lifestyle from that of a middle-class, ambitious career-minded
Western woman to a woman with a more traditional Eastern diet,
lifestyle and values. So here are some simple, practical guidelines
that you can follow to help you to cut your risk of prostate cancer

and probably many other non-communicable or degenerative diseases, and improve the health of all of us and our home, Planet Earth, at the same time.

TEN SIMPLE GUIDELINES

1. Make good food ingredients your top priority when it comes to spending money. Keep as closely as you can to the diet and lifestyle recommendations set out in this book and in *The Plant Programme,* and wherever and whenever possible be prepared to pay extra for organically grown food produced as naturally as possible, ideally to the standards of the Soil Association, or grow your own. This sends the clearest possible message to government and the food industry.

2. Eat only those foods which human adults have evolved to eat. Most crucially, leave out dairy produce which is designed for baby calves, goats or lambs. Also refuse to eat food depleted of nutrients or otherwise altered by food processing, including food which contains artificial chemical additives such as colouring and flavouring agents, preservatives and emulsifiers or food which has been chemically altered, for example fats which have been hydrogenated. Refuse to be bamboozled by marketing and advertising, look for the 'weasel words' and separate them in your mind from the underlying facts. Be suspicious – check labels and demand information. Make eating good nutritious meals based on wholesome nutritional ingredients your top priority when it comes to your time.

3. Try to be less materialistic. Buy fewer new cars or clothes – don't be a fashion victim. In fact, try to cut down on buying *things* generally.

4. Be concerned and take action to improve the environment for everybody. There are many chemicals being introduced that we can do nothing about as individuals. Collectively, we can reduce the impact of chemicals on the environment by reducing our use of materials such as perfumed deodorants and aftershaves, soft plastics, detergents, cleaning products and house and garden chemicals, and man-made fibres. Remember how in the past we were sold 'wonder' chemicals such as DDT and PCBs which have turned out to cause serious problems to the health of man, animals and the environment and which are still with us. What chemicals are we using today that scientists

will have a similar view of in the future? Press for more research into the environment, nutrition and human health, with more medical research on epidemiology aimed at prevention.

5. Try to understand some basic science. Usually it is your money that scientists are spending directly or indirectly and you need to understand what they are doing. Ensure scientists contribute more to the public understanding of science by asking questions. If you do not understand the answer do not be embarrassed to repeat your question until you get a satisfactory answer. If a scientist cannot explain their work properly it is their problem, not yours. It is essential that a well-informed body of opinion exists if science is to be directed for the benefit of humankind rather than lead to our downfall. Books that will 'fire you up' are *Silent Spring* by Rachel Carson, *Our Stolen Futures* by Colborn, Dumanski and Myers and *Planetary Overload* by AJ McMichael. If you want to become more involved as lay members of the boards of scientific organisations, write in and offer your services.

6. Learn to understand your basic anatomy and, depending on your age, discuss with your doctor whether you should have regular PSA tests and other examinations (*see* Chapter 1).

7. If you are diagnosed with prostate cancer – use all the tools at your disposal to fight back. For your orthodox treatment ensure you are treated at a centre of excellence which uses a specialist cancer team led by a surgeon, radiotherapist and chemotherapist. Work with your doctors and be an involved and constructive participant in overcoming your illness, not a passive victim.

8. Follow my diet and lifestyle recommendations closely and avoid man-made chemicals as much as possible. This includes minimising the use of prescriptions available from doctors and pills from pharmacists. If you are prescribed or recommended drugs, demand to know precisely how they work and what the side effects are. Take them only if you are satisfied with the explanation and convinced there is no alternative. If your physician cannot explain how the drugs work and give examples of their successes and failures, be sceptical.

9. Use methods such as meditation, hypnotherapy, visualisation and yoga to cope with any emotional distress and to

develop the most positive approach possible. But do not rely on positive thinking alone. It is changing your body chemistry by changing your diet and lifestyle that is the crucial thing to do. Talk to your friends and family members and allow their help and support into your life, but if they find difficulty in coping, understand that they are distressed. Forgive them and allow them back into your life as soon as they feel able to return.

10. Prostate cancer is NOT an automatic death sentence. Remember the experience of the men whose stories I recounted in Chapter 1 – as well as my own experience with breast cancer. Keep reminding yourself that it is possible to overcome even advanced cancer.

TOWARDS A HAPPY ENDING

I am delighted that in the four years since *Your Life in Your Hands* was first published so many people have told me how helpful they have found it, and that no credible science has been published to persuade me to change even one word of my advice to prostate-cancer and breast-cancer sufferers. I hope that this new book will be used widely to help men to reduce their risk of suffering from prostate cancer. For those already suffering from the condition, I hope it will provide help and empowerment to work with your medical professionals to overcome your illness.

Knowledge is power. In this book I have tried to empower all men to deal with prostate cancer, individually and as a society, by trying to share with them the knowledge that I have gained on the subject of prostate and breast cancer as a scientist and as a five-times breast-cancer sufferer.

Notes

WELCOME

1. Plant, Jane, 2000. *Your Life in Your Hands.* Virgin Books. The second, revised edition (2003) contains all of the first edition, unchanged, together with additional sections updating each chapter.
2. Plant, Jane and Tidey, Gill, 2002. *The Plant Programme.* Paperback edition. Virgin Books.
3. Kradjian, Robert D., 1994. *Save Yourself From Breast Cancer.* Berkley Publishing.
4. Plant, Jane and Tidey, Gill, 2003. *Understanding, Preventing and Overcoming Osteoporosis.* Virgin Books.
5. Waxman, Jonathan, 2001. *The Prostate Cancer Book.* London: Vermillion.
6. Medical Report: Prostate Cancer. *ICON,* 2002, 1 (5), 8–10.

1. PROBLEMS WITH THE PROSTATE?

1. Plant, Jane, 2000. *Your Life in Your Hands.* Virgin Books. The second, revised edition (2003) contains additional sections updating each chapter.
2. Plant, Jane A. and Moore, P.J., 1979. Geochemical mapping and interpretation in Britain. *Phil Trans Roy Soc, London,* B288, 95–112.
3. Plant, Jane A., Smith, D., Smith, B. and Williams, L., 2000. Environmental Geochemistry at the Global Scale. Geological Society Special Issue.
4. Finkelman, R.B., Belkin, H.E., Centena, J.A. and Zheng, B., 2003. Geological Epidemiology: Coal Combustion from China. In *Geology and Health – closing the gap.* Skinner, H.C.W. and Berger, A.R. (eds). Oxford University Press.
5. Eaton, Lynn, 2003. World cancer rates set to double by 2020. *British Medical Journal,* 326, 728.
6. Peto, R. and others, 2000. Smoking, smoking cessation and lung cancer in the UK since 1950. *BMJ,* 321, 323–9.
7. Raleigh, V.S., 1999. World population and health in transition. *BMJ,* 319, 981B4.
8. Packham, D.E., 1999. Impacts of Commercialisation and Privatisation on Capabilities for Scientific Advice, Oracles or Scapegoats? IPMS Conference notes, October; see also: Packham, David and Tasker, Mary, 1997. Industry and the academy – a Faustian contract. *Industry and Higher Education,* April 1997, 85–90.
9. http://www.cancer.med.umich.edu/prostcan/
10. Waxman, Jonathan, 2001. *The Prostate Cancer Book.* London: Vermillion.
11. http://www.nci.nih.gov/cancerinfo/wyntk/prostate
12. Waxman, Jonathan, 2001. *Op. cit.*
13. http://www.cancerresearchuk.org/aboutcancer/specificcancers/prostatecancer
14. http://www.pcacoalition.org/education/facts_figures.php
15. Plant, Jane and Tidey, Gill, 2002. *The Plant Programme. Op. cit.*
16. Coulter, Angela, 2002. Patients' views of the good doctor. *BMJ,* 325, 668–669.
17. *Ibid.*
18. Donaldson, Liam, 2003. Expert patients usher in a new era of opportunity for the NHS. *BMJ,* 326, 1279–1280.

19. Plant, Jane and Tidey, Gill, 2003. *Op. cit.*
20. Wilkins, David, 2003. Patient's response to the research. *BMJ*, 326, 1313.
21. Waern, M. and five others, 2002. Burden of illness and suicide in elderly people: case control study. *BMJ*, 324, 1355–1357.
22. Stone, Mike, 2003. What patients want from their doctors. *BMJ*, 326, 1294.
23. Berry, D.C., Michas, I.C., Gillie, T. and Forster M., 1997. What do patients want to know about their medicines, and what do doctors want to tell them? A comparative study. *Psychol Health*, 12, 467–480; Berry, D.C., Knapp, P. and Raynor, D.K., 2002. Provision of information about drug side effects to patients. *Lancet*, 359, 853–854.
24. Waxman, Jonathan, 2001. *Op. cit.*
25. http://www.nccn.org/patient_gls/_english/_prostate/
26. Gask, Linda and Usherwood, Tim, 2002. ABC of psychological medicine: The consultation. *BMJ*, 324, 1567.
27. Herxheimer, Andrew and Ziebland, Sue, 2003. DIPEx: fresh insights for medical practice. *Journal of the Royal Society of Medicine*, 95, (5), 209–210.
28. Cox, Peter and Brusseau, Peggy, 1992. *Superliving A Beginner's Guide to Medspeak*, Vermillion; Rule, Ashley, 2003. Shocking language. *BMJ*, 327, 422.
29. Watts, Geoff, 2003. Second coming for patient power. *BMJ*, 326, 520.
30. Plant, Jane, 2003. *Your Life in Your Hands*, *Op. cit.* pp. 246–248.
31. Medical Report: Prostate Cancer. *ICON*, 2002, 1 (5), 8–10.
32. *Ibid.*; Waxman, Jonathan, 2001. *Op. cit.*
33. Waxman, Jonathan, 2001. *Op. cit.*
34. Medical Report: Prostate Cancer. *Op. cit.*
35. Waxman, Jonathan, 2001. *Op. cit.*
36. *Ibid.*
37. http://www.nci.nih.gov/cancerinfo/wyntk/prostate
38. Medical Report: Prostate Cancer. *Op. cit.*
39. Wilt, Timothy J., 2002. Treatment options for benign prostatic hyperplasia. *BMJ*, 324, 1047–1048.
40. Kirby, R.S. and seven others, 2003. Efficacy and tolerability of doxazosin and finasteride, alone and in combination, in treatment of symptomatic benign prostatic hyperplasia: the Prospective European Doxazosin and Combination Therapy (PRE-DICT) trial. *Urology*, 61 (1), 119–126.
41. Lee, E., 2002. Comparison of tamulosin and finasteride for lower urinary tract symptoms associated with benign prostatic hyperplasia in Korean patients. *J Int Med Res*, 30 (6), 584–590.
42. Wilt, Timothy J., 2002. *Op. cit.*
43. Brookes, Sara T., Donovan, Jenny L., Peters, Tim J., Abrams, Paul and Neal, David E., 2002. Sexual dysfunction in men after treatment for lower urinary tract symptoms: evidence from randomised controlled trial. *BMJ*, 324, 1059–1061.
44. Waxman, Jonathan, 2001. *Op. cit.*; Medical Report: Prostate Cancer. *Op. cit.*
45. Medical Report: Prostate Cancer. *Op. cit.*
46. http://www.nccn.org/patient_gls/_english/_prostate/
47. Waxman, Jonathan, 2001. *Op. cit.*
48. Medical Report: Prostate Cancer. *Op. cit.*
49. http://www.cancer.med.umich.edu/prostcan/
50. http://www.nccn.org/patient_gls/_english/_prostate/
51. Waxman, Jonathan, 2001. *Op. cit.*
52. http://www.cancer.med.umich.edu/prostcan/
53. http://www.cancer.org/docroot/NWS/content/NWS_1_1x_Prostate_Screening_Test_Results_Vary_Over_Time.asp
54. http://www.nlm.nih.gov/medlineplus/news/fullstory_13465.html
55. http://www.nccn.org/patient_gls/_english/_prostate/
56. *JAMA*, 289, 2695–2700.
57. Stuttaford, Thomas, 2003. Cancer: the four tests. *The Times (T2)*, 24 October 2003.

58. Chapple, A. and five others, 2002. Why men with prostate cancer want wider access to prostate specific antigen testing: qualitative study. *BMJ*, 325, 737–739.
59. *Ibid.*
60. Chapple, A. and five others, 2002. Is 'watchful waiting' a real choice for men with prostate cancer? A qualitative study. *BJU (Urol Int)*, 90, 257–264.
61. *Journal of the National Cancer Institute*, 1 October 2003, reported in *The Times (T2)*, 7 October 2003.
62. Donovan, J.L., Frankel, S.J., Neal, D.E. and Hamdy, F.C., 1999. Dilemmas in treating early prostate cancer: the evidence and a questionnaire survey of consultant urologists in the United Kingdom. *BMJ*, 318, 299–300.
63. Duckworth, Martin J., 2002. Right to choose is important. *BMJ*, 324, 1392.
64. Josefson, Deborah, 2002. PSA screening leads to overdiagnosis, study says. *BMJ*, 325, 61.
65. Lu-Yao, Grace, Albertsen, Peter C., Stanford, Janet L. and others. 2002. Natural experiment examining impact of aggressive screening and treatment on prostate cancer mortality in two fixed cohorts from Seattle area and Connecticut. *BMJ*, 325, 740–743.
66. http://www.cancer.med.umich.edu/prostcan/
67. *Urology*, 2003, 61, 1177–1180; http://www.nlm.nih.gov/medlineplus/news/fullstory _13258.html
68. Medical Report: Prostate Cancer. *Op. cit.*
69. Perron, Linda, Moore, Lynne, Bairati, Isabelle, Bernard, Paul-Marie and Meyer, Francois, 2002. PSA screening and prostate cancer mortality. *Canadian Medical Association Journal*, 166 (5), 586–591.
70. http://www.cancer.med.umich.edu/prostcan/
71. Thompson, Ian, Leach, Robin J., Pollock, Brad H. and Naylor, Susan L., 2003. Prostate cancer and prostate-specific antigen: the more we know, the less we understand. *J Nat Cancer Inst*, 95, 1027–1028.
72. Yamey, Gavin and Wilkes, Michael, 2002. The PSA storm. *BMJ*, 324, 431.
73. Cramer, Scott D. and 13 others, 2003. Association between genetic polymorphisms in the prostate-specific antigen gene promoter and serum prostate-specific antigen levels. *J Nat Cancer Inst*, 95, 1044–1053.
74. http://www.post-gazette.com/healthscience/20030716prostateheal.asp
75. *Ibid.*
76. http://www.nlm.nih.gov/medlineplus/news/fullstory_13363.html.
77. http://www.nccn.org/patient_gls/_english/_prostate/
78. *Ibid.*
79. Gottlieb, Scott, 2003. Prostate specific antigen test must be repeated before biopsy. *BMJ*, 326, 1231.
80. *JAMA*, 289, 2695–2700.
81. http://www.nccn.org/patient_gls/_english/_prostate/
82. Waxman, Jonathan, 2001. *Op. cit.*
83. *Canadian Medical Association Journal*, 2002, 166, 1399–1406.
84. http://www.nccn.org/patient_gls/_english/_prostate/
85. Medical Report: Prostate Cancer. *Op. cit.*; Waxman, Jonathan, 2001. *Op. cit.*
86. http://www.cancer.med.umich.edu/prostcan/
87. http://www.nccn.org/patient_gls/_english/_prostate/
88. http://www.nccn.org/patient_gls/_english/_prostate/3_stages.htm
89. http://www.prostatelab.com/grading.htm
90. *Ibid.*
91. http://www.cancer.med.umich.edu/prostcan/
92. http://www.nccn.org/patient_gls/_english/_prostate/
93. *Cancer*, 2002, 94, 3135–3141.
94. Spurgeon, David, 2002. Scientists develop more sensitive grading system for prostate cancer. *BMJ*, 324, 1476.

95. http://www.nccn.org/patient_gls/_english/_prostate/
96. Waxman, Jonathan, 2001. *Op. cit.*
97. http://www.nccn.org/patient_gls/_english/_prostate/
98. Medical Report: Prostate Cancer. *Op. cit.*
99. Waxman, Jonathan, 2001. *Op. cit.*
100. http://www.nccn.org/patient_gls/_english/_prostate/
101. *Ibid.*
102. *Ibid.*
103. Spurgeon, David, 2003. Advanced scanning techniques help doctors stage prostate cancer. *BMJ*, 326, 1418.
104. *New England Journal of Medicine*, 2003, 348, 2491–2499.
105. http://www.nccn.org/patient_gls/_english/_prostate/
106. http://www.cancer.org
107. Stuttaford, Thomas, 2003. *Op. cit.*
108. *Ibid.*
109. http://www.nccn.org/patient_gls/_english/_prostate/
110. Waxman, Jonathan, 2001. *Op. cit.*
111. *Ibid.*
112. http://www.fgcu.edu/chp/deadlytomen/info.html
113. Kirwan, C.C., Nath, E., Byrne, G.J. and McCollum, C.N., 2003. Prophylaxis for venous thromboembolism during treatment for cancer: questionnaire survey. *BMJ*, 327, 597–598.
114. Waxman, Jonathan, 2001. *Op. cit.*
115. *Ibid.*
116. *Ibid.*
117. Medical Report: Prostate Cancer. *Op. cit.*
118. http://www.nccn.org/patient_gls/_english/_prostate/
119. Gottlieb, Scott, 2002. Watchful waiting as good as surgery for prostate cancer. *BMJ*, 325, 613; Lenzer, Jeanne, 2002. The operation was a success (but the patient died). *BMJ*, 325, 664.
120. Medical Report: Prostate Cancer. *Op. cit.*
121. Waxman, Jonathan, 2001. *Op. cit.*
122. http://www.shot.demon.co.uk
123. Waxman, Jonathan, 2001. *Op. cit.*
124. http://www.nccn.org/patient_gls/_english/_prostate/
125. Ask the nurses. *ICON*, 2002, 1, 7.
126. UK National Radiological Protection Board, http://www.nrpb.org/radiation-topics/risks/exposure.htm
127. Shiralkar, A. and five others, 2003. Doctor's knowledge of radiation exposure: questionnaire study. *BMJ*, 327, 371–372.
128. Medical Report: Prostate Cancer. *Op. cit.*
129. Waxman, Jonathan, 2001. *Op. cit.*
130. http://www.nccn.org/patient_gls/_english/_prostate/
131. http://www.cancer.med.umich.edu/prostcan/
132. Waxman, Jonathan, 2001. *Op. cit.*
133. *Ibid.*
134. *Ibid.*
135. *Ibid.*
136. http://www.nccn.org/patient_gls/_english/_prostate/
137. *Ibid.*
138. Waxman, Jonathan, 2001. *Op. cit.*
139. http://www.nccn.org/patient_gls/_english/_prostate/
140. http://www.cancer.med.umich.edu/prostcan/
141. Waxman, Jonathan, 2001. *Op. cit.*
142. *Ibid.*

143. http://www.nccn.org/patient_gls/_english/_prostate/
144. Alternative Therapy, British Medical Association, 1986.
145. *New Scientist*, 27 August 1987.
146. Vickers, A. and Zollman, C., 1999. ABC of complementary medicine: Acupuncture. *BMJ*, 973–976.
147. Medical Report: Prostate Cancer. *Op. cit.*; http://www.nccn.org/patient_gls/_english/_prostate/
148. Waxman, Jonathan, 2001. *Op. cit.*
149. *Ibid.*
150. http://www.nccn.org/patient_gls/_english/_prostate/
151. The best way to live with cancer. *The Times*, 11 September 2003.
152. Ross, J.R. and five others, 2003. Systematic review of role of bisphosphonates on skeletal morbidity in metastatic cancer. *BMJ*, 327, 469.
153. Waxman, Jonathan, 2001. *Op. cit.*
154. Chapple, A. and Ziebland, S., 2002. 'I take the piss out of life, because it's the only way to get through it': what jokes do for men with testicular cancer [Abstract]. In: BSA Medical Sociology Group Annual Conference, 27–29 September 2002. Durham: BSA, 2002.
155. See, for example, section on cytotoxic (cell poisoning) drugs in the British National Formulary, 1998.
156. Josefson, Deborah, 2002. Doctors warned to be wary of new drugs. *BMJ*, 324, 1113.
157. Garattini, Silvio and Bertele, Vittorio, 2002. Efficacy, safety, and cost of new anticancer drugs. *BMJ*, 325, 269–271.
158. http://www.nccn.org/patient_gls/_english/_prostate/
159. *Ibid.*
160. http://www.cancer.gov/
161. Modified after: Chemotherapy and You: A Guide to Self-Help During Cancer Treatment. Information about what to expect during chemotherapy and what patients can do to take care of themselves during and after treatment. *NIH Publication* 99–1136; http://www.cancer.gov/cancerinfo/chemotherapy-and-you (There are, however, other recommendations in this booklet with which I do not agree.)
162. http://grants1.nih.gov/grants/guide/rfa-files/RFA-DK-01-008.html
163. Suicide cells. *The Times (T2)*, 10 October 2003.
164. http://www.news.harvard.edu/gazette/2001/05.10/gleevec.html
165. Pagan Westphal, Sylvia, 2003. Behind the mask. *New Scientist*, 19 July 2003.
166. Drug companies delve deep to advance the battle against cancer. *The Times*, 27 October 2003.
167. Waxman, Jonathan, 2001. *Op. cit.*
168. *Ibid.*; http://www.nccn.org/patient_gls/_english/_prostate/
169. Coulter, Angela, 2003. Killing the goose that laid the golden egg. *BMJ*, 326, 1280.
170. *Ibid.*
171. Ernst, E., 2003. Herbal medicines put into context. *BMJ*, 327, 881–882.
172. Waxman, Jonathan, 2001. *Op. cit.*
173. Dyer, Owen, 2003. Aspirin could be used to prevent cancer. *BMJ*, 326, 565.
174. Flower, Rod, 2003. What are all the things that aspirin does? *BMJ*, 327, 572–573.
175. UK limits use of aspirin by under 16s. *BMJ*, 2002, 324, 1294.
176. Bartram, Thomas, 1998. *Bartram's Encyclopedia of Herbal Medicine*. London: Robinson; http://www.prostatepointers.org/cmyers/pf0696.html
177. Astralagus. *ICON*, 2002, 1 (3), 23.
178. http://www.anticancerherb.com/aboutcarctol.htm
179. Medical Report: Prostate Cancer. *Op. cit.*
180. De La Taille, A. and five others, 1999. Effects of a phytotherapeutic agent, PC-SPES, on prostate cancer: a preliminary investigation on human cell lines and patients. *Br J Urol Int*, 84, 845–850.

181. Ernst, Edzard (ed.), 2001. *The Desktop Guide to Complementary and Alternative Medicine: an evidence-based approach.* Mosby.
182. Waxman, Jonathan, 2001. *Op. cit.*
183. Bartram, Thomas, 1998. *Op. cit.*
184. Medical Report: Prostate Cancer. *Op. cit.*
185. http://www.nci.nih.gov/cancerinfo/wyntk/prostate
186. Medical Report: Prostate Cancer. *Op. cit.*
187. Greenwald, Peter, 2002. Cancer chemoprevention. *BMJ*, 324, 714–718.

2. CELLS BEHAVING BADLY

1. http://bioscience.igh.cnrs.fr/2001/v6/d/hansen/2.asp
2. Weinberg, Robert A., 1996. How cancer arises. *Scientific American*, Special Issue, What you need to know about Cancer, September, 275, (3), 62–70.
3. Woolf, Neville, 1998. *Pathology, Basic and Systemic.* W.B. Saunders Publishing Co. Chapter 28, p. 274, Figure 28-3.
4. Thissen, J.-P., Ketelslegers, J.-M. and Underwood, L.E., 1994. Nutritional regulation of the insulin-like growth factors. *Endocrine Reviews*, 15 , 80–101; Holly, J.M.P., Gunnell, D.J. and Davey Smith, G., 1999. Growth hormone, IGF-I and cancer. Less intervention to avoid cancer? More intervention to prevent cancer? *J Endocrinol*, 162, 321–330.
5. Davey Smith, George, Gunnell, David and Holly, Jeff, 2000. Cancer and insulin-like growth factor-I. *BMJ*, 321, 847–848; Holly, J.M.P., 1999. *Op. cit.*
6. http://www.intouchlive.com/cancergenetics/onco.htm
7. Oliver, S.E., Gunnell, D.G., Donovan, J. and others, 2004. Screen-detected prostate cancer and the insulin-like growth factor axis: Results of a population-based case-control study. *International Journal of Cancer*, 108, 887–892.
8. Reuters, 4 August 1999.
9. Ludwig, T., Fisher, P., Ganesan, S. and Efstratiadis, 2001. Tumorigenesis in mice carrying a truncating BRCA1 mutation. *Genes and Development*, 15 (10), 1188–1193; Xu, X., Wagner, K.U., Larson, D. and others, 1999. Conditional mutation of BRCA1 in mammary epithelial cells results in blunted ductal morphogenesis and tumour formation. *Nature Genetics*, 22 (1), 37–43; Paull, T.T., Cortez, D., Bowers, B., Elledge, S.J. and Gellert, M., 2001. Direct DNA binding by BRCA1. *Proceedings of the National Academy of Sciences of the USA*, 98 (11), 6086–6091.
10. Jensen, R.A., Thompson, M.E., Jetton, T.L. and others, 1996. BRCA1 is secreted and exhibits properties of a granin. *Nature Genetics*, 12, 303–308; http://www.mc.vanderbilt.edu/cancer/research/roster/jensen.html
11. Waxman, Jonathan, 2001. *Op. cit.*
12. http://www.cancer.med.umich.edu/prostcan/
13. http://www.mercola.com/2002/apr/27/sv40.htm
14. Waxman, Jonathan, 2001. *Op. cit.*
15. Murray, R.K., Granner, D.K., Mayes, P.A. and Rodwell, V.W., 1990. *Harper's Biochemistry.* Appleton and Lange Norwalk, CT, p. 653.
16. Weinberg, Robert A., 1996. *Op. cit.*
17. Jain, R.K., 1994. Barriers to drug delivery in solid tumours. *Scientific American*, July, 271 (1), 58–65.
18. Davey Smith, George, 2000. *Op. cit.*
19. Lichtenstein, P., Holm, N.V., Verkasalo, P.K. and others, 2000. Environmental and heritable factors in the causation of cancer – analyses of cohorts of twins from Sweden, Denmark, and Finland. *New England Journal of Medicine*, 343, 78–85.
20. Hursting, S.D., Slaga, T.J., Fischer, S.M., DiGiovanni, J. and Phtang, J.M., 1999. Mechanism-based cancer prevention approaches: targets, examples, and the use of transgenic mice. *Journal of the National Cancer Institute*, 35, 2031–2038.
21. Cheeseman, K.H. and Slater, T.F., 1993. *Free Radicals in Medicine.* Churchill Livingston.
22. *Ibid.*

23. Holly, J.M.P., 1999. *Op. cit.*
24. Gann, P.H., Hennekens, C.H., Ma, J., Longcope, C. and Stampfer, M.J., 1996. Prospective study of sex hormone levels and risk of prostate cancer. *J Nat Cancer Inst*, 88, 1118–1126.
25. Waxman, Jonathan, 2001. *Op. cit.*
26. http://grants1.nih.gov/grants/guide/rfa-files/RFA-DK-01-008.html
27. *Ibid.*
28. Miller, W.R. and Sharpe, R.M., 1998. Environmental oestrogens and human reproductive cancers. *Endocrine-Related Cancer*, 5, 69–96.
29. *Ibid.*
30. Yu, H. and Rohan, T., 2002. Role of the insulin-like growth factor family in cancer development and progression. *J Natl Cancer Inst*, 92, 1472–1489.
31. Rose, Steven, with Mileusnic, Radmila, 1999. *The Chemistry of Life*. Fourth (revised) edition. Penguin Books.
32. Voet, Donald and Voet, Judith, 1995. *Biochemistry*. Second edition. John Wiley & Sons, Inc.
33. Outwater, J.L., Nicholson, A. and Barnard, N., 1997. Dairy products and breast cancer: the IGF-I, estrogen, and bGH hypothesis. *Medical Hypotheses*, 48, 453–461.
34. Baserga, R., Resnicoff, M. and Dews, M., 1997. The IGF-I receptor and cancer. *Endocrine*, 7, 99–102; Resnicoff, M. and Baserga, R., 1998. The role of the insulin-like growth factor I receptor in transformation and apoptosis. *Annals of the New York Academy of Sciences*, 842, 76–81.
35. Loeb, L.A., 1991. Mutator phenotype may be required for multistage carcinogenesis. *Cancer Research*, 51, 3075–3079; Orr-Weaver, T.L. and Weinberg, R.A., 1998. A checkpoint on the road to cancer. *Nature*, 392, 223–224.
36. Tedeschi, B., Spadoni, G.L., Sanna, M.L. and others, 1993. Increased chromosome fragility in lymphocytes of short normal children treated with recombinant human growth hormone. *Human Genetics*, 91, 459–463.
37. Cianfarani, S., Tedeschi, B., Germani, D. and others, 1998. In vitro effects of growth hormone (GH) and insulin-like growth factor I and II (IGF-I and -II) on chromosome fragility and p53 protein expression in human lymphocytes. *European Journal of Clinical Investigation*, 28, 41–47.
38. Oliver, S.E., 2004. *Op. cit.*; Gunnell, D. and 10 others, 2003. Are diet–prostate-cancer associations mediated by the IGF axis? A cross-sectional analysis of diet, IGF-I and IGFBP-3 in healthy middle-aged men. *British Journal of Cancer*, 88, 1682–1686; Holly, J.M.P., 1999. *Op. cit.*
39. Chan, J.M. and seven others, 1998. Plasma insulin-like growth factor-I and prostate cancer risk: a prospective study. *Science*, 279, 563–566; Harman, S.M., Metter, E.J., Blackman, M.R., Landis, P.K. and Carter, H.B., 2000. Serum levels of insulin-type growth factor I (IGF-I), IGF II, IGF-binding protein-3, and prostate-specific antigen as predictors of clinical prostate cancer. *J Clin Endocrinol Metab*, 85, 4258–4265; Stattin, P., and nine others, 2000. Plasma insulin-like growth factor-I, insulin-like growth factor-binding proteins, and prostate cancer risk: a prospective study. *J Natl Cancer Inst*, 92, 1910–1917; Chokkalingam, A.P. and 12 others, 2001. Insulin-like growth factors and prostate cancer: a population-based case-control study in China. *Cancer Epidemiology Biomarkers and Prevention*, 10, 421–427.
40. Rajah, R., Valentinis, B. and Cohen, P., 1997. Insulin-like growth factor (IGF)-binding protein-3 induces apoptosis and mediates the effects of transforming growth factor-β1 on programmed cell death through a p53- and IGF-independent mechanism. *Journal of Biological Chemistry*, 272, 12181–12188.
41. Oliver, S.E., 2004. *Op. cit.*
42. Yu, H. and Rohan, T., 2002. *Op. cit.*
43. *Ibid.*
44. Cariani, E., Dubois, N., Lasserre, C., Briand, P. and Brechot, C., 1991. Insulin-like growth factor II (IGF-II) mRNA expression during hepatocarcinogenesis in transgenic

mice. *Journal of Hepatology*, 13, 220–226; Schirmacher, P., Held, W.A., Yang, D. and others, 1993. Reactivation of insulin-like growth factor II during 1998 hepatocarcinogenesis in transgenic mice suggests a role in malignant growth. *Cancer Research*, 52, 2549–2556; Christofori, G., Naik, P. and Hanahan, D., 1994. A second signal supplied by insulin-like growth factor II in oncogene-induced tumorigenesis. *Nature*, 369, 414–418.

45. *Ibid.*
46. Loeb, L.A., 1991. *Op. cit.*
47. Barres, B.A., Hart, I.K., Coles, H.S.R. and others, 1992. Cell death and control of cell survival in the oligodendrocyte lineage. *Cell*, 70, 31–46; Harrington, E.A., Bennett, M.R., Fanidi, A. and Evan, G.I., 1994. c-Myc-induced apoptosis in fibroblasts is inhibited by specific cytokines. *EMBO Journal*, 13, 3286–3295.
48. Davey Smith, George, 2000. *Op. cit.*
49. Oliver, S.E., Barrass, B., Gunnell, D.J. and others, 2004. Serum insulin-like growth factor-I is positively associated with serum prostate-specific antigen in middle-aged men without evidence of prostate cancer. *Cancer Epidemiol Biomarkers Prev*, 13, 163–165.
50. Chokkalingam, A.P. and seven others, 2002. Insulin-like growth factors and risk of benign prostatic hyperplasia. *Prostate*, 52, 98–105.
51. Oliver, S.E., Gunnell, D.G., 2004. *Op. cit.*
52. Yao, S.L., Lu-Yao, G., 2002. Understanding and appreciating overdiagnosis in the PSA era. *J Natl Cancer Inst*, 94, 958–960.
53. Oliver, S.E., Gunnell, D.G., 2004. *Op. cit.*
54. Holly, J.M.P., 1999. *Op. cit.*
55. Jiang, Wen G., Matsumoto, Kunio and Nakamura, Toshikazu (eds), 2001. *Growth Factors and their Receptors in Cancer Metastasis*. Dordrecht: Kluwer Academic Publishers.
56. Yu, H. and Rohan, T., 2002. *Op. cit.*
57. Holly, J.M.P., 1999. *Op. cit.*
58. E.g. http://www.ucop.edu/srphome/bcrp/progressreport/abstracts/innov/3CB-0186.html
59. Yu, H. and Rohan, T., 2002. *Op. cit.*
60. http://www.preventcancer.com/pdf/InsulinGrowth266.html
61. Outwater, J.L. and others, 1997. *Op. cit.*
62. Gunnell, D. and 10 others, 2003. *Op. cit.*

3. THE THIRD STRAWBERRY

1. Forbes, Alec, 1984. *The Bristol Diet*. Century.
2. http://www.nci.nih.gov/cancerinfo/wyntk/prostate
3. http://www.who.int/nut/malnutrition-worldwide.htm
4. *Cancer Incidence in Five Continents*, 1997. Vol. VII, published by the IARC (International Agency for Research on Cancer).
5. Anon, 2003. Cancer now biggest cause of death in UK men. *BMJ*, 326, 1052.
6. Eaton, Lynn, 2003. World Cancer rates set to double by 2020. *BMJ*, 326, 728.
7. Medical Report: Prostate Cancer. *ICON*, 2002, 1 (5), 8–10.
8. Parkin, D.M., Whelan, S.L., Ferlay, J., Raymond, L. and Young, J., 1997. *Cancer in five Continents*. Vol. VII. Lyon: IARC Press.
9. Minino, A.M., Arias, E., Kochanek, K.D., Murphy, S.L. and Smith, B.L., 2002. *Deaths: Final Data for 2000. National vital statistics reports*. Hyattsville, Maryland: National Center for Health Statistics.
10. http://www.rense.com/general/dair.htm
11. http://www.cancer.med.umich.edu/prostcan/
12. Waxman, Jonathan, 2001. *Op. cit.*; http://www.cancer.med.umich.edu/prostcan/
13. Medical Report: Prostate Cancer. *Op. cit.*
14. http://www.cancer.med.umich.edu/prostcan/

15. Oishi, K., Yoshida, O. and Schroeder, F.H., 1995. The geography of prostate cancer and its treatment in Japan. *Cancer Surveys*, 23, 267–280.
16. Chan, J.M., Stampfer, M.J., Giovannucci, E. and others, 1998. Plasma insulin-like growth factor-I and prostate cancer risk: a prospective study. *Science*, 279, 563–566; Hankinson, S.E., Willett, W.C., Colditz, G.A. and others, 1998. Circulating concentrations of insulin-like growth factor-I and risk of breast cancer. *Lancet*, 351, 1393–1396; Toniolo, P., Bruning, P.F., Akhmedkhanov, A. and others, 2000. Serum insulin-like growth factor-I and breast cancer. *International Journal of Cancer*, 88, 828–832; Ma, J., Pollak, M.N., Giovannucci, E. and others, 1999. Prospective study of colorectal cancer risk in men and plasma levels of insulin-like growth factor (IGF)-I and IGF-binding protein-3. *Journal of the National Cancer Institute*, 91, 620–625. Giovannucci, E., Pollak, M., Platz, E.A. and others, 2000. Insulin-like growth factor I (IGF-I), IGF-binding protein-3 and the risk of colorectal adenoma and cancer in the nurses' health study. *Growth Hormone & IGF Research*, 10, S30–S31.
17. *Proceedings of the European Cancer Conference*, September 23, 2003, quoted in *The Times (Public Agenda)*, 30 September 2003.
18. Mayor, Susan, 2003. UK improves cancer control. *BMJ*, 326, 72.
19. *The Atlas of Cancer Mortality in the People's Republic of China.*
20. Pike, M.C., Kolonel, L.N., Henderson, B.E. and others, 2002. Breast cancer in a multiethnic cohort in Hawaii and Los Angeles: risk factor-adjusted incidence in Japanese equals and in Hawaiians exceeds that in whites. *Cancer Epidemiology Biomarkers and Prevention*, 11 (9), 795–800.
21. http://www.hawaii.edu/crch/ProfileKolonel.htm
22. World Cancer Research Fund, 1997. *Food, nutrition and the prevention of cancer: a global perspective*. Washington, DC: American Institute of Cancer Research; Gunnell, D.L. and 10 others, 2003. Are diet–prostate-cancer associations mediated by the IGF axis? A cross-sectional analysis of diet, IGF-I and IGFBP-3 in healthy middle-aged men. *British Journal of Cancer*, 88, 1682–1686.
23. http://www.prostatepointers.org/cmyers/pf0696.html
24. *Ibid.*
25. Plant, Jane and Tidey, Gill, 2003. *Understanding, Preventing and Overcoming Osteoporosis*. Virgin Books.
26. Campbell, T.C. and Junshi, C., 1994. Diet and chronic degenerative disease perspectives from China. *American Journal of Clinical Nutrition*, 59 (Suppl.), 1153S–1161S.
27. *Statistical Abstracts of the US*, 1994 edition.
28. Campbell, T.C., quoted in http://www:milksucks.com/osteo.html; Robbins, John, 1987. *A Diet for a New America*. Stillpoint Publishing; McDougall, John, 2000. *The McDougall Program for Women*.
29. Plant, Jane and Tidey, Gill, 2003. *Op. cit.*
30. Frassetto, L.A., Todd, K.M., Morris, R.C., Jr and Sebastian, A., 2000. Worldwide incidence of hip fracture in elderly women: relation to consumption of animal and vegetable foods. *J Geront: Med Sci*, 55A, (10), M585–M592.
31. Forbes, Alec, 1984. *Op. cit.*
32. Cramer, D.W. and others, 1989. Galactose consumption and metabolism in relation to the risk of ovarian cancer. *Lancet*, 2, 66–71.

4. MILK IS A FOUR-LETTER WORD

1. Cox, Peter and Brusseau, Peggy, 1995. *LifePoints For Kids*. Bloomsbury.
2. The Royal Society, 2000. Endocrine-disrupting chemicals. *Document* 06/00. The Royal Society.
3. *Statistical Abstracts of the US*, 1994 edition.
4. Charatan, Fred, 2003. Book Review: Fat Land: How Americans Became the Fattest People in the World, by Greg Critser. *BMJ*, 326, 229.
5. *Ibid.*
6. http://www.13.waisays.com/cancer2.htm

7. le Huerou-Luron, I. and others, 1998. Source of dietary protein influences kinetics of plasma gut regulatory peptide concentration to feeding in preruminant calves. *Comparative Biochemistry and Physiology: A – Molecular and Integrative Physiology*, 119 (3), 817–824.

8. Koldovski, O. and others, 1995. Milk-borne hormones: possible tools of communication between mother and suckling. *Physiological Research*, 1995. 44 (6), 349–351; Koldovsky, O. and others, 1994. Hormonally active peptides in human milk. *Acta Paediatrica* Suppl., 402, 89–93; Lehy, T. and others, 1990. Promoting effect of bombesin on the cell proliferation in the rat endocrine pancreas during the early post natal period. *Regulatory Peptides*, 27 (1), 87–96; Pollack, P.F., 1989. Effects of enterally- and parenterally- administrated bombesin on intestinal luminal tryptic activity and protein in the suckling rat. *Experienta*, 45 (4), 385–388; Lazarus, L.H. and others, 1986. An immunoreactive peptide in milk contains bombesin-like bioactivity. *Experienta*, 42 (7), 822–823; Jahnke, G.D. and others, 1984. A bombesin immunoreactive peptide in milk. *Proc Natl Acad Sci USA.*, 81 (2), 578–582.

9. Berseth, C.I. and others, 1990. Postpartum changes in pattern of gastrointestinal regulatory peptides in human milk. *Am J Clin Nutr*, 51 (6), 985–990.

10. Markwalder, R. and others, 1999. Gastrin-releasing peptide receptors in the human prostate: relation to neoplastic transformation. *Cancer Research*, 59 (5), 1152–1159; Festuccia, C. and others, 1998. In vitro regulation of pericellular proteolysis in prostatic tumor cells treated with bombesin. *International Journal of Cancer*, 75 (3), 418–431; Krongrad, A. and others, 1997. Endopeptidase 24.11 activity in the human prostate cancer cell lines LNCaP and PPC-1. *Urological Research*, 25 (2), 113–116; Jungwirth, A. and others, 1997. LHRH antagonist Cetrolix (SB-75) and bombesin-antagonist RC-3940-II inhibit the growth of androgen-independent PC-3 prostate cancer in nude mice. *Prostate*, 32 (3), 164–172; Larran, J. and others, 1996. In vitro characterization of bombesin and calcitonin on the proliferation of PC3, DK145 and LNCaP cancer prostatic cell lines. *International Journal of Developmental Biology*, 1996 (Suppl. 1), 275S–276S; Aprickian, A.G. and others, 1996. Bombesin specifically induces intracellular calcium mobilization via gastrin-releasing peptide receptors in human prostatic cancer cells. *Journal of Molecular Endocrinology*, 16 (3), 297–306; Bologna, M. and others, 1989. Bombesin stimulates growth of human prostatic cancer cells in vitro. *Cancer*, 63 (9), 1714–1720; Wasilenko, W.J. and others, 1996. Effects of the calcium influx inhibitor carboxyamido-triazole on the proliferation and invasiveness of human prostate tumor cell lines. *Int J Cancer*, 68 (2), 259–264.

11. Burns, D.M. and others, 1999. Breast cancer cell-associated endopeptidase EC24.11 modulates proliferative response to bombesin. *British Journal of Cancer*, 79 (2), 214–220; Bold, R.J. and others, 1998. Bombesin stimulates in vitro growth of human breast cancer independent of estrogen receptor status. *Anticancer Research*, 18 (16A), 4051–4056; Miyazaki, M. and others, 1998. Inhibition of growth of MDA-MB-231 human breast cancer xenografts in nude mice by bombesin/gastrin-releasing peptide (GRP) antagonists RC-3940-II and RC-3095. *European Journal of Cancer*, 34 (5), 710–717; Nelson, J. and others, 1991. Bombesin stimulates proliferation of human breast cancer cells in culture. *Br. J. Cancer*, 63 (6), 933–936; Giacchetti, S. and others, 1990. Characterization, in some human breast cancer cell lines, of gastrin-releasing peptide-like receptors which are absent in normal breast epithelial cells. *Int J Cancer*, 46 (2), 293–298; Weber, C.J. and others, 1989. Gastrin-releasing peptide, calcitonin gene-related peptide, and calcitonin-like immuno-reactivity in human breast cyst fluid and gastrin-releasing peptide-like immunoreactivity in human breast carcinoma cell lines. *Surgery*, (6), 1134–1139 (disc.1139–1140).

12. Takeyama, M. and others, 1989. Enzyme immunoassay of gastrin-releasing peptide (GRP)-like immunoreactivity in milk. *Int J Pept Protein Research*, 34 (1), 70–74.

13. Ducroc, R. and others, 1995. Immunoreactive substance P and calcitonin-gene-related peptide (CGRP) in rat milk and in human milk and infant formulas. *Am J Clin Nutr*, 62 (3), 554–558.

14. Lembeck, F. and others, 1979. Substance P as neurogenic mediator of antidromic vasodilation and neurogenic plasma extravasation. *Arch Pharmacol*, 310 (2), 175–183.

15. Khare, V.K. and others, 1998. The neuropeptide/mast cell secretagogue substance P is expressed in cutaneous melanocyticlesions. *Journal of Cutaneous Pathology*, 25 (1), 2–10.

16. Ducroc, R., 1995. *Op. cit.*

17. Faulkner, A., 1998. Insulin-like growth factor 1 concentrations in milk and plasma after growth hormone treatment. *Biochemical Society Transactions*, 26 (4), 386; Silanikove, N. and others, 1998. Metabolic and productive response of dairy cows to increased ion supplementation at early lactation in warm weather. *Journal of Dairy Research*, 65 (4), 529–543; Ginjala, V. and others, 1998. Determination of transforming growth factor-beta 1 (TGF-beta 1) and insulin-like growth factor-1 (IGF-1) in bovine colostreum samples. *Journal of Immunoassay*, 19 (2–3), 195–207; Schober, D.A. and others, 1990. Perinatal expression of type 1 IGF receptors in porcine small intestine. *Endocrinology*, 126 (2), 1125–1132.

18. Rao, R.K. and others, 1998. Luminal stability of insulin-like growth factor-1 and -2 in developing rat gastrointestinal tract. *Journal of Pediatric Gastroenterology and Nutrition*, 26 (2), 179–185.

19. Untergasser, G. and others, 1999. Proliferative disorders of the aging human prostate: involvement of protein hormones and their receptors. *Experimental Gerontology*, 34 (2), 275–287; Xu, Z.D., 1999. Hammerhead ribozyme-mediated cleavage of the human insulin-like growth factor-2 ribonucleic acid in vitro and in prostate cancer cells. *Endocrinology*, 140 (5), 2134–2144; Marelli, M.M. and others, 1999. Luteinizing hormone-releasing hormone agonists interfere with the antagonic activity of the insulin-like growth factor system in androgen-dependent prostate cancer cells. *Endocrinology*, 140 (1), 329–334; Lamharzi, N. and others, 1998. Growth hormone-releasing hormone antagonist MZ-5-156 inhibits growth of DY-145 human androgen-independent prostate carcinoma in nude mice and suppresses the levels and mRNA expression of insulin-like growth factor-2 in tumors. *Proc Natl Acad Sci USA*, 95 (15), 8864–8868; Wang, Y.Z. and others, 1998. Sex hormone-induced prostatic carcinogenesis in the noble rat: the role of insulin-like growth factor-1 (IGF-1) and vascular endothelial growth factor (VEGF) in the development of cancer. *Prostate*, 35 (3), 165–177.

20. Parisot, J.P. and others, 1999. Altered expression of the insulin-like growth factor-1 receptor in a tamoxifen-resistant human breast cancer cell line. *Br J Cancer*, 79 (5–6), 693–700; Sciacca, L. and others, 1999. Insulin receptor activation by insulin-like growth factor-2 in breast cancers: evidence for a new autocrine/paracrine mechanism. *Oncogene*, 18 (15), 2471–2479; Grothey, A. and others, 1999. The role of insulin-like growth factor and its receptor in cell growth transformation, apoptosis, and chemoresistance in solid tumors. *Journal of Cancer Research and Clinical Oncology*, 125 (3–4), 166–173; Perks, C.M. and others, 1999. Activation of integrin and ceramide signalling pathways can inhibit the mitogenic effect of insulin-like growth factor-1 (IGF-1) in human breast cancer cell lines. *Br J Cancer*, 79 (5–6), 701–706; de Cupis, A. and others, 1998. Responsiveness to hormone, growth factor and drug treatment of a human breast cancer cell line: comparison between early and late cultures. *In Vitro Cellular and Developmental Biology – Animal*, 34 (10), 836–843; Kobari, M. and others, 1998. The inhibitory effect of an epidermal growth factor receptor specific tyrokinase inhibitor on pancreatic cancer cell lines was more potent than inhibitory antibodies against the receptors for EGF and IGF-1. *International Journal of Pancreatology*, 24 (2), 85–95; Gooch, J.L. and others, 1998. Interleukin 4 inhibits growth and induces apoptosis in human breast cancer cells. *Cancer Res*, 58 (18), 4199–4205; Choki, I. and others, 1998. Osteoblast-derived growth factors enhance adriamycin-cytostasis of MCF-7 human breast cancer cells. *Anticancer Res*, 18 (16A), 4213–4224; Jackson, J.G. and others, 1998. Insulin receptor substrate-1 is the predominant signaling molecule activated by insulin-like growth factor-1,

insulin, and interleukin-4 in estrogen receptor-positive human breast cancer cells. *Journal of Biological Chemistry*, 273 (16), 9994–10003; Westley, B.R. and others, 1998. Interactions between the oestrogen and IGF signalling pathways in the control of breast epithelial cell proliferation. *Biochemical Society Symposium*, 63, 35–44; Surmacz, E. and others, 1995. Overexpression of insulin receptor substrate 1 (IRS-1) in the human breast cancer cell line MCF-7 induces loss of estrogen requirements for growth and transformation. *Clinical Cancer Research*, 1 (11), 1429–1436.

21. He, Y., 1999. Comment on the association between insulin-like growth factor-I (IGF-I) and bone mineral density: further evidence linking IGF-I to breast cancer risk. *Journal of Cellular Endocrinology and Metabolism*, 84, 1760.

22. Perks, C. M. and Holly, J.M.P., 2000. Insulin-like growth factor binding proteins (IGFBPs) in breast cancer. *Journal of Mammary Gland Biology and Neoplasia*, 5, 75–84.

23. Murphy, M.S. and others, 1998. Growth factors and the gastrointestinal tract. *Nutrition*, 14 (10), 771–774; Buts, J.P., 1998. Bioactive factors in milk. (in French.) *Archives de Pédiatrie*, 5 (3), 298–306.

24. Shen, W.H. and others, 1998. Stability and distribution of orally administered epidermal growth factor in neonatal pigs. *Life Sciences*, 63 (10), 809–820; Rao, R.K. and others, 1998. Bovine milk inhibits proteolytic degradation of epidermal growth factor in human gastric and duodenal lumen. *Peptides*, 19 (3), 495–504; McCuskey, R.S. and others, 1997. Effect of milk-borne epidermal growth factor on the hepatic microcirculation and Kupfer cell function in suckling rats. *Biology of the Neonate*, 7 (3), 202–206; Oguchi, S. and others, 1997. Growth factors in breast milk and their effect on gastrointestinal developement. *Chang Hua Min Kuo Hsiao Erh Ko I Hsuek Tsa Chih*, 38 (5), 332–337.

25. Zhau, H.J. and others, 1996. Androgen-depressed phenotype in human prostate cancer. *Proc Natl Acad Sci USA*, 93 (26), 15152–15157.

26. Salomon, D.S. and others, 1999. Cripto: a novel epidermal growth factor (EGF)-related peptide in mammary gland developement and neoplasia. *Bioessays*, 21 (1), 61–70; Chou, Y.C. and others, 1999. Induction of mammary carcinomas by N-methyl-N-nitrosurea in ovariectomized rats treated with epidermal growth factor. *Carcinogenesis*, 20 (4), 677–684; Kurtz, A. and others, 1998. Local control of mammary gland differentation: mammary-derived growth inhibitor and pleiotrophin. *Biochemical Society Symposium*, 63, 51–69; Taylor, M.R. and others, 1997. Lactadherin (formerly BA46); a membrane-associated gycoprotein expressed in human milk and breast carcinomas, promotes Arg-Gly-Asp (RGD)-dependent cell adhesion. *DNA and Cell Biology*, 16 (7), 861–869.

27. Thornburg, W. and others, 1984. Gastrointestinal absorption of epidermal growth factor in suckling rats. *American Journal of Physiology*, 246, G80–G85.

28. http://www.prostatepointers.org/cmyers/pf0696.html

29. Gaull, G.E. and others, 1985. Significance of growth modulators in human milk. *Pediatrics*, 75 (2), 142–145.

30. Delgrange, E. and others, 1997. Sex related differences in the growth of prolactinomas : a clinical and proliferation marker study. *Journal of Clinical Endocrinology and Metabolism*, 82 (7), 2102–2107.

31. Leav, I. and others, 1999. Prolactin receptor expression in the developing human prostate and in hyperplastic, dysplastic, and neoplastic lesions. *American Journal of Pathology*, 154 (3), 863–870; Horti, J. and others, 1998. A phase 2 study of bromocriptine in patients with androgen-independent prostate cancer. *Oncology Reports*, 5 (4), 893–896; Franklin, R.B. and others, 1997. Prolactin regulation of mitochondrial aspartate aminotransferase and proteinkinase C. *Molecular and Cellular Endocrinology*, 127 (1), 19–25; Janssen, T. and others, 1996. In vitro characterization of prolactin-induced effects on proliferation in the neoplastic LNCaP, DU145, and PC3 models of the human prostate. *Cancer*, 77 (1), 144–149; Janssen, T. and others, 1995. Organ culture of human tissue as study model of hormonal and pharmalogical regulation of benign prostatic hyperplasia and of prostatic cancer. *Acta*

Urol Belg, 63 (1), 7–14; Oliver, R.T. and others, 1995. New directions with hormone therapy in prostate cancer: possible benefit from blocking prolactin and use of hormone treatment intermittently in combination with immunotherapy. *Eur J Cancer*, 31A (6), 859–860; Rana, A. and others, 1995. A case for synchronous reduction of testicular androgen, adrenal androgen and prolactin for the treatment of advanced carcinoma of the prostate. *Eur J Cancer*, 31A (6), 871–875.

32. Vonderhaar, B.K., 1998, Prolactin: The forgotten hormone of human breast cancer. *Pharmacology and Therapeutics*, 79 (2), 169–178; Das, R. and others, 1996. Involvement of SHC, GRB2, SOS and RAS in prolactin signal transduction in mammary epithelial cells. *Oncogene*, 13 (6), 1139–1145; Mershon, J. and others, 1995. Prolactin is a local growth factor in rat mammary tumors. *Endocrinology*, 136 (8), 3619–3623; Ginsberg, E. and others, 1995. Prolactin secretion by human breast cancer cells. *Cancer Res*, 55 (12), 2591–2595; Fuh, G. and others, 1995. Prolactin receptor antagonists that inhibit the growth of breast cancer cell lines. *J Biol Chem*, 270 (22), 13133–13137.

33. Hinuma, S. and others, 1998. A prolactin-releasing peptide in the brain. *Nature*, 393 (6682), 272–276.

34. Smith, S.S. and others, 1986. Presence of luteinising hormone-releasing hormone (LHRH) in milk. *Endocrinol Exp*, 20 (2–3), 147–153; Koldovsky, O., 1989. Search for the role of milk borne biologically active peptides for the suckling. *J Nutr*, 119 (11), 1543–1551; Nair, R.M. and others, 1987. Studies on LHRH and physiological fluid amino acids in human colostreum and milk. *Endocrinologia Experimentalis*, 21 (1), 23–30.

35. White, M.E. and others, 1986. Milk progesterone concentrations following simultaneous administration of buserelin and cloprostenol in cattle with normal corporal lutea. *Canadian Journal of Veterinary Research*, 50 (2), 285–286; Dinsmore, R.P. and others, 1989. Effect of gonadotropin-releasing hormone on clinical response and fertility in cows with cystyic ovaries, as related to milk progesterone concentration and days after parturition. *Journal of the American Veterinary Medical Association*, 195 (3), 327–330.

36. Berseth, C.I. and others, 1990. Postpartum changes in pattern of gastrointestinal regulatory peptides in human milk. *Am J Clin Nutr*, 51 (6), 985–990.

37. *Ibid.*

38. Flood, J.F. and others, 1991. Increased food intake by neuropeptide Y is due to an increased motivation to eat. *Peptides*, 12 (6), 1329–1332.

39. Slebodzinski, A.B. and others, 1998. Triiodothyronine (T3), insulin and characteristics of 5/-monodiodinase (5/-MD) in mare's milk from parturition to 21 days post-partum. *Reproduction Nutrition Development*, 38 (3), 235–244.

40. Fujimoto, N. and others, 1997. Upregulation of the estrogen receptor by triiodothyronine in rat pituitary cell lines. *Journal of Steroid Biochemistry and Molecular Biology*, 61 (1–2), 79–85.

41. Tenore, A. and others, 1980. Thyroidal response to peroral TSH in suckling and weaned rats. *American Journal of Physiology*, 238 (5), E428–430.

42. Amarant, T. and others, 1982. Luteinising hormone-releasing hormone and thyrotropin-releasing hormone in human and bovine milk. *European Journal of Biochemistry*, 127 (3), 647–650; Baram, T. and others, 1977. Gonadotropin-releasing hormone in milk. *Science*, 198 (4314), 300–302.

43. Koike, K. and others, 1997. The pituitary folliculo-stellate cell line TtT/GF augments basal and TRH-induced prolactin secretion by GH3 cells. *Life Sci*, 61 (25), 2491–2497; Tyson, J.E. and others, 1975. The influence of prolactine secretion on human lactation. *J Clin Endocrinol Metab*, 40 (5), 764–773.

44. Grochowska, R. and others, 1999. Stimulated growth hormone (GH) release in Friesian cattle with respect to GH genotypes. *Reproduction Nutrition Development*, 39 (2), 171–180; Bourne, R.A. and others, 1977. Serum growth hormone concentrations after growth hormone or thyroid-releasing hormone in cows. *Journal of Dairy Science*, 60 (10), 1629–1635.

45. Chomczinsky, P. and others, 1993. Stimulatory effect of thyroid hormone on growth hormone gene expression in a human pituitary cell line. *J Clin Endocrinol Metab*, 77 (1), 281–285; Reynolds, A.M., 1991. The effects of chronic exposure to supra-physiological concentrations of 3,5,3/triiodo-L-thyronine (T3) on cultured GC cells. *Journal of Cellular Physiology*, 149 (3), 544–547.

46. Koldovsky, O., 1989. *Op. cit.*; Buts, J.P., 1998. *Op. cit.*

47. Faulkner, A., 1998. *Op. cit.*; Baldini, E. and others, 1994. In vivo cytokinetic effects of recombinant human growth hormone (rhGH) in patients with advanced breast carcinoma. *Journal of Biological Regulators and Homeostatic Agents*, 8 (4), 113–116; Scheven, B.A. and others, 1991. Effects of recombinant human insulin-like growth factor-1 and -2 (IGF) and growth hormone (GH) on the growth of normal adult human osteoblast-like cells and human osteogenic sarcoma cells. *Growth Regulation*, 1 (4), 160–167; Hodate, K. and others, 1990. Plasma growth hormone, insulin-like growth factor-1, and milk production response to exogenous human growth hormone-releasing factor analogs in dairy cows. *Endocrinologia Japonica*, 37 (2), 261–273.

48. Koldovsky, O., 1989. *Op. cit.*; Buts, J.P., 1998. *Op. cit.*

49. Westrom, B.R. and others, 1987. Levels of immunoreactive insulin, neurotensin, and bombesin in porcine colostreum and milk. *J Pediatr Gastroenterol Nutr*, 6 (3), 460–465; Ehman, R. and others, 1985. Bombesin, neurotensin and pro-gamma-melanotropin in immunoreactants in human milk. *Regulatory Peptides*, 10 (2–3), 99–105.

50. Shutt, D.A. and others, 1985. Comparison of total and free cortisol in bovine serum and milk colostreum. *J Dairy Sci*, 68 (7), 1832–1834.

51. Vaarala, O. and others, 1998. Cow milk feeding induces antibodies to insulin in children – a link between cow milk and insulin-dependent diabetes mellitus? *Scandinavian Journal of Immunology* 47 (2), 131–135; Slebodzinsky, A.B., 1998. *Op. cit.*; Westrom, B.R., 1987. *Op. cit.*

52. Ferrando, T. and others, 1990. Beta-endorphin-like and alpha-MSH-like immunoreac-tivities in human milk. *Life Sci*, 47 (7), 633–635.

53. http://www.13.waisays.com/cancer2.htm

54. Reiter, E. and others, 1999. Effects of pituitary hormones on the prostate. *Prostate*, 38 (2), 159–165; Lamharzi, N. and others, 1998. Luteinising hormone-releasing hormone (LH-RH) antagonist Cetrorelix inhibits growth of DU-145 human androgen-independent prostate carcinoma in nude mice and suppresses the levels and mRNA expression of IGF-2 in tumors. *Regulatory Peptides*, 77 (1–3), 185–192; Jungwirth, A., 1997. *Op. cit.*; Maezawa, H. and others, 1997. Potentiating effect of buserelin acetate, an LHRH agonist, on the proliferation of ventral prostatic epithelial cells in testosterone-treated castrated rats. *Int J Urol*, 4 (4), 411–416; Hsing, A.W. and others, 1993. Serological precursers of cancer serum hormones and risk of subsequent prostate cancer. *Cancer Epidemiology Biomarkers and Prevention*, 2 (1), 27–32; Garde, S. and others, 1993. Effect of prostatic inhibiting peptide on prostate cancer cell growth in vitro and in vivo. *Prostate*, 7 (2), 183–194.

55. Maruuchi, T. and others, 1998. Effects of gonadotropin-releasing hormone agonist on rat ovarian adenocarcinoma cell lines in vitro and in vivo. *Japanese Journal of Cancer Research*, 89 (9), 977–983; Kuroda, H. and others, 1998. Human chorionic gonadot-rophin (hCG) inhibits cisplatin-induced apoptosis in ovarian cancer cells: possible role of up-regulation of IGF-1 by hCG. *Int J Cancer*, 76 (4), 571–578; Kurbacher, C.M. and others, 1995. Influence of luteinising hormone on cell growth and CA 125 secretion of primary epithelial ovarian carcinomas in vitro. *Tumour Biology*, 16 (6), 374–384; Manetta, A. and others, 1995. Inhibition of growth of human ovarian cancer in nude mice by luteinising hormone-releasing hormone antagonist Cetrorelix (SB-75). *Fertility and Sterility*, 63 (2), 282–287.

56. Bosland, M.C., 1996. Hormonal factors in carcinogenesis of the prostate and testis in humans and in animal models. *Progress in Clinical and Biological Research*, 394, 309–352.

57. Chapman, S. and others, 1992. Changes in adult cigarette consumption per head in 128 countries, 1986–1990. *Tobacco Control*, 1, 281–284.
58. http://www.who.int
59. Chapman, S., 1992. *Op. cit.*
60. http://www.who.int
61. http://www.13.waisays.com/cancer2.htm
62. Underwood, L.E., D'Ercole, J.A. and Van Wyk, J.J., 1980. Somatomedin-C and the assessment of growth. *Ped Clin N Amer*, 27, 4, 771–782; Perdue, J.F., 1984. Chemistry, structure and function of insulin-like growth factors and their receptors: a review. *Can J Biochem Cell Bio*, 62, 1237–1245.
63. Evidence for a zinc uptake transporter in human prostate cancer cells which is regulated by prolactin and testosterone. *J Biol Chem*, 274, 17499–504.
64. Medical Report: Prostate Cancer. *ICON*, 2002, 1(5), 8–10.
65. http://vvv.com/healthnews/milk.html
66. Pollack, Michael, 2003. Cancer, aging and IGF physiology. Meeting of the Royal Society of Medicine in London in October 2003, entitled 'Biology of IGF-I: its interaction with insulin in health and malignant states'.
67. Lonning, Per Eystein, 2003. IGF-I and breast cancer. Meeting of the Royal Society of Medicine in London in October 2003, entitled 'Biology of IGF-I: its interaction with insulin in health and malignant states'.
68. Yee, Doug, 2003. Targeting the IGF system for anti-tumour therapy. Meeting of the Royal Society of Medicine in London in October 2003, entitled 'Biology of IGF-I: its interaction with insulin in health and malignant states'.
69. Rudman and others, 1990. *New England Journal of Medicine*, 323.
70. Chan, J.M., Stampfer, M.J., Giovannucci, E. and others, 1998. Plasma insulin-like growth factor-I and prostate cancer risk: a prospective study. *Science*, 279, 563–566; Hankinson, S.E., Willett, W.C., Colditz, G.A. and others, 1998. Circulating concentrations of insulin-like growth factor-I and risk of breast cancer. *Lancet*, 351, 1393–1396; Ma, P., Pollak, M.N., Giovannucci, E. and others, 1999. Prospective study of colorectal cancer risk in men and plasma levels of insulin-like growth factor (IGF)-I and IGF-binding protein-3. *J Natl Cancer Inst*, 91, 620–625.
71. Chan, J.M. and others, 1998. *Op. cit.*; Hankinson, S.E. and others, 1998. *Op. cit.*; Ma, P. and others, 1999. *Op. cit.*
72. Holly, J.M.P., Gunnell, D.J. and Davey Smith, G., 1999. Growth hormone, IGF-I and cancer. Less intervention to avoid cancer? More intervention to prevent cancer? *Journal of Endocrinology*, 162, 321–330.
73. Chan, J.M. and others, 1998. *Op. cit.*
74. Pollack, M.N. and others, 1998. IGF-1 Risk Factor for Prostate Cancer. *Science*, 279, 563–566.
75. Pollack, Michael, 2003. *Op. cit.*
76. Pollack, M.N., Huynh, H.T. and Lefebvre, S.P., 1992. Tamoxifen reduces serum insulin-like growth factor 1 (IGF-1). *Br Cancer Res Treat*, 22, 91–100.
77. Holly, Jeff, 1998. Insulin-like growth factor-1 and new opportunities for cancer prevention. *Lancet*, 351, 9113, 9 May, 1373–1375.
78. Maison, P., Balkau, B., Simon, D., Chanson, P., Rosselin, G. and Eschwege, E., 1998. Growth hormone as a risk for premature mortality in healthy subjects: data from the Paris prospective study. *BMJ*, 316, 1132–1133.
79. *Ibid.*
80. Robbins, John, 1987. *A Diet for a New America*. Stillpoint Publishing.
81. http://www.dhn.csiro.au/crctissue.html
82. Mepham, T.B. and others, 1994. Safety of milk from cows treated with bovine somatotropin. *Lancet*, 334, November 19, 1445–1446; Mepham, T.B. and Schonfield, P.N., 1995. *Health Aspects of BST Milk*, prepared for the International Dairy Federation Nutrition Week conference in Paris, France, June 1995.
83. Plant, Jane, 2003. *Your Life in Your Hands*. Second edition. Virgin Books.

84. Xian, C., 1995. Degradation of IGF-1 in the adult rat gastrointestinal tract is limited by a specific antiserum of the dietary protein casein. *J Endocrinol*, 146, (2), 1 August, 215; Thornburg, W., 1984. *Op. cit.*

85. The European Commission. Health and Consumer Protection. Scientific Committee on Veterinary Measures Relating to Public Health – Outcome of discussions. http://europa.eu.int/comm/dg24/health/sc/scv/out19_en.html

86. Allen, N.E. and others, 2000. Hormones and diet: low insulin-like growth factor-1 but normal bioavailable androgens in vegan men. *Brit J Canc*, 83 (1), 95–97.

87. Simpson and others, http://www.nal.usda.gov/ttic/tektran/glimpse/data/000007/75/0000077539 .html

88. Miller, M.A., Hildebrand, J.R., White, T.C., Hammond, B.G., Madson, K.S. and Collier, R.J., 1989. Determination of insulin-like growth factor-1 (IGF-1) concentrations in raw pasteurised and heat treated milk. *Journal of Dairy Science*, 72, Supplement 1, 186–187.

89. Outwater, J.L., Nicholson, A. and Barnard, N., 1997. Dairy products and breast cancer; the IGF-1 estrogen, and bGH hypothesis. *Medical Hypotheses*, 48, 453–461.

90. The European Commission. *Op. cit.*

91. http://www.cancernetwork.com/journals/oncnews/n0007hh.htm

92. Chan, J.M., Stampfer, M.J., Ma, J., Gann, P.H., Gaziano, J.M. and Giovannucci, E.L., 2001. *Am J Clin Nutr*, 74, 549–554.

93. Hansen, C.M., Binderup, L., Hamberg, K.J. and Carlberg, C., 2001. Vitamin D and cancer: effects of 1,25 (OH)2D3 and its analogs on growth control and tumorigenesis. *Frontiers in Bioscience*, 6, d820–848.

94. Barnard, Neal D. 2002. Milk Consumption and Prostate Cancer, http://www.pcrm.org/health/Dairy_and_Prostate_Cancer/d_p_article.html

95. Hansen, C.M., 2001. *Op. cit.*

96. Nickerson, T. and Huynh, H., 1999. Vitamin D analogue EB 1089-induced prostate regression is associated with increased gene expression of insulin-like growth factor binding proteins. *J Endocrinol*, 160, 223–229.

97. http://bioscience.igh.cnrs.fr/2001/v6/d/hansen/2.asp

98. http://www.rense.com/general/dair.htm

99. Feldman, David, 2002. Pathways of Vitamin D Action to Inhibit Prostate Cancer Cell Growth. http://www.annieappleseedproject.org/nutgenprotin.html

100. Seol, J.G. and five others, 1998. Telomerase activity in acute myelogenous leukemia: clinical and biological implications. *Br J Haematology*, 100, 156–165; Savoysky, E. and seven others, 1996. Down-regulation of telomerase activity is an early event in the differentiation in HL-60 cells. *Biochem Biophys Res Commun*, 226, 329–334; Albanell, J. and five others, 1996. Telomerase activity is repressed during differentiation of maturation-sensitive but not resistant human tumor cell lines. *Cancer Res*, 56, 1503–1508.

101. Gross, C., Stamey, T.A., Hancock, S. and Feldman, D., 1998. Treatment of early recurrent prostate cancer with 1,25-Dihydroxyvitamin D3 (Calcitriol). *J Urol*, 159, 2035–2040.

102. Results of the Physicians Study presented at the American Association for Cancer Research in San Francisco, April 4, 2000.

103. Barretto, A.M., Schwartz, G.G., Woofruff, R. and Cramer, S.C., 2000. 5-hydroxyvitamin D-3, the prohormone of 1,25-dihydroxyvitamin D-3, inhibits the proliferation of primary prostatic epithelial cells. *Cancer Epidemiol Biomarkers Prev*, 9, (3), 265–270.

104. Health Topics from The Dr Gabe Mirkin Show. Box 10, Kensington MD 20895.

105. See also Plant, Jane and Tidey, Gill, 2003. *Understanding, Preventing and Overcoming Osteoporosis*. Virgin Books.

106. Medical Report: Prostate Cancer. *Op. cit.*

107. Giovannucci, E, 1999. Nutritional factors in human cancers. *Advances in Experimental Medicine and Biology*, 472, 29–42.

108. Giovannucci, E, 1998. Dietary influences of 1,25(OH)2 vitamin D in relation to prostate cancer: a hypothesis. *Cancer Causes and Control*, 9 (6), 567–582.

109. Medical Report: Prostate Cancer. *Op. cit.*

110. Chan, J.M. and others, 1998. *Op. cit.*; Harman, S.M. and others, 2000. Serum levels of insulin-type growth factor 1 (IGF-I), IGF II, IGF-binding protein-3, and prostate-specific antigen as predictors of clinical prostate cancer. *J Clin Endocrinol Metab*, 85, 4258–4265; Stattin, P. and others, 2000. Plasma insulin-like growth factor-I insulin-like growth-binding proteins, and prostate cancer risk: a prospective study. *J Natl Cancer Inst*, 92, 1910–1917; Chokkalingam, A.P. and others, 2001. Insulin-like growth factors and prostate cancer: a population-based case-control study in China. *Cancer Epidemiol Biomarkers Prev*, 10, 421–427; Chan, J.M. and others, 2002. Insulin-like growth factor-I (IGF-I) and IGF binding protein-3 as predictors of advanced-stage prostate cancer. *J Natl Cancer Inst*, 94, 1099–1106; Mantzoros, C.S. and others, 1997. Insulin-like growth factor 1 in relation to prostate cancer and benign prostatic hyperplasia. *Br J Cancer*, 76, 1115–1118; Wolk, A. and others, 1998. Insulin-like growth factor 1 and prostate cancer risk: a population-based, case-control study. *J Natl Cancer Inst*, 90, 911–915.

111. Holly, J.M.P., 1999. *Op. cit.*

112. Schuurman, A.G. and others, 1999. Animal products, calcium and protein and prostate cancer risk in The Netherlands Cohort Study. *Br J Cancer*, 80 (7), 1107–1113; Giovannucci, E., 1999. *Op. cit.*; Giovanucci, E., 1998. *Op. cit.*; Willet, W.C., 1997. Nutrition and Cancer. *Salud Publica de Mexico*, 39 (4), 298–309; De Stefani, E. and others, 1995. Tobacco, alcohol, diet and risk of prostate cancer. *Tumori*, 81 (5), 315–320; Le Marchand, L. and others, 1994. Animal fat consumption and prostate cancer: a prospective study in Hawaii. *Epidemiology*, 5 (3), 276–282; Talamini, R. and others, 1992. Diet and prostate cancer: a case control study in northern Italy. *Nutrition and Cancer*, 18 (3), 277–286; La Vecchia, C. and others, 1991. Dairy products and the risk of prostatic cancer. *Oncology*, 48 (5), 406–410; Mettlin, C. and others, 1989. Beta-carotene and animal fats and their relationship to prostate cancer risk. A case control study. *Cancer*, 64 (3), 605–612; Snowdon, D.A., 1988. Animal product consumption and mortality because of all causes combined, coronary heart disease, stroke, diabetes, and cancer in Seventh-day Adventists. *Am J Clin Nutr*, 48 (3 Suppl.), 739–748; Talamini, R. and others, 1986. Nutrition, social factors, and prostate cancer in a northern Italian population. *Br J Cancer*, 53 (6), 817–821; Rose, D.P. and others, 1986. International comparisons of mortality rates for cancer of the breast, ovary, prostate, and colon, and per capita food consumption. *Cancer*, 58 (11), 2263–2271.

113. Mannisto, S. and others, 1999. Diet and the risk of breast cancer in a case control study: does the threat of disease have an influence on recall bias? *Journal of Clinical Epidemiology*, 52 (5), 429–439; Outwater, J.L., 1997. *Op. cit.*; Gaard, M. and others, 1995. Dietary fat and the risk of breast cancer: a prospective study of 25,892 Norwegian women. *Int J Cancer*, 63 (1), 13–17; Decarli, A. and others, 1986. Environmental factors and cancer mortality in Italy: correlational exercise. *Oncology*, 43 (2), 116–126; Rose, D.P., 1986. *Op. cit.*; Shimada, A. and others, Ecological approach to the eating habits and the cancer mortality of Brazilian people. (in Japanese.) *Gan No Rinsho*, 32 (6), 631–640; La Vecchia, C. and others, 1986. Age at first birth, dietary practises and breast cancer mortality in various Italian regions. *Oncology*, 43 (1), 1–6; Talamini, R., 1984. *Op. cit.*

114. Outwater, J.L., 1997. *Op. cit.*

115. Leonard, Rodney E., 1995. Codex at the Crossroads: Conflict on Trade Health. *Nutrition Week*, 25, 26, 14 July, 4–5. *Nutrition Week* is published by the Community Nutrition Institute, 910 17th Street, N.W., Suite 413, Washington DC 20006; The European Commission. *Op. cit.*

116. Heaney, R.P. and seven others, 1999. Dietary changes favorably affect bone remodelling in older adults. *J Am Diet Assoc*, 99, 1228–1233.

117. Chan, J.M. and Giovannucci, E.L., 2001. Dairy products, calcium and vitamin D and risk of prostate cancer. *Epidemiol Rev*, 23, 87–92.

118. Bradford Hill, A., 1965. The environment and disease: association or causation? *Proceedings of the Royal Society of Medicine*, 58, 295–300.

119. Holly, J.M.P., 1999. *Op. cit.*

120. *Ibid.*

121. World Cancer Research Fund, 1997. *Food, nutrition and the prevention of cancer: a global perspective*. Washington, DC: American Institute of Cancer Research

122. Gunnell, D.L. and 10 others, 2003. Are diet–prostate-cancer associations mediated by the IGF axis? A cross-sectional analysis of diet, IGF-I and IGFBP-3 in healthy middle-aged men. *Br J Cancer*, 88, 1682–1686.

123. Mucci, L.A. and six others, 2001. Are dietary influences on the risk of prostate cancer mediated through the insulin-like growth factor system? *BJU Int*, 87, 814–820

124. Allen, N.E., Appleby, P.N., Davey, G.K. and Key, T.J., 2000. Hormones and diet: low insulin-like growth factor-I but normal bioavailable androgens in vegan men. *Br J Cancer*, 83, 95–97.

125. Outwater, J.L., 1997. *Op. cit.*

126. http://www.shef.ac.uk/uni/academic/a-c/csi/1997/pir2.html

127. Clevenger, C.V., Chang, W.P., Ngo, W. and others, 1995. Expression of prolactin and prolactin receptor in human breast carcinoma. Evidence for an autocrine/paracrine loop. *Am J Pathol*, 146, 695–705.

128. Struman, I., Bentzien, F., Lee, H. and others, 1999. Opposing actions of intact and N-terminal fragments of the human prolactin/growth hormone family members on angiogenesis: an efficient mechanism for the regulation of angiogenesis. *Proc Natl Acad Sci USA*, 96, 1246–1251.

129. Lawrence R., 1994. *Breastfeeding – A Guide to the Medical Profession*, Fourth edition, Mossby, USA.

130. e.g. http://www.inter-medico.com/prolactin.html

131. Lawrence R., 1994. *Op. cit.*

132. Holly, J.M.P., 1999. *Op. cit.*

133. Clark, P.A. and Rogol, A.D., 1996 Growth hormones and sex steroid interactions at puberty. *Endocrinology and Metabolism Clinics of North America*, 25, 665–681.

134. Chan, J.M., 1998. *Op. cit.*

135. De Mellow, J.S.M., Handelsman, D.J. and Baxter, R.C., 1987. Short-term exposure to insulin-like growth factors stimulates testosterone production by testicular interstitial cells. *Acta Endocrinologica*, 115, 483–489.

136. Giudice, L.A., 1992. Insulin-like growth factors and ovarian follicular development. *Endocrine Reviews*, 13, 641–669.

137. Westley, B.R. and May, F.E.B., 1994. Role of insulin-like growth factors in steroid modulated proliferation. *Journal of Steroid Biochemistry and Molecular Biology*, 51, 1–9; Marcelli, M., Haidacher, S.J., Plymate, S.R. and Birnbaum, R.S., 1995. Altered growth and insulin-like growth factor-binding protein-3 production in PC-3 prostate carcinoma cells stably transfected with aconstitutively active androgen receptor complementary deoxyribonucleic acid. *Endocrinology*, 136, 1040–1048.

138. Culig, Z., Hobisch, A., Cronauer, M.V. and others, 1994. Androgen receptor activation in prostate tumor cell lines by insulin-like growth factor-I, keratinocyte growth factor, and epidermal growth factor. *Cancer Res*, 54, 5474–5478.

139. Holly, J.M.P., 1999. *Op. cit.*

140. The European Commission. *Op. cit.*

141. Allen, N.E., 2000. *Op. cit.*; Chan, J.C., 1998. *Op. cit.*

142. Kradjian, R.D., 1994. *Save Yourself from Breast Cancer*, Berkley Books, New York.

143. http://www.afpafitness.com/milkdoc.htm

144. Anyon, C.P. and Clarkson, K.G., 1971. A cause of iron-deficiency anaemia in infants. *N Z Med J*, 74, 24–25.

145. American Academy of Pediatrics Committee on Nutrition (1992). The use of whole cows' milk in infancy. *Pediatrics*, 89, 1105–1109.
146. Anon, 2003. UK supports exclusive breast feeding for six months. *BMJ*, 326, 1052.
147. Clyne, P.S. and Kulczycki, A. 1991. Human breast milk contains bovine IgG. Relationship to infant colic? *Pediatrics*, 87 (4), 439–444.
148. Wilson, J.F., Lahey, M.E. and Heiner, D.C., 1974. Studies on iron metabolism. V. Further observations on cow's milk-induced gastrointestinal bleeding in infants with iron-deficiency anaemia. *J Pediatr*, 84, 335–344.
149. Bahna, S.L., 1987. Milk allergy in infancy. *Ann Allergy*, 59, 131.
150. Dunea, G., 1982. Beyond the etheric. *BMJ*, 285, 428–429.
151. Kretchmer, N., 1981. The Significance of Lactose Intolerance. In: Paige, D.M. and Bayless, T.M., eds, *Lactose Digestion: Clinical and Nutritional Implications*. Johns Hopkins University Press.
152. http://www.fda.gov/fdac/features/2001/401_food.html. This article (Food Allergies: When Food Becomes the Enemy, by Ray Formanek Jr) originally appeared in the July-August 2001 issue of *FDA Consumer*, and contains revisions made in September 2002.
153. http://www.ifst.org/hottop19.htm
154. Taylor, S.L., 1992. Chemistry and detection of food allergens. *Food Technology*, 46 (5), 146–152.
155. http://www.ifst.org/hottop19.htm
156. Martin, Peter, 2002. Milk: Nectar or Poison? *Sunday Times Magazine*, July 21, 2002.
157. Scott, F.W., 1990. Cow milk and insulin-dependent diabetes mellitus: is there a relationship? *Am J Clin Nutr*, 51, 489–491.
158. Chiodini, R.J. and Hermon-Taylor, J., 1993. The thermal resistance of Mycobacterium paratuberculosis in raw milk under conditions simulating pasteurisation. *J Vet Diagn Invest*, 5, 629–631; Grant, I.R., Ball, H.J. and Rowe, M.T., 1996. Inactivation of Mycobacterium paratuberculosis in cows' milk at pasteurisation temperatures. *Appl and Env Microbiology*, 62, 631–636.
159. The Institute of Food Science & Technology Position Statement, 1998. Food Science & Technology Today, 12 (4), 223–228, September. http://www.ifst.org/hottop23.html
160. *Financial Times* for the weekend 20–21 November 1999.
161. http://www.defra.gov.uk/animal/tb/stats/stats_nov2003.htm
162. The Institute of Food Science & Technology Position Statement http://www.ifst.org/hottop2.html. Hard copies available from IFST, 5 Cambridge Court, 210 Shepherds Bush Road, London, W6 7NJ.
163. EU Directive 70/524 February 1999.
164. US FDA websites: http://vm.cfsan.fda.gov/~ear/m190-11.html; http://vm.cfsan.fda.gov/~ear/
165. Ingersoll, Bruce, 1990. Technology and Health: FDA Detects Drugs in Milk but Fails to Confirm Results. *Wall Street Journal*, 6 February pB6; Ingersoll, Bruce, 1990. Politics and Policy: GAO Says FDA Can't Substantiate Claims About Milk. *Wall Street Journal*, 21 November pA16; Ingersoll, Bruce, 1990. Technology & Health: FDA Plans a Nationwide Test of Milk for Antibiotics, Other Drug Residues. *Wall Street Journal*, 28 December p10.
166. European Commission. *Op. cit.*
167. Plant, Jane and Tidey, Gill, 2003. *Op. cit.*
168. *Robbins, John, 1987. A Diet for a New America.* Stillpoint Publishing.

5. THE FOOD FACTORS

1. World Cancer Research Fund and American Institute for Cancer Research, 1997. *Food, Nutrition and the Prevention of Cancer: a Global Perspective*. Washington DC: American Institute for Cancer Research. (http://www.aicr.org/report2.htm)
2. http://www.pcrm.org/health/Dairy_and_Prostate_Cancer/d_p_article.html

3. Plant, Jane, 2003. *Your Life in Your Hands.* Second edition. Virgin Books; Plant, Jane and Tidey, Gill, 2002. *The Plant Programme.* Paperback edition. Virgin Books.
4. Smith-Warner, S.A. and Giovannucci, E., 1999. Fruit and Vegetable Intake and Cancer. In: Heber, D., Blackburn, G.L. and Go, V.L.W., eds. *Nutritional Oncology.* San Diego: Academic Press. 153–183.
5. American Institute for Cancer Research, 2000. Press Release (August 31, 2000) from the AICR Annual Research Conference 2000: New Methods in Clinical Trials Lending New Insights on Diet-cancer Connection, Expert Says.
6. Greenwald, Peter, 2002. Cancer chemoprevention. *BMJ*, 324, 714–718.
7. National Cattlemen's Beef Association, 1999. Conjugated Linoleic Acid and Dietary Beef – An Update. *Beef Facts: Nutrition*, Series No. FS/N 016.
8. Ip, C., Scimeca, J.A. and Thompson, H.J., 1994. Conjugated linoleic acid. A powerful anticarcinogen from animal fat sources. *Cancer*, 74, 1050–1054.
9. Steinhart, Carol, 1996. Conjugated linoleic acid: the good news about animal fat. *Journal of Chemical Education*, 73, A302. (http://jchemed.chem.wisc.edu/Journal/ Issues/1996/Dec/absA302.html)
10. Campbell, T.C. and Junshi, C., 1994. Diet and chronic degenerative disease perspectives from China. *American Journal of Clinical Nutrition*, 59 (Suppl.), 1153S–1161S.
11. Waxman, Jonathan, 2001. *The Prostate Cancer Book.* London: Vermillion.
12. *Ibid.*
13. Campbell, T.C., 1994. *Op. cit.*
14. *Food Chemical News*, April 29, 1996.
15. Medical Report: Prostate Cancer. *ICON*, 2002, 1 (5), 8–10.
16. Pritchard, K.I. and others, 1996. Increased thromboembolic complications with concurrent tamoxifen and chemotherapy in a randomized trial of adjuvant therapy for women with breast cancer. *Journal of Clinical Oncology*, 14 (10), 2731–2738.
17. Gooderham, M.J., Adlercreutz, H., Sirpa, T.O., Wahala, K. and Holub, B.J., 1996. A soy protein isolate rich in genistein and daidzein and its effects on plasma isoflavone concentrations, platelet aggegation, blood lipids and fatty acid composition of plasma phospholipid in normal men. *J Nutr*, 126, 2000–2006.
18. Greenwald, Peter, 1996. Chemoprevention of Cancer. *Scientific American*, Special Issue, What you need to know about Cancer, September, 275, (3), 96–99.
19. Setchell, K.D.R., 1998. Phyto-oestrogens: the biochemistry, physiology and implications for human health of soy isoflavones. *Nutrition*, 68, 1333S–1346S.
20. Kurzer, M.S. and Xu, X., 1999. Dietary phytoestrogens. *Annual Reviews of Nutrition*, 17, 353–381.
21. Conil, Christopher and Conil, Jean. *New Tofu Recipes.*
22. Shurtleff, William and Aoyagi, Akiko, 1975. *The Book of Tofu.* Autumn Press Inc.
23. Conil, Christopher. *Op. cit.*
24. Kurzer, M.S., 1999. *Op. cit.*
25. Adlercreutz, H., 1995. Phyto-oestrogens: epidemiology and a possible role in cancer protection. *Environmental Health Perspectives*,103 (Supppl 7), 103–112; Adlercreutz, H., Mazur, W., Bartels, P. and others, 2000. Phyto-oestrogens and prostate disease. *J Nutr*, 130, 658S–659S.
26. http://www.ifst.org/hottop34.htm
27. Adlercreutz, H. and others, 2000. *Op. cit.*
28. Zhou, J.-R., Gugger, E.T., Tanaka, T., Guo, Y., Blackburn, G.L. and Clinton, S.K., 1999. Soy-bean phytochemicals inhibit the growth of transplantable human prostate carcinoma and tumor angiogenesis in mice. *J Nutr*, 129, 1628–1635; Davis, J.N., Singh, B., Bhuiyan, M. and Sarkar, F.H., 1998. Genistein-induced upregulation of p21WAF1, downregulation of cyclin B, and induction of apoptosis in prostate cancer cells. *Nutr Cancer*, 32, 123–131; The Royal Society, 2000. Endocrine-disrupting chemicals. *Document 06/00.* The Royal Society; Setchell, K.D.R., 1998. *Op. cit.*
29. Robbins, John, 1987. *A Diet for a New America.* Stillpoint Publishing; Kradjian, R.M., 1994. *Save Yourself from Breast Cancer.* New York: Berkley Books; McDougall, John,

2000. *The McDougall Program for Women*; Lee, John R., 1999. *Natural Progesterone.* Second revised edition. Jon Carpenter; Plant, Jane and Tidey, Gill, 2003. *Understanding, preventing and overcoming osteoporosis.* Virgin Books; Fox, Douglas, 2001. Hard cheese. *New Scientist*, 15 December 2001, 42–45.

30. http://wayne.unl.edu/00aprilcolumn.htm
31. Martin, Peter, 2002. Milk: Nectar or Poison? *Sunday Times Magazine*, July 21, 2002, 46–54.
32. http://www.nationaldairycouncil.org/lvl04/nutrilib/digest/dairydigest_710.htm
33. Steinhart, Carol, 1996. *Op. cit.*
34. Website of the American Cancer Society, http://www.cancer.org/docroot/eto/content/eto_5_3x_soybean.asp?siteare a=&viewmode=print
35. Gottlieb, Scott, 2003. Men should eat nine servings of fruit and vegetables a day. *BMJ*, 326, 1003.
36. UK Ministry of Agriculture, Fisheries and Food advice as reported in the *Sunday Times*, 1999.
37. Willet, W.C., 1994. Micronutrients and cancer risk. *Am J Clin Nutr*, 59, (suppl), 1162S–5S. See also: Willett, Walter C., Colditz, Graham A. and Mueller, Nancy A., 1996. Strategies for Minimising Cancer Risk. *Scientific American*, Special Issue, What you need to know about Cancer, September, 275, (3), 88–95.
38. Greenwald, Peter, 1996. *Op. cit.*
39. Huang, M.-T., Asawa T., Ho C.-T., Rosen R.T., eds, 1994. *Food phytochemicals for cancer prevention I – fruits and vegetables.* Washington, DC: American Chemical Society; Ho, C.-T., Osawa, T., Huang, M.-T. and Rosen, R.T., eds, 1994. *Food phytochemicals for cancer prevention II – teas, spices, herbs.* Washington, DC: American Chemical Society; American Institute for Cancer Research, ed., 1996. *Dietary phytochemicals in cancer prevention and treatment.* New York: Plenum Press; Liu, R.H. and Espinosa, A., 2000. Bio-active Compounds from Fruits and Vegetables in the Prevention of Cancer. In: *Agriculture in the New Century: Managing Bio-Resources and Bio-Diversity*, National Taiwan University, Taipei, Taiwan, 53–59.
40. Greenwald, Peter, 2002. *Op. cit.*
41. Alpha-Tocopherol Beta-Carotene Cancer Prevention Study Group, Heinonen, O.P., Huttunen, J.K. and Albanes, D., 1994. The effect of vitamin E and beta-carotene on the incidence of lung cancer and other cancers in male smokers. *New England Journal of Medicine*, 330, 1029–35; Omenn, G.S., Goodman, G.E., Thornquist, M.D., Balmes, J., Cullen, M.R. and Glass, A., 1996. Effects of a combination of beta carotene and vitamin A on lung cancer and cardiovascular disease. *N Engl J Med*, 334, 1150–1155.
42. Medical Report: Prostate Cancer. *ICON*, 2002, 1 (5), 8–10.
43. Levy, J., Bosin, E., Feldman, B., Giat, Y., Miinster, Danilenko M. and Sharoni, Y., 1995. Lycopene is more potent inhibitor of human cancer cell proliferation than either A-carotene or B-carotene. *Nutr Cancer*, 24, 257–266.
44. Gunnell, D.L. and 10 others, 2003. Are diet–prostate-cancer associations mediated by the IGF axis? A cross-sectional analysis of diet, IGF-I and IGFBP-3 in healthy middle-aged men. *British Journal of Cancer*, 88, 1682–1686.
45. Mucci, L.A. and six others, 2001. Are dietary influences on the risk of prostate cancer mediated through the insulin-like growth factor system? *BJU Int*, 87, 814–820.
46. Giovannucci, E., 1999. Tomatoes: tomato-based products, lycopene and cancer: review of the epidemiological literature. *J Nat Cancer Inst*, 91, 317–331.
47. Willett, Walter C., 1996. *Op. cit.*
48. Ortega, R.M. and others, 1996. Functional and psychic deterioration in elderly people may be aggravated by folate deficiency. *J Nutr*, 126, 1992–1999.
49. http://www.flax.com.fda
50. Hambridge, K. M., Casey, C. E. and Krebs, N. F., 1986. Zinc. In: *Trace Elements in Human and Animal Nutrition*, Fifth Edition, Mertz, W., Ed. Academic Press, Inc., London.

51. Medical Report: Prostate Cancer. *Op. cit.*
52. McCusker, R.H., 1998. Controlling insulin-like growth factor activity and the modulation of insulin-like growth factor binding protein and receptor binding. *Journal of Dairy Science*, 81, 1790–1800.
53. Greenwald, Peter, 1996. *Op. cit.*
54. Coghlan, Andy, 1999. Crunch Time for Cancer. *New Scientist*, 13 November, 264, 2212.
55. Pinto, J.T., Qiao, C.H., Xing, J. and others, 1999. Effects of garlic thioallylic derivatives on growth, glutathione concentration, and polyamine formation of human prostate carcinoma cells in culture. *Am J Clin Nutr*; see also: Li, G., Qiao, C.H., Lin, R.I. and others, 1995. Antiproliferative effects of garlic constituents in cultured human breast cancer cells. *Oncology Reports*, 2, 787–791.
56. http://www.3mistral.co.uk/garlic/cancer.htm; see also: http://www.mskcc.org/rande/pharmacology/189.html
57. Inside Story. *Which?* April 2002, 4.
58. Doll, R. and Peto, R., 1981. *The Causes of Cancer: quantitative estimates of avoidable risks of cancer in the United States today*. New York: Oxford University Press.
59. Lang, T. and Clutterbuck, C., 1991. *P is for Pesticides*. Ebury Press, Random Century Group.
60. Mittelstaedt, Martin, 2002. Data point to breast-cancer risk. *Globe and Mail*, 22 November 2002, A5.
61. McMichael, A.J., 1993. *Planetary Overload – Global Environmental Change and the Health of the Species*. Cambridge University Press.
62. Royal Commission on Environmental Pollution, 2002. *A Short Report on the Environmental Effects of Civil Aircraft in Flight*. Royal Commission on Environmental Pollution.
63. Bristow, Amanda, 2002. *Which?*, April 2002, 22–23.
64. *ICON*, September 2002.
65. Hunter, David J. and Willett, Walter C., 1993. Diet and body build: diet, body size and breast cancer, *Epidemiologic Reviews*, 15, 1, 110–132.
66. http://www.eurocbc.org/page641.html; http://www.ciwf.co.uk/Trust/FF/farm_facts_fish_farming.htm
67. Simpson and others. Effect of exogenous estradiol on plasma concentrations of somatotropin, insulin-like growth factor 1, insulin-like growth factor-binding protein activity, and metabolites in ovariectomised Angus and Brahman cows. http://www.nal.usda.gov/ttic/tektran/glimpse/data/000007/75/0000077539.html
68. The Globe and Mail, 31 July 1999.
69. Hendler, S.S., 1990. *The Doctors' Vitamin and Mineral Encyclopaedia*. Simon and Schuster, New York.
70. Hetzel, B.S. and Maberly, G.F., 1986. Iodine, In: *Trace Elements in Human and Animal Nutrition*, Fifth Edition, Mertz, W., Ed. Academic Press, Inc., London.
71. Johnson, C., 1999, Environmental controls in iodine deficiency disorders (IDD), *Earthworks*, 9 November, p. 3, British Geological Survey.
72. http://www.prostatepointers.org/cmyers/pf0696.html
73. *Ibid.*
74. *Ibid.*; *American Heart Association Cookbook*, fifth edition, 1995. New York: Times Books, Random House; Pritikin, Nathan, 1979. *The Pritikin Program for Diet and Exercise*. New York: Bantam Books; Ornish, D., 1990. *Dr Dean Ornish's Program for Reversing Heart Disease*. New York: Ballantyne Books.
75. www.annieappleseedproject.org/nutgenprotin.html
76. Kohlmeier, L. and others, 1997. Adipose tissue trans fatty acids and breast cancer in the European Community Multicenter Study on Antioxidants, Myocardial Infarction, and Breast Cancer. *Cancer Epidemiology Biomarkers and Prevention*, 6, (9), 705–710.
77. Koletzko, B., 1992. Trans fatty acids may impair biosynthesis of long-chain polyunsaturates and growth in man. *Acta Paediatrica*, 81, 302–306.

78. Dupont, J., White, P.J., Johnston, K.M. and others, 1989. Food safety and health effects of canola oil. *J Am Coll Nutr*, 8, 360–375.
79. Simopoulos, A.P., 1991. Omega-3 fatty acids in health and disease and in growth and development. *Am J Clin Nutr*, 54, 438–463.
80. Quoted in Small, Meredith F., 2002. The happy fat. *New Scientist*, Aug 2002, 34–37.
81. *Ibid.*
82. Ingram, A.J. and others, 1995. Effects of a flaxseed and flax oil diet in a rat–5/6 renal ablation model. *American Journal of Kidney Disease*, February 25, 2, 320–329.
83. Obermeyer, W.R., Musser, S.M., Betz, J.M. and others, 1995. Chemical studies of phytoestrogens and related compounds in dietary supplements – flax and chaparral. *Proceedings of the Society for Experimental Biology and Medicine*. See also Obermeyer, W.R., Warner, C., Casey, R.E. and Musser, S., 1993. Flaxseed lignans isolation metabolism and biological effects. *Fed Am Soc Exp Biol J*, A863.
84. Trichopoulos, Dimitrios, Li, Frederick P. and Hunter, David J., 1996. What Causes Cancer? *Scientific American*, Special Issue, What you need to know about Cancer, September, 275, (3), 80–85.
85. http://www.findarticles.com/cf_0/m0FKA/5_62/62702338/p1/article. jhtml?term = turmeric%2C + Liz + Brown
86. Steinmetz, K.A. and Potter, J.D., 1991. Vegetables, fruit, and cancer, II. Mechanisms. *Cancer Causes Control*, 2, 427–442; Lam, L.K.T., Zhang, J., Hasegawa, S. and others, 1994. Inhibition of chemically induced carcinogenesis by citrus liminoids. In: Huang, M-T. *Op. cit.*, 209–219; Zheng, G.Q., Zhang, J., Kenney, P.M. and Lam, L.K.T., 1994. Stimulation of glutathione S-transferase and inhibition of carcinogenesis in mice by celery seed oil constituents. In: Huang, M.-T. *Op. cit.*, 230–238.
87. Nakatani, N., 1994. Chemistry of antioxidants from Labiatae herbs. In: Ho, C.-T. *Op. cit.*, 144–153.
88. Ho, C.-T., Ferraro, T., Chen, Q and others, 1994. Phytochemicals in teas and rosemary and their cancer-preventive properties. In: Ho, C.-T. *Op. cit.*, 2–19.
89. Kikuzaki, H. and Nakatani, N., 1993. Antioxidant effects of some ginger constituents. *Journal of Food Science*, 58, 1407–1410.
90. Zheng, G.Q., Kenney, P.M. and Lam, L.K.T., 1993. Potential anticarcinogenic natural products isolated from lemongrass oil and galanga root oil. *Journal of Agricultural and Food Chemistry*, 41, 153–156; Zheng, G.Q., Kenney, P.M. and Lam, L.K.T., 1992. Anethofuran, carvone, and limonene: potential cancer chemopreventive agents from dill weed oil and caraway oil. *Planta Medica*, 58, 338–341; Zheng, G.Q., Kenney, P.M., Zhang, J. and others, 1993. Chemoprevention of benzo[a]pyrene-induced forestomach cancer in mice by natural phthalides from celery seed oil. *Nutr Cancer*, 19, 77–86; Zheng, G.Q., Kenney, P.M. and Lam, L.K.T., 1992. Sesquiterpenes from clove (Eugenia caryophyllata) as potential anticarcinogenic agents. *Journal of Natural Products*, 55, 999–1003; Zheng, G.Q., Kenney, P.M. and Lam, L.K.T., 1992. Myristicin: a potential cancer chemopreventive agent from parsley leaf oil. *J Agric Food Chem*, 40, 107–110.
91. http://www.pcrm.org/health/Dairy_and_Prostate_Cancer/d_p_article.html;   World Cancer Research Fund. *Op. cit.*
92. *Journal of the American Diabetic Association*, May 2001; http://www.wadsworth.com/ nutrition_d/special_features/news/nutu1201.ht ml.
93. Thompson, L.U., 1994. Antioxidants and hormone-mediated health benefits of whole grains. *Critical Reviews in Food Science and Nutrition*, 34, 473–497.
94. Thompson, L.U., 1992. Potential health benefits of whole grains and their components. *Contemp Nutr*, 17 (6), 1–2.
95. Elson, C.E. and Yu, S.G., 1994. The chemoprevention of cancer by mevalonate-derived constituents of fruits and vegetables. *J Nutr*, 124, 607–614.
96. *Ibid.*
97. Fox, Douglas, 2002. Bread to blame for plague of pimples. *New Scientist*, 7 December 2002.
98. Forbes, Alec, 1984. *The Bristol Diet*, Century.

99. *Ibid.*
100. Ingram, A.J., 1995. *Op. cit.*
101. http://www.dorway.com/badnews.html
102. http://www.stevia.net; http://www.holisticmed.com/sweet/
103. Lee, S. and others, 1999. Monitoring of Drinking Water in Terms of Natural Organic Matter and Disinfection By-products. Proc 2nd Intern. Symp. On Advanced Env. Monitoring, Kwangju, Korea.
104. Anon, 2003. News, In brief: Pesticide residues found in Indian bottled water. 2003. *BMJ*, 326, 352.
105. Herrick, D., 1996. Cryptosporidium and Giardia: Should you be concerned? *Water Well Journal*, 50, 4, 49, 44–46.
106. Jankun, Jerzy, Selman, Steven H., Swiercz, Rafal and Skrzypczak-Jankun, Ewa, 1997. Why drinking green tea could prevent cancer. *Nature*, 387, 15 June, 561; see also: Greenwald, Peter, 1996. *Op. cit.*
107. Jankun, Jerzy, 1997. *Op. cit.*
108. Meiers and others, 2001. The Anthocyanidins Cyanidin and Delphinidin are potent inhibitors of the epidermal growth-factor receptor. *J Agric Food Chem*, 49, 958–962.
109. http://www.annieappleseedproject.org/nutgenprotin.html, reporting on a conference on nutritional genomics and proteomics in cancer prevention in September 2002, at the USNIH, Bethesda.
110. Campion, K., 1986. *Vegetarian Encyclopaedia*. Century Hutchinson Ltd, London.
111. Jankun, Jerzy, 1997. *Op. cit.*
112. Oliver, S.E., Gunnell, D.G., Donovan, J. and others, 2004. Screen-detected prostate cancer and the insulin-like growth factor axis: Results of a population-based case-control study. *International Journal of Cancer*, 108, 887–892.
113. http://research.kib.ki.se/e-uven/public/51419.html
114. ENDS Report.
115. http://www.vegansociety.com/html/info/info28.html
116. http://www.vegansociety.com
117. Royal College of Physicians, 2002. *Nutrition and patients: a doctor's responsibility.*

6. THE LIFESTYLE FACTORS

1. Berger, Abi, 2002. Science commentary: What does zinc do? *BMJ*, 325, 1062–1063.
2. Josefson, Deborah, 2002. Popping a multivitamin daily can keep disease at bay. *BMJ*, 324, 1544.
3. Campbell, T.C. and Junshi, C., 1994. Diet and chronic degenerative disease perspectives from China. *American Journal of Clinical Nutrition*, 59 (Suppl.), 1153S–1161S.
4. Greenwald, Peter, 1996. Chemoprevention of Cancer. *Scientific American*, Special Issue, What you need to know about Cancer, September, 275 (3), 96-99.
5. Olivotto, Ivo, Hoffer, Abram and Lesperance, Mary, 2002. In *Breast Cancer Research and Treatment*, http://www.nlm.nih.gov/medlineplus/news/fullstory_10706.html
6. Bender, David A., 2002. Daily doses of multivitamin tablets. *BMJ*, 325, 173–174.
7. *Annals of Internal Medicine*, July 1, 2003; http://www.nlm.nih.gov/medlineplus/news/fullstory_13210.html
8. Kmietowicz, Zosia, 2003. Food watchdog warns against high doses of vitamins and minerals. *BMJ*, 326, 1001.
9. http://www.nlm.nih.gov/medlineplus/news/fullstory_13219.html
10. Spallholz, J.E., Stewart, J.R., 1989. Advances in the role of minerals in immunobiology. Center for Food and Nutrition, Texas Tech University, Lubbock 79409. *Biol Trace Elem Res Mar*, 19 (3) 129–151.
11. Redbook, April, 1989, v172, n6, p. 96 (5).
12. Veith, R., 1999. Vitamin D supplementation, 25-hydroxyvitamin D concentrations, and safety. *American Journal of Clinical Nutrition*, 69, 842–856; Chesney, R.W., 1989. Vitamin D: Can an upper limit be defined? *J Nutr*, 119 (12 Suppl), 1825–1828; http://www.cc.nih.gov/ccc/supplements/vitdref.html

13. Oakley, Godfrey P., 2002. Delaying folic acid fortification of flour. *BMJ*, 324, 1348–1349.
14. Reynolds, Edward, 2002. Fortification of flour with folic acid. *BMJ*, 324, 918.
15. Niki, E., Noguchi, N., Tsuchihashi, H. and others, 1995. Interaction among vitamin C, vitamin E and beta-carotene. *Am J Clin Nutr*, 62 (Suppl), 1322S–1326S.
16. Craig, Winston J., 2002. Phytochemicals: Guardians of Our Health, http://www.andrews.edu/NUFS/phyto.html, 03/12/02.
17. Monographs on the Evaluation of the Carcinogenic Risk of Chemicals to Man, 1982. Geneva: World Health Organization, International Agency for Research on Cancer, 1972–present. (Multivolume work). V29, 282.
18. Anon, 2003. Growing problems: Endocrine disruptors under the spotlight. *ENDS Report*, 336, 20–23.
19. Vikse, R. and others, 1999. Heterocyclic amines in cooked meat. *Tidsskr Nor Laegeforen*, 119 (1), 45–49.
20. Skog, K. and others, 1997. Polar and non-polar heterocyclic amines in cooked fish and meat products and their corresponding pan residues. *Food Chemical Toxicology*, 35 (6), 555–565.
21. Anon, 2002. 'Minerva'. *BMJ*, 325, 1250.
22. http://www.who.int/inf/en/pr-2002-51.html
23. JIFSTAN/NCFST Acrylamide in Food Workshop, 1989. White paper for Working Group 5: Risk Communication. National Research Council, National Academy of Sciences (NRC-NAS). *Improving Risk Communication*. National Academy Press, Washington DC.
24. Fleck, Fiona, 2002. Experts launch action on staple foods. *BMJ*, 325, 120.
25. Anon, 2002. Acrylamide clues found in Asparagine. *ICON*, 1 (6), 24.
26. Anon, 1997. Acrylamide. Toxic Air Contaminant Identification. List Summaries – ARB/SSD/SES. September 1997.
27. website of the US Environmental Protection Agency, http://www.epa.gov/ttn/atw/hlthef/acrylami.html
28. *Ibid.*
29. http://ntp-server.niehs.nih.gov/htdocs/Chem_H&S/NTP_Chem7/Radian79-06-1.html
30. http://www.nsc.org/library/chemical/Acrylami.htm
31. Anon, 1997. *Op. cit.*
32. Advisory Committee on Hazardous Substances. *Sixth Annual Report* (2001–2002). Department for Environment, Food and Rural Affairs; The Royal Commission on Environmental Pollution, 2003. Chemicals in products: safeguarding the environment and human health. *Report* 24.
33. website of the US Environmental Protection Agency. *Op. cit.*
34. http://ntp-server.niehs.nih.gov/htdocs/Chem_H&S/NTP_Chem7/Radian79-06-1.html
35. http://www.foodstandards.gov.uk/multimedia/webpage/acrylamide_study_faq
36. Inside Story. *Which?* April 2002, 4.
37. Waxman, Jonathan, 2001. *The Prostate Cancer Book*. London: Vermillion.
38. White, Craig A. and Macleod, Una, 2002. ABC of psychological medicine: Cancer. *BMJ*, 325, 377–380.
39. Walsh, Kiri, King, Michael, Jones, Louise, Tookman, Adrian and Blizzard, Robert, 2002. Spiritual beliefs may affect outcome of bereavement: prospective study. *BMJ*, 324, 1551–1554.
40. White, Craig A. 2002. *Op. cit.*
41. *Ibid.*
42. *Ibid.*
43. Petticrew, Mark, Bell, Ruth and Hunter, Duncan, 2002. Influence of psychological coping on survival and recurrence in people with cancer: systematic review. *BMJ*, 325, 1066–1069.

44. Ernst, Edzard (ed.), 2001. *The desktop guide to complementary and alternative medicine.* Mosby.
45. http://www.nccn.org/patient_gls/_english/_prostate/
46. King, Michael and five others, 2002. Effectiveness of teaching general practitioners skills in brief cognitive behaviour therapy to treat patients with depression: randomised controlled trial. *BMJ*, 324, 947.
47. Heason, P., Deep Relaxation available from 37 Tollerton Lane, Tollerton, Nottingham.
48. *European Journal of Cancer*, 2003, 39, 1562–1567; quoted in *BMJ*, 327, 402.
49. Based on Holland, J C., 1996. Cancer's Psychological Challenges. *Scientific American*, Special Issue, What you need to know about Cancer, September, 275, (3), 158–161.
50. Bartram, Thomas, 1998. *Bartram's Encyclopedia of Herbal Medicine.* London: Robinson.
51. *Cancer Epidemiology Biomarkers & Prevention*, July 2003; http://www.nlm.nih.gov/medlineplus/news/fullstory_13352.html
52. Oliver, S.E., Gunnell, D.G., Donovan, J. and others, 2004. Screen-detected prostate cancer and the insulin-like growth factor axis: Results of a population-based case-control study. *International Journal of Cancer*, 108, 887–892.
53. Signorello, L.B., Kuper, H., Lagiou, P. and others, 2000. Lifestyle factors and insulin-like growth factor 1 levels among elderly men. *European Journal of Cancer Prevention*, 9, 173–178.
54. Chan, J.M., Stampfer, M.J., Giovannucci, E., 1998. Plasma insulin-like growth factor-I and prostate cancer risk: a prospective study. *Science*, 279, 563-566; Stattin, P., Bylund, A., Rinaldi, S. and others, 2000. Plasma insulin-like growth factor-I, insulin-like growth factor-binding proteins, and prostate cancer risk: a prospective study. *J Natl Cancer Inst*, 92, 1910–1917.
55. *Cancer Epidemiology*, July 2003, *Op. cit.*
56. Plant, Jane and Tidey, Gill, 2003. *Understanding, Preventing and Overcoming Osteoporosis.* Virgin Books.
57. Goodman-Gruen, D. and Barrett-Connor, E., 1997. Epidemiology of insulin-like growth factor-I in elderly men and women. The Rancho Bernardo Study. *American Journal of Epidemiology*, 145, 970–976; Kaklamani, V.G., Linos, A., Kaklamani, E., Markaki, I. and Mantzoros, C., 1999. Age, sex, and smoking are predictors of circulating insulin-like growth factor 1 and insulin-like growth factor-binding protein 3. *Journal of Clinical Oncology*, 17, 813–817.
58. Levy, Len, 1998. Biomed II: Exposure to low-level benzene, p. 76. In: Institute for Environment and Health, Annual Report.
59. Pearson, J.K., 2000. The Air Quality Challenge, American Society of Automotive Engineers and HMSO.
60. North Atlantic Treaty Organisation, 1988. International Toxicity Equivalency Factor (I-TEF) method of risk assessment for complex mixtures of dioxins and related compounds. Pilot study on international information exchange on dioxins and related compounds. *CCMS Report* Number 176, Environmental Protection Agency, Washington DC, USA.
61. EPA Dioxin Reassessment Summary, 1994 4//94 – Vol. 1, CER/ORD Publication Centre, USEPA.
62. MAFF, 1997. Dioxins and PCBs in Retail Cows' Milk in England. *Food Surveillance Information Sheet*, No. 136, Ministry of Agriculture, Fisheries and Food, London.
63. Tanabe, S., 1988. PCB problems in the future: foresight from current knowledge. *Environmental Pollution*, 50, 5–28.
64. Department of the Environment, 1989. Dioxins in the Environment. *Pollution Paper*, No. 27, HMSO, London.
65. MAFF, 1997. Dioxins and Polychlorinated Biphenyls in Fish Oil Dietary Supplements and Licensed Medicines. *Food Surveillance Information Sheet*, No 106, Ministry of Agriculture, Fisheries and Food, London.
66. MAFF, 1996. Dioxins in Human Milk. *Food Surveillance Information Sheet*, No 88, Ministry of Agriculture, Fisheries and Food, London.

67. MAFF, 1996. Polychlorinated Biphenyls in Food – UK Dietary Intakes. *Food Surveillance Information Sheet*, No 89, Ministry of Agriculture, Fisheries and Food, London.

68. The Environment Agency, March 2000. *Endocrine-disrupting substances in the environment: The Environment Agency's Strategy*, The Environment Agency, Bristol, UK.

69. Miller, W.R. and Sharpe, R.M., 1998. Environmental oestrogens and human reproductive cancers. *Endocrine-Related Cancer*, 5, 69–96; Plant, J.A. and Davis, D.L., 2003. Breast and prostate cancer: sources and pathways of endocrine-disrupting chemicals (EDCs). In *Geology and Health*. Skinner, H.C.W. and Berger, A.R. (eds). OUP. 95–99.

70. Toppari, J., Larsen, J.C., Christiansen, P. and others, 1996. Male reproductive health and environmental xenoestrogens. *Environmental Health Perspectives*, 104, 741–803.

71. The Royal Commission on Environmental Pollution, 2003. *Op. cit.*; Annual Reports of the (UK) Chemical Stakeholders Forum, 2002, and The Advisory Committee on Hazardous Substances, 2002; Miller, W.R. and Sharpe, R.M., 1998. Environmental oestrogens and human reproductive cancers. *Endocrine-Related Cancer*, 5, 69–96.

72. *Environmental Endocrine Disruptors: A Handbook of Property Data*, John Wiley & Sons Inc..

73. Colborn, T., Dumanoski, D. and Myers, J.P., 1996. *Our Stolen Futures*, Dutton, Penguin Books, USA.

74. Webb, S.F., 2000. Risk assessment approaches for pharmaceuticals. In: International Seminar: Pharmaceuticals in the Environment, Technological Institute, Section on Environmental Technology, Brussels, 2000.

75. Kolpin, D.A., Furlong, E.T., Meyer, M.T. and others, 2002. Pharmaceuticals, hormones, and other organic wastewater contaminants in US streams, 1999–2000: a national reconnaissance. *Environmental Science & Technology*, 36, 1202–1211.

76. McQuillan, D., Mullany, J., Parker, J. and others, 2000. Drug Residues in Ambient Water: Initial Surveillance in New Mexico, USA. December 2000 Progress Report, http://www.nmenv.state.nm.us/gwb/drugs.html; Morelli, J., 2000. Are Our Medicines Tainting the Environment? http://webmd.lycos.com/content/article/25/1728_58159?

77. McQuillan, D., 2000. *Op. cit.*

78. The Royal Commission on Environmental Pollution, 2003. *Op. cit.*

79. Hamburger Umwelt Institute, 1997. Poor Design Practices – gaseous emissions form complex products.

80. Brown, S.K. and Cheng, M., 2000. Volatile Organic Compounds (VOCs) in New Car Interiors. Presented at the 15th International Clean Air & Environment Conference Sydney, 26–30 November 2000.

81. http://www.le.ac.uk/ieh

82. Dyson, T., 1999. Prospects for feeding the world. *BMJ*, 319, 988–991.

83. McMichael, A.J., 1993. *Planetary Overload.* Cambridge University Press.

84. Wolford, S.T. and Argoudelis, C.J., 1979. Measurement of estrogens in cow's milk, human milk and dairy products. *Journal of Dairy Science*, 62 (9), 1458–63.

85. Reuters, 8 October 1998.

86. McMurry, Laura M., Oethinger, Margaret, Levy, Stuart B., 1998. Triclosan targets lipid synthesis. *Nature*, 394, 6693, 531–532.

87. Trichopoulos, Dimitrios, Li, Frederick P. and Hunter, David J., 1996. What Causes Cancer? *Scientific American*, Special Issue, What you need to know about Cancer, September, 275, 3, 80–85.

88. Waxman, Jonathan, 2001. *Op. cit.*

89. www.ananova.com/news/story/sm_800400.html.

7. INFORMATION, MISINFORMATION AND MONEY

1. Campbell, T.C. and Junshi, C., 1994. Diet and chronic degenerative disease perspectives from China. *American Journal of Clinical Nutrition*, 59, Suppl., 1153S–1161S.

2. Plant, Jane, 2000 and 2003. *Your Life in Your Hands*. Virgin Books; Plant, Jane and Tidey, Gill, 2001. *The Plant Programme*. Virgin Books; Plant, Jane and Tidey, Gill, 2003. *Understanding, Preventing and Overcoming Osteoporosis*. Virgin Books.

3. Marwick, Charles, 2003. Food industry obfuscates healthy eating message. *BMJ*, 327, 121.
4. Martin, Peter, 2002. Milk: Nectar or Poison? *Sunday Times Magazine*, 21 July 2002, 46–54.
5. http://www.cafod.org.uk
6. Anon, 2003. UK supports exclusive breast feeding for six months. *BMJ*, 326, 1052.
7. Laurens, Claire, 2003. Baby milk company fined for advertising direct to consumers. *BMJ*, 327, 307.
8. http://www.nationaldairycouncil.org
9. Plant, Jane, 2000 and 2003. *Op. cit.*
10. Kradjian, R.M., 1994. *Save Yourself from Breast Cancer*. Berkley Books, New York.
11. Outwater, J.L. and others, 1997. Dairy products and breast cancer: the IGF-1, estrogen and bGH hypothesis. *Medical Hypotheses*, 48, 453–461.
12. European Commission, Scientific Committee on Vetinerary Measures Relating to Public Health. 1999. Report on Public Health Aspects of the Use of Bovine Somatotropin, 15–16 March.
13. Yu, H. and Rohan, T., 2002. Role of the insulin-like growth factor family in cancer development and progression. *J Natl Cancer Inst*, 92, 1472–1489.
14. http://www.milksucks.com/osteo.html
15. Martin, Peter, 2002. *Op. cit.*
16. *Ibid.*
17. *Ibid.*
18. Bristow, A., 2002. Organic processed food. *Which?* April 2002, 22–23.
19. *Ibid.*
20. Inside Story. *Which?* April 2002, 4.
21. Smith, Richard, 2003. Do patients need to read research? *BMJ*, 326, 1307.
22. *Ibid.*
23. Corrie, Pippa, Shaw, Justin and Harris, Roy, 2003. Rate limiting factors in recruitment of patients to clinical trials in cancer research: descriptive study. *BMJ*, 327, 320–321.
24. Baum, M., 2002. The ATAC (arimidex, tamoxifen, alone or in combination) adjuvant breast cancer trial in postmenopausal patients: factors influencing the success of patient recruitment. *European Journal of Cancer*, 38, 1684–1686.
25. Wald, Nicholas J. and Morris, Joan K., 2003. Teleoanalysis: combining data from different types of study. *BMJ*, 327, 616-618.
26. Waxman, Jonathan, 2001. *The Prostate Cancer Book*. London: Vermillion.
27. Research muddled by political pressures. *The Times (Public Agenda)*, 19 August 2003.
28. Chaturvedi, P., 2003. Medical community may be partly responsible for cancer misery. *BMJ*, 326, 1146.
29. Kmietowicz, Zosia, 2002. Research spending on cancers doesn't match their death rates. *BMJ*, 325, 920.
30. Plant, J.A., Turner, K.T. and Highley, D.E., 1998. Minerals and the environment. Proceedings of Minerals '98 Conference, June 1998; Republished in the *Mineralogical Society Bulletin* No.119, July 1998, 3–11; *Mineral Planning* 77, December 1998, 3–8; *IM&M Journal*, December 1998, 1, 12, 331–336.
31. Getz, Linn, Sigurdsson, Johann A. and Hetlevik, Irene, 2003. Is opportunistic disease prevention in the consultation ethically justifiable? *BMJ*, 327, 498.
32. Smith, Richard, 2003. Editor's choice: The screening industry. *BMJ*, 326, 26 April 2003.
33. Mason, Andrew C., 2003. Screening in private sector has knock on effects in public sector in two tier health systems. *BMJ*, 326, 1457-1458.
34. Gottlieb, Scott, 2003. US drug sales continue to rise. *BMJ*, 326, 518.
35. Gottlieb, Scott, 2002. Drug companies maintain 'astounding' profits. *BMJ*, 324, 1054.
36. Kjaergard, Lise L. and Als-Nielsen, Bodil, 2002. Association between competing interests and authors' conclusions: epidemiological study of randomised clinical trials published in the *BMJ*. *BMJ*, 325, 249–252.
37. Eaton, Lynn, 2003. Readers want transparency in link between doctors and drug firms. *BMJ*, 326, 1352.

38. *BMJ*, 31 May 2003.
39. Mayor, Susan, 2002. Researchers claim clinical trials are reported with misleading statistics. *BMJ*, 324, 1353.
40. *JAMA*, 2003, 389, 454–465, quoted by Hopkins Tanne, Janice, 2003. Industry is deeply involved in funding US research. *BMJ*, 326, 179.
41. Tonks, Alison, 2002. Authors of guidelines have strong links with drugs industry. *BMJ*, 324, 383.
42. Spurgeon, David, 2002. Doctors accept $50 a time to listen to drug representatives. *BMJ*, 324, 1113.
43. Josefson, Deborah, 2002. Doctors warned to be wary of new drugs. *BMJ*, 324, 1113.
44. Aronson, Jeffrey, 2003. Anecdotes as evidence. *BMJ*, 326, 1346.
45. Aronson, J.K., ed., 2001. *Side Effects of Drugs Annual*. Amsterdam: Elsevier.
46. Altman, D.G. and others, 2001. The revised CONSORT statement for reporting randomised trials: explanation and elaboration. *Ann Intern Med*, 134, 663–694.
47. Eaton, Lynn, 2003. 'Yellow card' announcement used to head off concerns, experts claim. *BMJ*, 327, 308.
48. Gottlieb, Scott, 2002. A fifth of Americans contact their doctor as a result of direct to consumer drug advertising. *BMJ*, 325, 854.
49. Anon, 2003. News: Drug companies want to inform patients. *BMJ*, 326, 1286.
50. Kmietowicz, Zosia, 2003. New Zealand GPs call for end to direct advertising. *BMJ*, 326, 1284.
51. Watson, Rory, 2003. EU health ministers reject proposal for limited direct to consumer advertising. *BMJ*, 326, 1284.
52. Mayor, Susan, 2002. GMC issues new guidance on clinical research. *BMJ*, 324, 384.
53. Marwick, Charles, 2002. US tackles drug company gifts to doctors. *BMJ*, 325, 795.
54. Mosconi, Paola, 2003. Declaration of competing interests is rare in Italian breast cancer associations. *BMJ*, 327, 344.
55. Herxheimer A., 2003. Relationships between the pharmaceutical industry and patients' organisations. *BMJ*, 326, 1208–1210.
56. Hirst J., 2003. Charities and patient groups should declare interests. *BMJ*, 326, 1211.
57. Clark, Jocalyn, 2003. A hot flush for Big Pharma. *BMJ*, 327, 400.
58. Writing Group for the Women's Health Initiative Investigators, 2002. Risks and benefits of estrogen plus progestin in healthy postmenopausal women. *JAMA*, 288, 321–333.
59. Moynihan, Ray, 2003. US seniors group attacks pharmaceutical industry 'fronts'. *BMJ*, 326, 351.
60. Lenzer, Jeanne, 2002. The operation was a success (but the patient died). *BMJ*, 325, 664.
61. Walsh, P.C., 2002. Surgery and the reduction of mortality from prostate cancer. *New England Journal of Medicine*, 347, 781–789.
62. Griffiths, Frances, 2003. Taking hormone replacement therapy. *BMJ*, 327, 820.
63. Clark, Jocalyn, 2003. *Op. cit.*
64. *N Engl J Med*, 349, 523–534.
65. *Lancet*, 362, 419–427.
66. Lenzer, Jeanne, 2002. *Op. cit.*
67. Moynihan, Ray, 2003. Blurring the boundaries. *BMJ*, 326, 1094.
68. *The Times*, Saturday August 9, 2003.
69. Bartlett, Christopher, Sterne, Jonathan and Egger, Matthias, 2002. What is newsworthy? Longitudinal study of the reporting of medical research in two British newspapers. *BMJ*, 325, 81.
70. Several versions of the poem, of which this is an extract, may be found on the internet; for example, http://www.madnessmansion.com/jimkc/txt/ambulanc.txt; http://www.public.asu.edu/tadams2/Quotes/Ambulance
71. McMichael, A.J. and Powles, J.W., 1999. Human numbers, environment, sustainability and health. *BMJ*, 319, 977–980.

To find out more about prostate cancer

1. BOOKS

The Prostate Cancer Book by Jonathan Waxman, published by Vermillion.
Prostate Problems by Jane Smith and Dr David Gillatt, published by Hodder and Stoughton.

2. BOOKLETS FROM THE US NATIONAL CANCER INSTITUTE*

Booklet About Prostate Cancer
'What You Need to Know about Prostate Cancer'

Booklet About Prostate Changes
'Understanding Prostate Changes: A Health Guide for All Men'

Booklets About Cancer Treatment
'Understanding Treatment Choices for Prostate Cancer: Know Your Options'
'Chemotherapy and You: A Guide to Self-Help During Treatment'
'Helping Yourself During Chemotherapy: 4 Steps for Patients'
'Radiation Therapy and You: A Guide to Self-Help During Treatment'
'Pain Control: A Guide for People with Cancer and Their Families'
'Get Relief From Cancer Pain'

Booklets About Living With Cancer
'Taking Time: Support for People With Cancer and the People Who Care About Them'
'Facing Forward: Life After Cancer Treatment'
'When Cancer Recurs: Meeting the Challenge'
'Advanced Cancer: Living Each Day'

3. USEFUL WEBSITES

The Prostate Cancer Charity (UK): http://www.prostate-cancer.org.uk
The National Cancer Institute (US): http://www.nci.nih.gov/cancerinfo/wyntk/prostate
  and http://cancer.gov
The National Comprehensive Cancer Network, in partnership with the American Cancer
  Society (US): http://www.nccn.org/patient_gls/_english/_prostate/
PSA Rising (US): http://www.psa-rising.com

4. FIND OUT ABOUT LOCAL PROSTATE-CANCER SUPPORT GROUPS

---

* http://www.nci.nih.gov/cancerinfo/wyntk/prostate.

5. FIND OUT ABOUT CENTRES THAT PROVIDE DIETARY ADVICE, SUPPORT COUNSELLING AND TRAINING IN RELAXATION AND OTHER COPING TECHNIQUES, SUCH AS THE BRISTOL CANCER HELP CENTRE (helpline 0117 980 9505, http://www.bristolcancerhelp.org)

And THE POSITIVE ACTION ON CANCER CHARITY (telephone 01373 455 255, http://www.pacproject.co.uk; offering a free counselling service to cancer patients and their families)

Index